FACE TO FACE WITH THE FACE

by the same author

Cranio-Sacral Integration – Foundation
ISBN 978 1 84819 098 6
eISBN 978 0 85701 078 0

FACE TO FACE WITH THE FACE

Working with the Face and the Cranial Nerves through Cranio-Sacral Integration

Thomas Attlee D.O., R.C.S.T.

ILLUSTRATED BY SAM WILSON
PHOTOGRAPHS BY LOUISE SAM

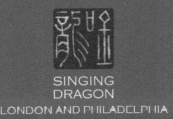

SINGING
DRAGON
LONDON AND PHILADELPHIA

First published in 2016
by Singing Dragon
an imprint of Jessica Kingsley Publishers
73 Collier Street
London N1 9BE, UK
and
400 Market Street, Suite 400
Philadelphia, PA 19106, USA

www.singingdragon.com

Library of Congress Cataloging in Publication Data
A CIP catalog record for this book is available from the Library of Congress

British Library Cataloguing in Publication Data
A CIP catalogue record for this book is available from the British Library

ISBN 978 1 84819 279 9
eISBN 978 0 85701 225 8

Printed and bound in Great Britain by Ashford Colour Press Ltd.

Contents

Thank you

to my family
Janice, Ashley, Ruskin

to all my students at the
College of Cranio-Sacral Therapy
over the past 30 years

to all the tutors
at the college

to Sam Wilson
for the illustrations

to Louise Sam
for the photographs

to Alice Paton
and Ashley Attlee
for modelling for the photos

to Jessica Kingsley
for publishing this book

to the production team
at Jessica Kingsley Publishers

Part I

Introduction

Chapter 1

Facial Torment – and Resolution

Fiona was forty-seven and had suffered a lifetime of countless recurrent ear infections, glue ear, severe deafness, extreme pain, burst ear drums, and inability to travel by air. She had been through countless courses of antibiotics, grommets, operations and other treatments without benefit – until she discovered cranio-sacral integration, and her life was transformed. She was able to hear again, was free of pain and was able to fly (by aeroplane, that is, not independently – cranio-sacral integration is not quite that miraculous!).

Eighty per cent of babies and children suffer middle ear infections,[1] often leading to glue ear, with potential repercussions on speech and language. Like Fiona, they may receive frequent prescriptions of antibiotics, sometimes grommets and possibly operations, none of which addresses the underlying cause and which may consequently lead to repeated episodes of the condition. Cranio-sacral integration is particularly effective at addressing the root of the issue and enabling dramatic changes, preventing recurrence, and abrogating or reducing the need for antibiotics and medical intervention. Loss of hearing can also arise from many other causes – sometimes resolvable through a more comprehensive understanding of the contributory factors.

Trigeminal neuralgia is widely regarded as the most excruciatingly painful condition known to the medical world,[2] with no clearly identified cause and limited means of treatment or management. Bell's palsy is a common cause of frustrating facial disturbance. Ménière's disease can be severely debilitating, with recurrent vertigo, tinnitus and deafness. Tinnitus itself is an interminable source of irritation, driving many people to distraction. Vertigo and labyrinthitis can be extremely disorientating. In everyday cranio-sacral practice, we repeatedly see that in many cases these conditions can be alleviated and resolved.

Many persistent tooth and jaw pains and temporo-mandibular joint disorders are not resolved through dentistry and orthodontics, but may respond to a cranio-sacral approach. Eyes are subject to squints, astigmatism, lazy eye, infections, and dry eye.

Obscure underlying facial sources can also be the undiagnosed cause of repeated headaches, recurrent migraines, neck pain, attention deficit hyperactivity disorder (ADHD), autism, exhaustion, chronic fatigue and severe debilitation.

So many conditions affecting the face – rhinitis, allergy, hypersensitivity, nasal congestion, and the agony of sinusitis – are so common that they are often taken for granted, accepted as normal. We live with these conditions, suffer in silence, manage them to some degree through constant medication – but they do not need to be merely managed, they can often be relieved to a large extent, and quality of life can be substantially enhanced. Through cranio-sacral integration, we often see profound transformations in so many persistent and apparently intractable conditions.

An integrative approach

For the most part, such conditions are treated locally and symptomatically. Cranio-sacral integration offers a different approach – by looking at the whole person, understanding that every part of the body affects and is affected by every other part, that local health is dependent on overall integration and fundamental vitality, and that underlying patterns of trauma arising from birth, childhood injury, accidents and traumatic incidents can predispose to a wide range of disturbances and dysfunctions later in life.

The cranio-sacral approach also recognizes that the body has an inherent potential for resolving health disturbances and restoring health, and engages with this inherent potential in order to help the body to re-establish its natural free mobility and fluent function.

We will be exploring the eyes, ears, nose, sinuses, mouth, teeth, jaw – the whole face, in the context of the whole person – gaining a clear understanding of each part and, most significantly, providing a practical means of resolving the many conditions affecting these areas in an exceptionally gentle, non-invasive, integrative manner, without the use of medication or surgery.

Dentistry

Dentists are undoubtedly a very valuable and welcome asset to society, saving us from a great deal of tooth pain, but there are also many conditions affecting the teeth and jaw which are not resolved through conventional dentistry and orthodontics. The integration of whole-person dentistry with cranial therapies is a rapidly developing field with major significance for the future of dental health care.

Since this is one of the most common areas of pain and disturbance to the face, we will start by looking at the teeth and jaw, how dentistry and orthodontics approach these disturbances, and how the combination of whole-person dentistry and cranio-sacral integration working together can be profoundly transformative. On this subject, I am very grateful for the two excellent chapters contributed by whole-person dentists Dr Granville Langly-Smith and Dr Wojciech Tarnowski.

Margaret suffered persistent pain in her jaw and in several teeth, often accompanied by severe headaches. Years of extensive dentistry had not helped. Her orthodontist wanted to embark on a comprehensive programme to restructure her jaw. Hoping to find an easier solution, Margaret tried cranio-sacral integration. Her symptoms were relieved very quickly and never recurred. The source of the condition was not in the teeth or jaw at all.

The whole person

Disturbances of the face can have profound effects on the whole person – leading to hyperactivity, learning difficulties, reduced academic ability, loss of mental clarity, poor motor function, asthma, eczema, migraine, depression, autism, severe debilitation, chronic fatigue and personality disorders. The facial origin of the condition will generally remain unidentified and undiagnosed outside of cranial therapies, but long-standing and apparently intractable conditions are resolvable.

Facial injury

Cranio-sacral integration can also be valuable in the reintegration of the face after injury or operations, and in resolving persistent pain, imbalance and discomfort following severe facial trauma from a car accident or an attack.

Cranial nerves

The twelve cranial nerves are responsible for neurological supply to the face. They also play a crucial part in our day-to-day function and in our survival, not only supplying the face and cranium, but also enabling the essential activity of the heart, lungs and digestive system. As we explore the face, we will therefore also examine the cranial nerves, understanding their vital role both in the face and elsewhere, and developing the means to enable and maintain their free and fluent function.

Early origins

Many conditions affecting the face can arise from birth, childhood injury, and long-forgotten accidents and incidents, such as a fall on the face at an early age – a factor which is seldom recognized, identified or addressed. Trauma, tension and stress are also held in the tissues, and their accumulation can be the factor that predisposes to many conditions.

Profound whole-person cranio-sacral integration

Cranio-sacral integration is a profound process. It engages with deep levels of health – quantum levels – releasing the deeply ingrained effects of trauma and injury held throughout the system, in body and mind, integrating the whole person, and establishing an underlying level of health and vitality so that specific conditions, whether affecting the face or anywhere else, can resolve in response to the body's inherent treatment potential.

The basic principles of cranio-sacral integration have been covered in a previous volume, *Cranio-Sacral Integration – Foundation*[3] (and are summarized briefly in this volume). This book explores the application of those principles to the specific area of the face.

Cranio-sacral integration always addresses the whole person, always enhances underlying health. Within that context, it is able to address specific circumstances affecting the face – working with the face to enable overall integration of the whole person, working with integration of the whole person to restore health to the face.

In order to work with the face, we need to look closely at its structure, function and dysfunction. We need to come face to face with the face (Figure 1.1).

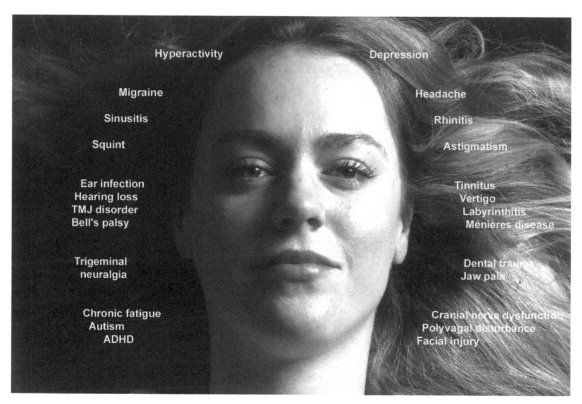

Hyperactivity

Depression

Migraine

Headache

Sinusitis

Rhinitis

Squint

Astigmatism

Ear infection
Hearing loss
TMJ disorder
Bell's palsy

Tinnitus
Vertigo
Labyrinthitis
Ménières disease

Trigeminal
neuralgia

Dental trauma
Jaw pain

Chronic fatigue
Autism
ADHD

Cranial nerve dysfunction
Polyvagal disturbance
Facial injury

1.1   Through cranio-sacral integration, we often see a profound transformation in many persistent and apparently intractable conditions

Part II

Dentistry and Cranio-Sacral Integration

Chapter 2

Dentistry, Orthodontics and Cranio-Sacral Integration

When you experience discomfort or concerns relating to your teeth or jaw, you will probably be inclined to go to a dentist. This is of course to be expected, and is appropriate for many dental issues. Modern dentistry brings substantial benefits and there are a great many excellent dentists carrying out very good work.

In everyday cranio-sacral practice, however, one encounters many patients with a variety of issues involving the teeth and jaw – persistent tooth pain, temporo-mandibular joint disturbances, facial pain – that have not been resolved through conventional dentistry.

It is also common to encounter patients with concerns as to whether the major dentistry or orthodontic treatment that has been recommended to them is appropriate or necessary. In order to establish an appropriate response to these circumstances which will be of greatest benefit to the patient, we need a thorough understanding of the often complex interactions that may be involved.

Local symptoms in the teeth, jaw, or temporo-mandibular joints (TMJ) may often arise from sources elsewhere in the body, and yet are generally (and understandably) treated as local disturbances – as a result of which a great deal of unnecessary and inappropriate dentistry and orthodontics may be carried out while the true source of the symptoms remains unidentified.

Conversely, disturbances to the teeth, jaw, or temporo-mandibular joints can have profound debilitating effects on the whole body and on general health. Often there may be no local symptoms in the teeth and jaw, rendering the source of the disturbance potentially difficult to trace – as a result of which such cases are often not recognized.

For effective health care, it is essential for the practitioner – dental practitioner, cranio-sacral therapist or any other practitioner – to acknowledge this two-way interaction and to develop the necessary skills to evaluate whether the situation will be most effectively addressed through dentistry, cranio-sacral therapy, or a combination of the two, and perhaps other therapies also.

Dental practice

Most dentists work within the conventional perspective for which they have been trained:

> As dentists we are taught to analyse body systems and body parts separately. We are taught to change one area at a time, but such approaches frequently ignore the interconnectedness of the systems in the human body.[1]

Conventional dentists and orthodontists carry out a great deal of excellent work – but they are trained to look at the teeth and jaw. They are not trained to look beyond that. They may therefore not identify disturbances elsewhere which may be contributing to dental symptoms, or leading to more serious health issues:

> Dental therapies for the most part fail to take into consideration areas of the body beyond dentition, the status of the maxillae and mandible, and their occlusion.[2]

They will therefore also tend to address dental issues within that local perspective – straightening teeth, extracting teeth, or jaw surgery – without acknowledgement of the underlying forces that may be causing the disturbance (compressed maxillae, cranial imbalances, whole-body twists, birth patterns) and the effects that those forces may be having both on the teeth and on general health.

They are also unlikely to be aware of the potentially detrimental effects that can be imposed on the body by localized treatment (such as extractions, bridges and braces) which does not take into account the wider perspective – potentially leading to unbalanced body systems, restricted mobility, and abnormal growth patterns in the jaw, with repercussions throughout the body and on general health.

As dentist John Laughlin reports:

> Dental procedures can potentially have debilitating, possibly long-term effects on a person's health, when those procedures interfere with the optimal functioning of the cranial complex.[3]

Interconnectedness

The teeth and jaw are an integral part of the rest of the body. If they are treated in isolation, without awareness of that interconnection, then the benefits may be limited and the effects potentially disruptive.

An uneven bite or malocclusion may lead to unbalanced muscle use – jaw muscles, throat muscles, neck muscles – with domino effects through the body. The malocclusion could, for example, result in tightness of the sterno-cleido-mastoid muscle on one side, leading to asymmetry of the head and neck, restriction of the temporal bone on the affected side, compression of the jugular foramen, impinging on the jugular vein, the spinal-accessory nerve and the vagus nerve, causing headaches, ear pain, tinnitus, respiratory, cardiac and digestive disturbances, neck and back pain, mental disorientation and a multitude of other possible symptoms.

Similarly, *an imbalance anywhere in the body* could result in unbalanced muscular pulls, leading to asymmetrical contraction of the sterno-cleido-mastoid muscle, leading to temporal bone restriction, mandibular imbalance, TMJ dysfunction, and an uneven bite, resulting in toothache, jaw pain, TMJ pain, clicking jaw, earache, tinnitus and a multitude of other symptoms.

Whole-person perspective

Ideally, dentistry is most effectively approached from a whole-person perspective, so that every patient can be evaluated within that whole-person understanding, and their situation can be addressed accordingly, with accurate identification of the underlying source, minimal extractions and surgery, and a more balanced, integrated and healthy resolution.

Unfortunately, despite the many excellent dentists in conventional practice, there are as yet very few dentists practising whole-person dentistry – incorporating an awareness of whole-body patterns, posture, nutrition, cranial restrictions, cranio-sacral mobility, and the inevitable interaction and interconnectedness of the teeth and jaw within the rest of the body. We will be hearing from two such whole-person dentists, Dr Granville Langly-Smith and Dr Wojciech Tarnowski, in subsequent chapters.

Ascending and descending patterns

Ascending patterns

From a whole-person dental perspective, disturbances affecting the teeth and jaw but arising from a primary source elsewhere in the body are described as *ascending patterns*. The source of the disturbance may be in the cranium, the pelvis, the spine, the feet, or anywhere else in the body. (An ascending pattern does not imply that there is no imbalance in the teeth or jaw, but that the imbalance in the jaw is arising as an adaptation or compensation for a primary imbalance elsewhere.)

Dr Kjell Bjørner, a Norwegian dentist of many years' experience, concluded in 1989 that many dental and occlusal problems are due to what he called 'Lock Foot':

> The more I work with patients who have an occlusal problem, the more clearly I see that cranio-mandibular dysfunction is often a result of orthopaedic faults of the ascending type, sometimes originating in the spine, the hips or, most frequently, the feet. The correction of 'Lock Foot' has become a matter of dental treatment.[4]

Descending patterns

Disturbances arising within the teeth and jaw as the primary source but affecting other parts of the body or affecting overall health are described as *descending patterns*. Symptoms may include headaches, skin rashes, earaches, gynaecological problems, asthma, eczema, postural collapse, disturbed motor function, reduced academic ability, irritability, neck pain, vertigo, hearing disturbances and chronic fatigue.

Descending patterns tend to remain unrecognized and misdiagnosed, partly because patients do not generally go to a dentist if their symptoms are not dental, and partly because most doctors, dentists and therapists are unaware of this possibility, and are therefore unlikely to identify the primary dental source when the symptoms do not involve the teeth and jaw.

There are many examples of transformations in function brought about through a whole-person dental approach which successfully identifies general health issues as having a source in the teeth and jaw, including reduced ADHD symptoms, improved social skills, ease of breathing, elimination of bedwetting, enhanced ease of learning, marked improvements in academic learning, increased self-esteem and increased energy.[5]

There is a very small number of dentists working with a whole-person perspective who might recognize these patterns, and a small number of cranial practitioners who have the necessary information to identify such situations correctly.

Simultaneous ascending and descending patterns

It is of course perfectly possible for ascending and descending patterns to be present simultaneously, creating a more complex picture. In fact, most patients will have multiple primary sources of disturbance, although not necessarily involving the teeth and jaw.

Stress

What is perhaps more readily recognized, and yet also seldom addressed effectively, is that a great many persistent dental and orthodontic issues arise as a result of stress, manifesting, for example, as teeth grinding or as a variety of forms of 'TMJ syndrome':

> TMJ syndrome is usually a symptom not a cause. Ninety per cent of cases are not primary temporo-mandibular joint disturbances. They

are usually a result of cranio-sacral system dysfunction, or stress.[6]

A great deal of dental and orthodontic work is carried out in an attempt to counteract the *repercussions* of stress – bite plates to protect worn teeth, building up worn teeth, restructuring of the jaw in an attempt to relieve the symptoms of 'TMJ syndrome'. Dentists may even acknowledge that the underlying cause is stress – and yet the stress itself is generally not addressed.

This is understandable. Dentists are trained to carry out dentistry, not stress management. But if the underlying cause is stress, then the appropriate and responsible approach (not just within dentistry but in all health care) is to address the stress by whatever means – stress management, mindfulness training, lifestyle, counselling, referral, cranio-sacral integration – rather than carrying out elaborate procedures to deal with the repercussions of stress while neglecting to address the underlying cause.

When stress is the cause of the disturbance, dental and orthodontic treatment is unlikely to be an effective solution and may not bring any benefits at all; at best it may merely be managing the effects, at worst it may lead to more significant health disturbances.

Many patients experience difficulties with tooth pain and temporo-mandibular joint disturbances persisting year after year despite extensive dental treatment, when the underlying cause is not being addressed. Addressing the stress factors (which is an integral part of cranio-sacral integration) can not only resolve such situations, but also save the patient from unnecessary dental and orthodontic treatment, and may also bring many other general health benefits.

Not assuming stress as a cause

On the other hand, it is not appropriate to assume that stress is the cause without proper investigation. We also need to recognize, for example, that some (but not many) teeth-grinding issues (which might appear to be stress-related) can be due to primary dental sources. Similarly, cases where there are multiple symptoms such as headache, neck pain, shoulder tension, irritability, exhaustion and general debilitation and which might appear to be stress-related, may be arising from an inflamed tooth or abscess. It is essential to identify these cases and address the dental disturbance rather than assuming a stress-related cause and undergoing extensive treatment for stress while neglecting the dental primary.

Accurate assessment

It is therefore necessary in every case to make an accurate assessment of the whole person – evaluating both local and distant causes, dental and whole-body patterns, acknowledging and addressing stress factors, accurately identifying the source of the issues – whether in the jaw, elsewhere in the cranium, elsewhere in the body, or in the psycho-emotional state – and for the practitioner (dental practitioner, cranio-sacral therapist or any other practitioner) to ensure that the patient receives treatment appropriate to their situation, rather than merely carrying out what he or she has been trained to do.

There is substantial evidence (as we will see in subsequent chapters) to show that a great many dental and jaw issues arise either from stress or from structural imbalances elsewhere in the system, and that they can be most effectively resolved through cranio-sacral therapy and stress management without the need for major dental work and orthodontics. Several experienced dentists have reported that cranio-sacral therapy resolves 90 per cent of the problems they see.[7]

In summary, cranio-sacral integration – which includes addressing stress factors, resolving structural imbalances and enhancing underlying health – can eliminate the need for much dentistry and orthodontics. But as cranio-sacral therapists, we also need to acknowledge and recognize primary dental issues, and we need to be able to distinguish dental sources and non-dental sources.

II

2

Chapter 3

Distinguishing Dental and Non-Dental Sources

Non-dental sources

Circumstances in which cranio-sacral integration can be the more appropriate treatment option are those where accurate whole-person diagnosis identifies that the primary source of the issues is *not* a dental or orthodontic issue requiring dental or orthodontic work. (This might seem obvious, but such distinctions are not always made.) Such circumstances include:

- stress
- trauma – local or general, recent or long-standing
- direct injury to the face
- cranio-sacral restrictions, strains or imbalances in the cranium, face, jaw, or teeth
- cranio-sacral restrictions, strains or imbalances anywhere in the body reflecting into the jaw and teeth
- various other considerations.

Stress

Where stress is the underlying cause, it is essential to address this as the main priority, rather than ignoring it or trying to address symptoms without acknowledging or addressing their underlying cause.

This point cannot be emphasized enough, since stress is the most common source of health issues, and yet it is for the most part not acknowledged or addressed adequately, not just in dentistry, but within health care as a whole. It is in some ways quite remarkable to observe the degree to which people (the public, as well as the medical professions) will pursue vastly invasive and expensive courses of treatment rather than acknowledge and address stress.

Trauma

It is also essential to identify and address trauma held in the system – whether due to birth trauma, injury, major accidents, shock, emotional patterning, dental trauma, or any other source. Trauma is not something exceptional or unusual; it does not have to be due to some particularly dramatic event. It is present in most people to some extent as a result of the ordinary processes of life – being born, growing up, school, work, relationships, accidents, injury, travelling along life's journey.

Trauma held in the system is fundamental to our state of health and wellbeing. It can be severely debilitating, influencing our response to everything around us. It undermines our underlying health and vitality, lowering our resistance, exacerbating our reactivity to minor health disturbances which might otherwise pass unnoticed, and leaving us susceptible to disease. It depletes our resources and is the underlying cause of many symptoms, health disturbances, diseases and discomforts. Once again this is something which is not usually acknowledged or addressed adequately in most health care.

Traumatized systems react more significantly to minor injuries, imbalances or disturbances – including minor tooth and jaw disturbances – which therefore become major health concerns. Untraumatized systems, or systems in which trauma has been resolved, accommodate and address the many minor imbalances and injuries that are an inevitable part of life, often to the extent that they are not even noticed.

It is sensible to release and resolve the underlying effects of day-to-day trauma which affect every one of us and which may be at the root of a patient's susceptibility to symptoms of all kinds, before embarking on extensive, elaborate and potentially invasive treatment in an attempt to address symptoms locally and separately within an over-reactive, traumatized system.

The resolution of trauma is of course a fundamental component of cranio-sacral integration.

Direct injury to the face

Even where the restriction or disturbance is directly to the teeth or jaw – such as an injury to the face – cranio-sacral integration of the area and of the effects of injury is the appropriate first option, not only because it is gentle and non-invasive and will often resolve any symptoms, but more significantly because it is *integrating* the tissues and the surrounding matrix within the context of the whole person, releasing trauma and disturbed forces in the affected area, thereby enhancing natural healing and repair rather than merely moving, repairing or reconstructing tissues on a mechanical, superficial and local level. Dental work may of course also be needed subsequent to, or in conjunction with, cranio-sacral treatment.

Time after time, we see patients who have suffered a fall on their face, perhaps in childhood, breaking their front teeth. The teeth have been repaired very skilfully but the patient may continue to suffer symptoms – including headaches, facial pain, sinusitis, loss of mental clarity, debilitation – ever afterwards, or perhaps arising later in life, as a result of the traumatic forces of the injury (and the subsequent dentistry) lodged in their teeth, their jaw, their face, and their whole being.

Cranio-sacral restrictions or imbalances

Cranio-sacral restrictions, tensions, strains or imbalances leading to dental, jaw or temporo-mandibular joint disturbance may involve any part of the body or any aspect of the cranio-sacral system.

They may arise as a result of injury, illness, infection, birth patterns, postural patterns, habit patterns, dental trauma, tension, stress, and many other sources. They may affect the teeth and jaw directly, or as compensatory adaptations to an injury elsewhere.

They involve not only the bony structure, but also muscles, fascia, soft tissues, nerve supply, blood supply and the flow of vitality and fundamental energy through the integrated matrix which constitutes the body.

They may be specifically identifiable within the anatomical structure, or they may be expressed as disturbances within the subtle matrix and in the overall balance and integration of the cranio-sacral system as a whole.

Overall integration of the cranio-sacral system invariably brings widespread health benefits, resolving disturbances throughout the body and on all levels, alleviating symptoms of all kinds, whether dental or otherwise, restoring and establishing healthy function and wellbeing.

Once again, it is logical to establish overall integration – which will generally resolve any specific disturbances – rather than undergoing invasive local treatment which ignores the wider perspective, with limited benefits.

The cranio-sacral restrictions or imbalances to be identified and addressed may include disturbances in:

- the teeth themselves – whether due to injury, falling on the face, dentistry, teeth grinding
- the face – particularly the maxillae, palatine bones, vomer, and zygomata
- the mandible, temporo-mandibular joints, temporal bones, sphenoid, and the cranium as a whole
- the tentorium, the intracranial membranes, the whole reciprocal tension membrane system down to the sacrum and coccyx
- the thoracic diaphragm and pelvic diaphragm
- the emotional centres
- the cervical, thoracic and lumbar spine, sacrum, coccyx, pelvis, sacroiliac joints, hips, knees, ankles and feet
- the muscles of mastication, and the medial and lateral pterygoid muscles in particular
- the muscles of the neck, throat, shoulders, back, pelvis, legs, and throughout the body

– in other words, the whole body, the whole cranio-sacral system, and the whole energetic matrix.

Once again, it must be emphasized that everything in the body – including the teeth and jaw – is interconnected, and any disturbance anywhere in the body can be responsible for symptoms anywhere else in the body, so complete integration is essential.

Further considerations

In any comprehensive assessment, there are also many other factors to consider, including:

- postural strain
- diet and nutrition
- toxicity
- emotional posturing
- habit patterns, often deeply ingrained
- lifestyle patterns – day-to-day dental care, day-to-day self-care.

Primary dental sources

Circumstances in which dentistry or orthodontic treatment can be the more appropriate option are those where accurate whole-person diagnosis identifies that the primary source of the issues is a dental or orthodontic disturbance.

This does not of course mean simply that there are symptoms in the teeth or jaw. There may be local dental symptoms – or there may not. There may be major systemic disturbances and widespread symptoms which would not usually be recognized as having a primary dental cause.

The pivotal factor is that, irrespective of where the symptoms may be, the situation specifically requires dentistry or orthodontics for whatever reason, and is not likely to be resolved by other means or through cranio-sacral integration alone. The crucial question is – how to identify such situations accurately?

Ascending and descending patterns

It is perhaps easier to understand how a foot or ankle injury can throw the whole body off balance and might lead to an uneven gait, an unbalanced pelvis, and consequent repercussions throughout the body up to the neck and head.

What is generally less readily recognized is that a maxillary or dental imbalance can have an equally significant effect on the rest of the body. Malocclusion, an uneven bite, or missing teeth, can lead to unbalanced pulls in the jaw muscles,

with a chain of effects potentially leading to a wide variety of symptoms throughout the rest of the body, or severely debilitating effects on mental function and energy levels.

Maxillary compression, maxillary arch distortion, mandibular retrusion, mandibular protrusion, entrapment of the mandible, temporo-mandibular disc displacement, loss of vertical dimension, worn teeth, abnormal growth patterns in the teeth maxillae or mandible, open bite, excessive overbite or overjet, crossbite, injuries to the teeth or face, tooth extractions, braces, bridges – all of these primary dental sources can lead to severe symptoms, locally or systemically, and can restrict cranio-sacral mobility, vitality and healthy function.

The consequent structural disturbances, deeply ingrained in the tissues and in the growth patterns, may be exerting a constant persistent imbalance which will maintain and perpetuate the disruption to health until the underlying structural cause in the dentition is resolved.

In such cases, cranio-sacral treatment will improve balance and integrity and enable the system to adapt around the structural imbalance. Often this may be enough, because a well-balanced fluently functioning integrated system may often cope with minor structural disturbances perfectly well. In other cases, however, this will not be enough and will only bring temporary relief, because the structural imbalances within the teeth and jaw can repeatedly reinstate the systemic imbalance and consequent symptoms, and may need specific whole-person dental treatment to bring about lasting change.

If a structural disturbance, such as worn or missing teeth, an underdeveloped maxilla, or a retruded mandible, is constantly exerting distorted forces into the jaw, the cranium, and the whole system 24 hours a day, then no amount of treatment through natural biodynamic forces is going to eliminate that structural aberration or resolve the underlying imbalance, because the pattern will continuously be reinstated by the imbalance in the teeth and by the day-to-day actions of chewing and talking – so the malocclusion needs to be addressed through dental intervention.

Cranio-sacral integration can still address the various other stresses and strains that may be contributing to the patient's discomfort, and rebalance the various repercussions of the unbalanced jaw. This will certainly enable the system to cope better and may perhaps eliminate symptoms completely. But cranio-sacral integration will not replace missing teeth or restore vertical dimension. So if the structural imbalance within the teeth and jaw is still there, then the symptoms may recur or persist. Such situations – in which cranio-sacral integration is not enough to enable the body to counteract the effects of a primary dental source – are not very common, but when they do arise, they need to be identified.

Primary dental sources which may require dental or orthodontic intervention include:

- missing teeth
- teeth growing out of position
- worn teeth
- loss of vertical dimension
- deeply ingrained maxillary and mandibular distortions
- temporo-mandibular disc displacements
- bridges and dentures which cross suture lines
- abscesses and cavitations.

These may arise from many different factors, including the following.

Factors involving the teeth

Extractions in childhood

Extractions are often carried out within conventional dentistry to reduce overcrowding or to make space for other teeth, when in fact the underlying cause is a disturbed maxilla or mandible – which may itself be causing many other symptoms that will not of course be addressed by extracting the tooth (as we will see later in the cases of Susan and George).

Such extractions can lead to distorted growth of other teeth, an uneven bite, tilting of adjacent teeth, other teeth growing into the space, or distorted growth of the maxillae and mandible, with arch length loss, and consequent inadequate space for the descending adult teeth, overclosure of the bite, and retrusion of the mandible – as well as failure to address the underlying disturbance.

Whole-person dentistry would involve accurate identification of the underlying cause of the overcrowding, an accurate assessment of the state of the maxillae and mandible, and appropriate treatment to restore the position and free mobility of the maxillae and mandible, so that the teeth can then grow into place naturally.

The following comments are from an experienced whole-person dentist:

> Many orthodontists believe that if the teeth are crowded, then the only thing to do is to remove them (usually the bicuspids). Such removal leads to elimination of the normal forces on the jaw.
>
> The underlying forces (tight muscles and fascia, etc.) which have created the disturbance in the first place are not addressed and continue to have their detrimental effect.[1]
>
> Removing teeth produces neuro-muscular imbalance, not only around the mouth and face, but consequently through the head, neck and whole body, with potential widespread disturbances such as back pain, as well as compression of the occipitomastoid suture, jugular foramen, and vagus nerve, with all their potential consequences on the heart, lungs and digestive system.[2]

In such cases, whole-person orthodontics may be needed in conjunction with cranio-sacral integration because the maxillary or mandibular distortions have by now become so long-standing and deeply ingrained, and because the teeth will have grown into the distorted jaw pattern.

Extractions in adulthood

Extraction of molars in adults is sometimes necessary (although it is preferable to save the tooth wherever possible). Where an extraction is essential, the space can be filled with a bridge or an implant. However, spaces are often left unfilled, perhaps because the patient cannot afford an implant or a bridge, and is unaware of the potential health consequences.

This can again lead to an uneven bite, distorted growth of adjacent teeth, and consequent muscular imbalances, with all the possible repercussions of TMJ syndrome, jaw pain, headaches, or multiple

II

3

symptoms whose origin is difficult to trace and often remains unidentified.

Where an unfilled space is leading to symptoms and health disturbances, the space needs to be filled.

Extractions, particularly of wisdom teeth, may also cause direct trauma or disturbance to the jaw, and in the case of upper wisdom teeth, disturbance of the palatine bones with their crucial connection to the sphenoid bone. Whilst many dentists will recommend removal of wisdom teeth, particularly if they are growing out of position, it is on the whole preferable only to remove them if there is a good reason to do so, if, for instance, they are actually causing symptoms or disturbance, since removal may lead to further disturbance and trauma and may be unnecessary (as we will see in a later example).

Crooked teeth

If a tooth is crooked, this may be a simple matter of an individual tooth growing in the wrong direction, in which case straightening it with dental appliances may address this effectively. However, it is always advisable to check for any underlying imbalance in the jaw or elsewhere which may be contributing to the crooked teeth and potentially resulting in more far-reaching effects.

Loss of vertical dimension

If teeth are missing, there may be a loss of vertical dimension – where the upper jaw and lower jaw close together excessively due to the absence of vertical support from the teeth (primarily the molars). This again may lead to distortion of the bite, unbalanced muscular pulls, and strain on the temporo-mandibular joint, with all their potential consequences and symptoms:

> Loss of vertical dimension can lead to ear infections, tinnitus, hearing loss, temporo-mandibular joint pain, face pain, headache, trigeminal neuralgia, sleep apnoea, sinus infection, jugular foramen impingement, vagal compression, equilibrium problems, and compression of cranial nerves IX, X and XI.[3]

It is necessary to replace or build up the teeth and restore the vertical dimension in order to re-establish an even bite.

Worn teeth

Wearing of the teeth may occur due to teeth grinding. Although the primary priority here is to address any stress factors and help the patient to desist from grinding their teeth, this in itself is not enough if the teeth are worn. Again, it is necessary to build up the worn teeth and restore the vertical dimension in order to maintain an even bite.

Grinding due to dental imbalance

Teeth clenching or grinding is almost always due to stress. It can occasionally also be due to a primary imbalance in the teeth or jaw. A malocclusion can lead to biting too forcefully in order to chew. A mandibular displacement, an open bite, or a temporo-mandibular joint disturbance may also lead to teeth clenching and over-forceful biting, in an attempt to compensate for the dental disturbance. In such cases it is necessary to restore the balance of the jaw in order to eliminate any persistent strain.

Teeth clenching and teeth grinding are common in children also. This is also probably due to stress factors but may sometimes be due to primary dental causes. It can interfere with the proper eruption and development of teeth, and may also manifest as ear infections or recurrent ear, nose and throat symptoms.

Sutural restriction, dentures, bridges

There are *sutures* within the maxillary complex, and in the mandible, whose mobility is essential to healthy function. Restriction of these sutures will impede the free mobility of the bones with potential ramifications on the whole cranio-sacral mechanism, and the expression of cranio-sacral motion and vitality. This can sometimes have devastating effects. It can lead to the now-familiar range of multiple symptoms – including headache, tension and irritability – but can also result in overwhelming sensations of compression and the feeling that life is closed down, locked up or walled in.

- The maxillae are two separate bones, with a midline sagittal suture between them (Figure 3.1).

- The maxillae also contain two pre-maxillary sutures, located between the posterior maxilla and the premaxilla on each side, passing between the lateral incisor and the canine (Figure 3.1).

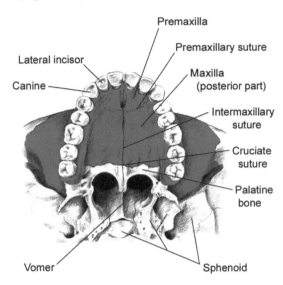

3.1 *Mobility of the sutures within the maxillary and premaxillary complex are essential to healthy function*

- The mandible also has a midline sagittal suture. The mandible is formed embryologically as two bones, and although the two bones become fused around the time of birth, intraosseous mobility around this midline suture is necessary for healthy function.

As dentist John Laughlin states:

> The most disturbing of dental therapies is the placement of a bridge that crosses the midline maxillary suture. Some of the symptoms that this can contribute to are depression, headache, irritability, sinusitis, and impaired reaction time.[4]

Release from appliances such as these will often provide immediate relief of apparently unrelated symptoms. Fixed orthodontic braces can have similar effects. Teenagers can suffer debilitating effects, but often don't express their discomfort. They may simply become irritable or depressed, so it is necessary to monitor such situations and ask them specifically.

Conventional dentistry does not on the whole allow for these sutures, so dentures and bridges may be constructed across the suture lines, limiting mobility with potential adverse consequences. In any patient with dentures or a bridge, it is necessary to check that it does not cross any of these sutures and, if necessary, arrange for the removal or adaptation of the appliance. There are always other ways of addressing the patient's needs more satisfactorily, for instance by incorporating a stress breaker.

Dentures may be partial or total, fixed or removable. If the dentures are removable, the effect of the dentures can be assessed through cranio-sacral palpation, monitoring the system with and without the dentures in place. If the dentures are causing disturbance, then the cranio-sacral mechanism is likely to seize up, close down, or become restricted when the dentures are in place, and become more fluent and mobile when the dentures are removed. Persistent symptoms can also arise due to worn or ill-fitting dentures.

Bridges which cross the sutures are more significant than dentures because they are more likely to be fixed, but the bridge can be cut at the suture line, or an alternative solution can be found, since the adverse effects of restricted sutures can again be devastating (as we will see subsequently).

With bridges and dentures which cross suture lines, it is quite likely that patients will not be aware of the relationship between the device and their symptoms. Many patients will only realize the connection when the bridge or denture is altered, at which point they may suddenly experience a transformation in their health and in their whole outlook on life, as if a heavy weight had been lifted.

Abscesses

Abscesses may not manifest as local discomfort in the tooth itself, but instead manifest as headaches, neck pain, exhaustion and debilitation – so the dental cause may not be apparent. When a patient is suffering persistent multiple symptoms such as these (symptoms which might well be mistaken for stress) and is not responding consistently to cranio-sacral treatment, the possibility of an abscess needs to be considered.

They will generally be identified and addressed within conventional dentistry, but are sometimes missed, particularly if the symptoms do not involve the teeth. If an abscess is suspected, a thorough dental check is the first priority.

Abscesses can also often respond well to homoeopathy. Homoeopathy is most effectively carried out within the context of the overall constitution of the individual, but even without a constitutional evaluation, tooth abscesses often respond well to the remedy *hepar sulphuris*. Other remedies such as *belladonna*, *myristica*, *bryonia* or *pulsatilla* may be more appropriate depending on the symptoms. They can also respond to cranio-sacral treatment, both to the system as a whole and to the individual tooth.

From a whole-person perspective, it is also valuable to identify any other factors anywhere in the system which might have contributed to the development of the abscess. These factors can range from postural and nutritional factors to cranio-sacral restrictions and general health. Abscesses need to be identified promptly and monitored so that the infection does not spread or fester.

Cavitations (NICOs)

Cavitations (Neuralgia Inducing Cavitational Osteonecrosis) are deep abscesses which the body has sealed off, so that the infection is festering within its own cavity (usually buried under a tooth or a crown), prevented from emerging to the surface. They are often difficult to identify because they are hidden, and they may again cause persistent undiagnosed discomfort and widespread symptoms and debilitation, often unrelated to the teeth, such as neck pain, headache, exhaustion or symptoms similar to post-viral syndrome. They are particularly difficult to identify because they are not generally visible on conventional X-rays and may only be discovered through more recent technology such as a Cavitat ultrasound scan (not generally available to most dentists) and through the acute awareness and alertness of the practitioner.

It is often postulated that the body, in its wisdom, will do whatever it needs to do in order to enable healing. This is a valuable principle, which emphasizes the powerful inherent healing potential which is fundamental to cranial therapy. But the body's own protective mechanisms can also sometimes be counterproductive. Cavitations are an interesting example. The body's way of dealing with them is to seal off the affected area in an attempt to protect itself by containing the infection – but this is likely to be detrimental to the body in the long term, leaving the infection to fester and leading to widespread adverse effects on health and potential metastases.

Factors involving the maxillae and mandible

The *maxillae* may be posteriorly compressed into the cranial base, laterally displaced, too small, or medially compressed so that the maxillary arch is too narrow or V-shaped.

As well as potentially causing all the usual disruptive ramifications through the rest of the body, maxillary restriction can also result in distorted growth of the teeth and crowded teeth. More significantly, it can trap the mandible, restricting growth and mobility of the lower jaw and teeth, with consequent disturbances of the temporal bones and the rest of the cranium, with further potential ramifications through the body.

The *mandible* may be too small, too large, displaced, protruded, retruded, trapped or underdeveloped, with similar consequences to the maxillary disturbances, additionally putting strain on the temporo-mandibular joint.

The repercussions of such patterns will be clearly demonstrated in the chapters by Dr Langly-Smith and Dr Tarnowski.

Conventional dentists (and the public at large) are often primarily concerned with the aesthetic appearance of the teeth, and may be unaware of the more profound ramifications of maxillary or mandibular disturbance – in fact may not be aware of the distortion at all.

Standard dentistry and orthodontics tend to try and adapt the teeth and the jaw to fit the malformation (extracting teeth, straightening teeth) – a process which is only addressing superficial factors. Whole-person dentistry and cranio-sacral integration seek to correct the underlying malformation, thereby resolving many other potential issues such as breathing and swallowing difficulties and more debilitating symptoms, so that the teeth can then grow as naturally as possible within a correctly balanced underlying jaw alignment, and any adjustment to the teeth and jaw can be minimized.

Causes of disturbance to the maxillae and mandible

These disturbances to the maxillae and mandible can arise from various causes:

- Abnormal growth patterns
  - undereruption of teeth, microdontia (small teeth), macrodontia (large teeth), crooked teeth, crossbite, losing milk teeth early
  - restricted development of the maxillae or mandible
  - intrauterine growth patterns
- Genetic factors
  - unbalanced genetic development
- Birth
  - compression or distortion – of the face, jaw, temporal bones, cranium, the whole system
  - especially in a back-to-back presentation, a face presentation, or with the overforceful use of forceps
  - trauma, shock
- Habit patterns
  - excessive prolonged use of a dummy (pacifier), or excessive prolonged thumb sucking – potentially contributing to an anterior open bite, with consequent strain on the TMJ
  - mouth breathing
  - teeth grinding – leading to worn teeth, or muscular imbalances
  - stress
  - postural habits
    - › leaning the jaw on the hands
    - › head and neck protruded forward or pulled back
    - › postural collapse
    - › overall whole-body posture
  - emotional posturing
    - › persistent determined or aggressive protrusion of the lower jaw
    - › fearful withdrawn tightness of the jaw and face
    - › resentful angry clenching of the teeth
- Injury
  - accidents to the teeth, jaw, face, cranium, or the body structure in general
  - falls on the face
  - injuries in childhood or adulthood
- Iatrogenic causes (due to dentistry)
  - tooth extractions, whether in childhood or adulthood
  - braces in childhood
  - substantial or prolonged dentistry in childhood, leading to stress, trauma, limited mobility, restricted growth, and restrictive habit patterns
  - dentistry adapting teeth and jaw to an unbalanced underlying structure
  - dental surgery and orthodontics without whole-person awareness.

Why might dental intervention be necessary in such patterns, rather than cranio-sacral integration alone?

At an early age, many of these disturbances may respond well to cranio-sacral integration, minimizing the development of subsequent distortions. But with some of these patterns, the structure of the teeth and jaw has been altered or disturbed in such a way that it cannot maintain healthy function without structural intervention.

These distorted patterns have often been present for many years before cranio-sacral treatment is sought. They are often deeply ingrained in the tissues. They are also maintained by consequent deeply embedded habit patterns in the use of the jaw muscles and other associated muscles. They are also further influenced by associated postural and psycho-emotional habit patterns affecting chewing, breathing, swallowing and facial expression.

Such deeply ingrained patterns may require the use of dental appliances in order to apply the consistent 24-hour-a-day corrective forces necessary to restore balanced and healthy function, to retrain the associated muscles, and to alter the deeply embedded habit patterns.

Together with cranio-sacral integration – in order to enable integration and the resolution of any unbalanced forces that may be affecting the

II

3

area and the system as a whole – dental appliances can be used to apply gentle but consistent corrective forces in order to restore balance and symmetry to the teeth and jaw, thereby enabling the teeth to grow into place naturally and, more significantly, enabling the healthy balanced function of the system as a whole, relieving or preventing the development of all the many symptoms that can arise from jaw disturbances.

Dental appliances are most effective when used in conjunction with cranio-sacral integration:

- Cranio-sacral integration can prepare the way beforehand by establishing balance of the system as a whole, and establishing mobility and responsiveness of the maxillae, mandible and surrounding tissues in particular.

- Regular cranio-sacral integration while the appliance is in place can also help the body to adapt to the gradual changes induced by the appliance, enabling quicker response, greater comfort, and a more effective outcome.

- Cranio-sacral integration can be invaluable in reintegrating and settling the system following the completion of any dental intervention.

Factors involving the temporo-mandibular joint

Many of the factors directly affecting the temporo-mandibular joint are secondary to maxillary and mandibular disturbance and have therefore been mentioned already. These include mandibular entrapment due to a small or narrow maxillary arch, overgrowth or underdevelopment of the mandible itself, distortion and displacement of the mandible due to injury or birth trauma, extractions, loss of vertical dimension, malocclusion, joint dislocation, disc displacement, temporal bone disturbance, and pterygoid muscle imbalance. There will be further exploration of the temporo-mandibular joint in Chapter 15.

Chapter 4

Integration of Dentistry with Cranio-Sacral Therapy

In treating patients with dental or jaw-related health issues, the most effective results are generally obtained through an intelligent and cooperative combination of cranio-sacral integration and whole-person dentistry:

> Dental therapy that considers the whole body can result in major benefits, especially when integrated with suitable cranial therapy.[1]

It is not, of course, a matter of choosing between them, nor believing that one or the other is better. It is a matter of finding the most effective treatment for each individual in order to enable the most positive outcome for the patient.

Ideally, every dental patient would be assessed from a whole-person perspective, whether by an appropriately trained whole-person dentist or an appropriately trained cranio-sacral therapist, in order to identify whether their dental symptoms are primary dental disturbances or secondary to other sources:

> In a perfect world, all dentists would be fully trained cranio-sacral healers and test their patients' cranial mechanics before and after every dental procedure.[2]

Even where the primary source is dental, it is advisable to use cranio-sacral integration before, after and in conjunction with the dental treatment – in order to ensure a clear and balanced system within which to carry out any dentistry, to help the body to adapt to changes as they occur, to address any trauma arising from the dentistry, and to bring the whole system into balance on completion of the dental work.

If dental or jaw work is carried out within an unbalanced cranio-sacral system, adapting the jaw and teeth to a misaligned cranium, then the dental work may be inappropriate, and may not be effective. It may produce the desired aesthetic effect, but fail to address other deeper components. If the system is then restored to a healthy and balanced state through cranio-sacral integration, the dental work may be found to be inappropriate to the newly balanced system:

> It is better to consider all external factors before performing occlusal or other invasive work.[3]

Cooperation between dentistry and cranio-sacral integration, along with whole-person awareness, is likely to enable the best outcome for patients, and would ideally proceed through the following course of events:

- Identify the primary source accurately (thereby avoiding unnecessary and inappropriate treatment, whether dental or cranio-sacral).
- Use cranio-sacral integration to bring the system as a whole (physical and psycho-emotional) into balance. This may be enough to resolve the issue, or it can lay the foundation for the dental work by establishing the most conducive circumstances for dental treatment.
- Utilize dentistry and orthodontics where appropriate to address any primary dental disturbances.
- Maintain regular cranio-sacral integration throughout any dental work in order to help the body to adapt to and integrate the dental changes as they occur.
- Use cranio-sacral integration to reintegrate the system around any dental work that has been carried out.

Why me?

Many people have significant dental imbalances and yet they go through life without any apparent symptoms, so why might it be necessary for some people to go through extensive dental and orthodontic treatment in order to resolve their health issues?

This is something which one encounters in all aspects of health care. Each case is individual, most cases involve multiple factors, and the reasons why some patients react in one way and other patients in another way are often complex and obscure, and can only be established through detailed assessment of the individual circumstances.

Disturbances to health are cumulative, so a variety of stresses and strains on the system from many different sources over many years may leave the person more susceptible to specific triggers. This is one reason why overall integration through cranio-sacral therapy can be so beneficial, clearing the patterns of injury, illness, trauma and tension that have accumulated throughout life, on all levels.

Stress and trauma can play a major part. If stress levels are low and underlying trauma is addressed, the body can cope with all manner of issues. If stress levels increase or if the system is traumatized or structurally unbalanced, minor imbalances and restrictions tend to become more apparent and more disruptive. This is fundamental to health in general.

There are also other specifically dental factors to consider, such as reactions to amalgam.

Amalgam

Amalgam is the most commonly used filling material for teeth, because it is cheap and easy to use. However, it contains mercury. Mercury is toxic, and it leaks out from fillings persistently throughout life:

> Evidence suggests that the presence of mercury amalgam or other metal fillings in the mouth interferes with the proper function of the nervous system. Electrical tests can show electrical readings in the mouth between metals.[4]

> Mercury constantly leaks from amalgam fillings even after twenty years.[5]

Some patients react significantly to the toxicity of mercury, suffering many years of persistent exhaustion, mental disorientation and depression, and they often report a dramatic transformation in their health and wellbeing following the removal of all their amalgam fillings. Others live with their amalgam fillings throughout life without any apparent adverse effects.

One more recently identified factor is that there are three distinct genome types which lead to differences in reaction to mercury. According to a report from the International Academy of Oral Medicine and Toxicology in March 2015:[6]

> An association was demonstrated between a specific genetic marker CPOX4, dental mercury, and neurobehavioural parameters.[7]

> CPOX4 genetic marker was identified as a factor for neurobehavioural issues in a study of children with dental amalgam tooth restorations.[8]

> A 2006 study found a correlation between individuals with APO-E4 and chronic mercury toxicity. The same study found that removal of dental amalgam fillings resulted in 'significant symptom reduction', and one of the symptoms listed was memory loss.[9]

> Research has additionally shown that dental mercury fillings can potentially play a role in immune system problems for genetically predisposed patients. Human studies have confirmed that genetic susceptibility to reactions from dental mercury is potentially related to chronic fatigue syndrome, multiple sclerosis, rheumatoid arthritis, amyotrophic lateral sclerosis, chemical sensitivities, and autism.[10,11]

Deciding whether to have your amalgam fillings removed or not may therefore be a matter of identifying your genome type (as well as addressing all the other cumulative factors that have contributed to your susceptibility).

The process of removing mercury fillings may lead to temporary (but sometimes prolonged) aggravation of symptoms due to the release of mercury into the system during the removal process. Whenever new fillings are needed, it is preferable to use white fillings (composite) rather than amalgam wherever possible.

Accurate identification of the source

Each situation is individual. Not everyone needs their amalgam fillings removed, nor does everyone need orthodontics. Many people will live quite comfortably with their amalgam fillings and with other dental imbalances. It is when patients are suffering symptoms that detailed identification of dental primaries and complete whole-person assessment become relevant – particularly when the symptoms are severe and long-term.

Whole-person dentistry

Many of the dental approaches described here – such as maxillary spreading – would not be acknowledged or utilized by the majority of dentists. They are the domain of whole-person dentistry, so if a significant primary dental disturbance is identified (other than minor disturbances which can readily be resolved by conventional dentistry) it is not enough simply to recommend to the patient that they need dentistry. It must be emphasized that what they need is whole-person dentistry from one of the small number of whole-person dentists available.

The majority of dentists are not particularly interested in whole-person dentistry. They have busy practices dealing with the many patients who want conventional dentistry, and they have no reason to give that up for a more time-consuming, demanding and specialized dedication to whole-person dentistry. Whole-person dentistry is for those dentists who wish to resolve the more persistent obscure health issues related to dental factors and to help those patients whose health is not resolved by simpler means. One should not therefore expect every dentist to embrace whole-person dentistry.

However, it would be beneficial to the health of the community in general if all dentists had some understanding of the principles of whole-person dentistry and of cranial work, so that they can:

- be aware that dental issues can arise from elsewhere in the body
- refer patients for whole-person dentistry where necessary

- be aware that dental issues can arise as a result of cranial restrictions, cranio-sacral imbalances and whole-person imbalances
- recognize the value of integrating cranio-sacral therapy with dentistry in order to enable more effective outcomes
- refer patients for cranio-sacral integration before, during and after dentistry
- recognize the significance of stress factors in many dental, jaw and temporo-mandibular joint conditions and refer accordingly
- avoid unnecessary and irrelevant dental work, especially in the field of TMJ syndrome.

As dentist John Laughlin concludes:

> Cranial therapy is beneficial for all dental patients, and should be included in most if not all dental regimens. The body needs to be viewed as an entire structure and the dental professional (dentist, orthodontist, or oral surgeon) must be encouraged to understand and consider this interrelatedness.[12]

It is a welcome development that an increasing number of dentists and orthodontists are taking an interest in cranio-sacral integration and whole-person dentistry and are working in conjunction with cranial practitioners.

It is to be hoped that the medical profession as a whole will also continue to develop a similar comprehensive understanding of whole-person health, the cranio-sacral system, the value of many alternative approaches to health, the potential for minimizing the more invasive methods of medication and surgery and their side effects, the role of stress in so many health issues, and the practical means of addressing these issues such as mindfulness and cranio-sacral integration.

Start early

In all malformations and imbalances, it is preferable to start treatment, both dental and cranio-sacral, as early as possible, within the bounds of what is practical.

As Harold Magoun (one of the earliest cranial osteopaths and a direct pupil of Sutherland) says:

> Much can be done in the early years for cases often sent to the orthodontist.[13]

Cranio-sacral integration at an early age

Ideally, baby care starts pre-conceptually, since the viability of both ovum and sperm, and the health and nutrition of the mother during pregnancy, play a significant part in the future health of the baby. Ideally, every baby would be checked cranio-sacrally at birth. Inevitably, in many cases, it is more common for many aspects of health care only to come into consciousness when symptoms arise.

Following birth, cranio-sacral integration would preferably start immediately, addressing any birth patterns, and restoring health and balance to the system from the start, when the system is at its most malleable and responsive, and establishing a strong and healthy vitality. In this way, developmental disorders can be ironed out before they become symptomatic, and many of the situations described previously would be resolved before they had even become apparent:

> In children it is advisable to spread the alveolar arches, upper and lower, as a matter of course, to help long term development – particularly if the arches are narrow, the nasal septum is deviated, or the teeth are coming down crooked.[14]

Following an accident or injury at any time in life, the sooner the repercussions are addressed through cranio-sacral integration the more effectively they can be resolved.

Unfortunately, most babies do not yet benefit from the advantage of high quality cranio-sacral integration at an early age. Consequently, many of these cases will only be brought for treatment when the child is older, when the symptoms have become more apparent, and the condition has become much more deeply entrenched – and often when substantial dental or orthodontic work has already been carried out.

Dentistry and orthodontics at an early age

When dental and orthodontic work are considered to be necessary, it is also best to start young, preferably around the age of four or five, before the adult teeth start to erupt:

> All orthodontics is best done as young as possible.[15]

> If treatment is started before the age of fifteen or sixteen, then the need for surgery or extraction is greatly reduced.[16]

It is possible, for example, to widen the maxillae with an expansion device and carry out other orthodontic work at any age, but it will be more responsive, and will require less treatment, at a younger age.

Children's systems are more malleable and adaptable. Early treatment enables quicker resolution of any imbalances or distortions. Establishing a healthy balanced structure at an early age enables the body to grow into a balanced healthy state, whereas neglecting imbalances leaves the distortions to become deeply embedded into the growth patterns, not only of the teeth and jaw but of the whole body. It may also leave the child to suffer prolonged symptoms and debilitation until the issues are addressed, and influence their social development and personality. The sooner any distortions are addressed, the more comfortable it will be for the child, the less treatment will be necessary, and the more satisfactory the final outcome.

Aesthetics

It is standard practice these days for teenagers to have their teeth straightened and to wear braces, for purely aesthetic reasons. This is of course beneficial, as it can enhance confidence and self-esteem.

When the situation is simple, and merely a matter of straightening teeth with a brace, this may be fairly straightforward. However, it is advisable to consider whether the crooked teeth might be due to the underlying infrastructure of the bones and to recognize the need for a whole-person perspective and for cranio-sacral integration. Otherwise, a localized approach may improve the aesthetic appearance, but may neglect other crucial factors affecting health and may lead to subsequent health disturbances. This will be clearly illustrated in subsequent chapters.

Chapter 5

Tooth Anatomy and Development, Dental Terminology, Classifications, Appliances

Dental development

Children develop twenty teeth, five in each quadrant of the mouth. Adult humans develop thirty-two teeth, eight in each quadrant.

Baby teeth

The deciduous teeth (also known as primary teeth, baby teeth, or milk teeth) are ascribed letters ABCDE (Figure 5.1):

Baby Teeth:

Upper teeth

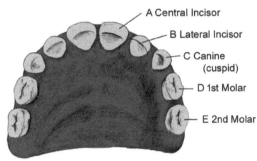

A Central Incisor
B Lateral Incisor
C Canine (cuspid)
D 1st Molar
E 2nd Molar

Lower teeth

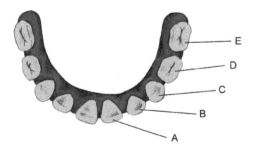

E
D
C
B
A

5.1   The deciduous teeth are ascribed letters A, B, C, D, E

A	Central incisor
B	Lateral incisor
C	Canine (cuspid)
D	First molar
E	Second molar

These deciduous teeth generally erupt between six months and two years old, roughly in order, starting with the lower incisors. There can, however, be many variations, and parents do not need to be unduly concerned if teeth do not emerge precisely at their expected time. Some babies are born with teeth already erupted (not comfortable for breastfeeding), others develop their teeth later than usual. Although it is not generally a cause for concern, it is sensible to make a whole-person cranio-sacral assessment to see if there are any underlying factors contributing to the delay in eruption of teeth.

The approximate age of eruption of the deciduous teeth is shown in the following table.

Age (months)	Tooth	Dental name
6–8	A (lower)	Central incisor (lower)
7–9	A (upper)	Central incisor (upper)
7–9	B	Lateral incisor (upper and lower)
17–22	C	Canine (upper and lower)
12–17	D	First molar (upper and lower)
24–33	E	Second molar (upper and lower)

Adult teeth

The adult teeth (also known as secondary teeth, or permanent teeth – if only they were!) are ascribed numbers 1–8 (Figure 5.2).

Within each quadrant of the mouth, they consist of:

1   Central incisor
2   Lateral incisor
3   Canine (eye tooth) – Cuspid (one point)
4   First premolar – Bicuspid (two points)
5   Second premolar – Bicuspid
6   First molar
7   Second molar
8   Third molar – Wisdom tooth

Adult Teeth:

Upper teeth

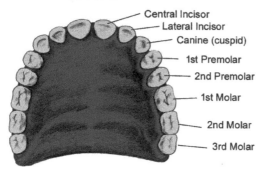

Lower teeth

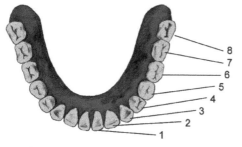

5.2   *The adult teeth are ascribed numbers 1–8*

Although most mammals share an almost identical arrangement of bones throughout the skeleton, when it comes to teeth, there is much greater variation. Non-mammals show even wider variation. One advantage of being a crocodile is that, not only do they have up to 80 teeth but, if any fall out, a new one replaces it, and each tooth can be replaced approximately 50 times. Sharks are even more prolific. A single shark may shed and replace 35,000 teeth in one lifetime. A single tooth can be replaced in a day, and a shark will commonly lose and replace one tooth each day. Furthermore, shark teeth do not suffer from cavities.[1]

All the human teeth, both deciduous and adult, are present or forming at birth, contained within the maxillae and mandible, awaiting their appropriate time to emerge (Figure 5.3).

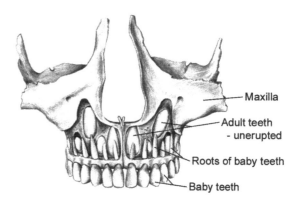

5.3   *Maxillae of a five-year-old child, with adult teeth already formed, waiting to erupt at the appropriate age*

The approximate age of eruption of the adult teeth is shown in the following table:

Age (years)	Position	Tooth
6–7	Upper 6	1st Molar – upper (not replacing anything)
	Lower 6	1st Molar – lower (not replacing anything)
7–8	Lower 1	Lower central incisor
	Lower 2	Lower lateral incisor
	Upper 1	Upper central incisor
8–9	Upper 2	Upper lateral incisor
9–10	Upper 4	1st Premolar – upper
	Lower 4	1st Premolar – lower
	Lower 3	Canines – lower
10–12	Upper 5	2nd Premolar – upper
11–12	Lower 5	2nd Premolar – lower
	Upper 3	Canines – upper
11–13	Lower 7	2nd Molars – lower
12–13	Upper 7	2nd Molars – upper
17–21	Upper/Lower 8	3rd Molars (wisdom teeth)

Tooth anatomy

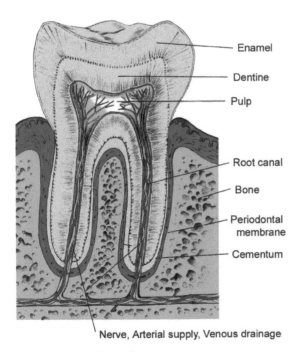

5 4 Anatomy of a tooth

Labels: Enamel, Dentine, Pulp, Root canal, Bone, Periodontal membrane, Cementum, Nerve, Arterial supply, Venous drainage

Dental terminology

Teeth are arranged in the form of an arch – an upper maxillary arch and a lower mandibular arch. Terminology to describe their relative surfaces and positions is as follows:

Mesial – nearer the midline (along the arch)

Distal – further from the midline (along the arch)

For the outer surfaces of the teeth:

Buccal – facing the cheek – in relation to the molars and premolars

Labial – facing the lips – in relation to the canines and incisors

For the inner surfaces of the teeth:

Lingual – facing the tongue – in relation to the lower teeth

Palatal – facing the palate – in relation to the upper teeth

Occlusal surface – the biting surface

Occlusion – closing the upper and lower teeth together

Malocclusion – the teeth not meeting as they should on biting together

TMJ (temporo-mandibular joint) – the joint between the mandible and the temporal bone on each side

Alveolar – relating to the tooth sockets

Alveolar process – the thickened ridge of bone within the mandible or maxilla which contains the tooth sockets

In healthy teeth and jaws:

- Perfectly healthy teeth are well balanced and symmetrical.
- The centreline between the upper incisors and the centreline between the lower incisors should be coincident (in alignment).
- In a healthy occlusion, the upper and lower teeth will come together in an even balanced symmetrical bite, the upper teeth slightly overlapping the lower teeth.

Overbite – the *vertical* overlap of the upper teeth over the lower teeth

An overlap of 2mm is healthy, with the upper teeth covering approximately an eighth of the lower teeth, so that seven eighths of the lower teeth is visible

Overjet – the *horizontal* protrusion of the upper teeth, protruding forward beyond the lower teeth

Common irregularities of bite or jaw position:

Excessive overbite – an overbite in excess of 2mm

Deep bite – a deep overbite, in which the upper teeth overlap the lower teeth substantially

Excessive overjet – the upper teeth project forward excessively beyond the lower teeth. This may be because:

- the maxillae are too far forward relative to the mandible
- the mandible is retracted relative to the maxillae

Underbite – the lower teeth protrude forward horizontally beyond the upper teeth

Crossbite – a lower tooth is outside its corresponding upper tooth (instead of inside)

This may be unilateral or bilateral, involving one tooth or several teeth

Crossbites may lead to a distortion in the position of the mandible, as it adapts to try and find a comfortable bite position within the distorted tooth arrangement, leading to strain on the temporo-mandibular joint

Open bite – the front teeth do not meet when the bite is closed (i.e. when the back teeth meet)

This may be congenital, or may arise through excessive use of a dummy (pacifier) or excessive thumb-sucking

Rotated tooth – a rotational distortion of an individual tooth

Torus palatinus – a ridge or bump in the middle of the hard palate

This may be due to bony growth, or due to the vomer pressing down on or protruding through the palate, or a combination of both

Vertical dimension – the height between the upper jaw and the lower jaw

The correct vertical dimension is usually maintained by the presence of healthy teeth (particularly the molars)

Loss of vertical dimension may occur as a result of missing teeth, worn teeth, or undererupted teeth

Vertical dimension is measured from the alveolar process of the mandible to the alveolar process of the maxillae

Bruxism – teeth grinding or clenching

Macrodontia – excessively large teeth

Microdontia – excessively small teeth

Crowded teeth – teeth for which there is inadequate space and which may therefore grow out of position

Edentulous – missing teeth, absence of teeth

Eruption – the emergence of a tooth

Overeruption – a tooth protruding too high

Undereruption – a tooth not emerging fully

Overclosure – the upper and lower jaws closing too fully

> This may be due to worn teeth, or undereruption of teeth, with consequent loss of vertical dimension

Protruded – positioned too far forward (e.g. the mandible)

Retruded – positioned too far back

Dislocation and displacements:

Dislocation of the jaw – dislocation of the mandibular condyle within the mandibular fossa of the temporal bone

Displacement of the disc (= dislocation of the disc) – displacement of the cartilaginous intra-articular disc between the mandibular condyle and the temporal bone within the TMJ

Self-reducing dislocation – the disc moves on opening the jaw, then moves back into place with a click or clunk on closing

Closed lock – the disc has displaced forward, usually as a result of injury, pulled by the lateral pterygoid muscle and is unable to move back into position

> This leads to reduced opening of the mouth

Trismus – a more extreme restriction to jaw opening (less than 4mm). This may arise as a result of muscle spasm, TMJ disturbance, inflammation, or injury

> It can also arise in response to factors affecting the jaw muscles or their nerve supply – surgery, radiation therapy, anaesthetics, infection, tetanus, tumours

Filling – the filling of a cavity or defect in a tooth

Amalgam – the most common material used for fillings, composed primarily of mercury and silver

Composite resin – white filling material, the preferred option due to its lack of mercury and its white appearance

Crown – a replacement for an excessively worn or absent tooth

Implant – a small metal device implanted into the bone of the jaw, as the base for a crown, after a tooth has been extracted

Restoration – restoring the structure of a tooth through the addition of restorative material. Includes fillings, crowns, bridges, veneers, etc.

Frenulum – the thin membrane which attaches the tongue to the floor of the mouth

Tongue tie (= ankyloglossia) – an excessively restrictive frenulum which limits free movement of the tongue

> Occurs in approximately 5 per cent of babies

Frenotomy (lingual) (= frenectomy) – a minor operation to cut the frenulum when it is overly restrictive

> This is often recommended if the frenulum is interfering with feeding or speech

> If the restricted frenulum is causing difficulties, frenotomy is best carried out as soon as possible after birth to enable healthy feeding

> It is usually and most easily carried out by cutting, but may preferably be performed by laser, since this minimizes bleeding and scar tissue

Gomphosis (plural: gomphoses) – the joint between a tooth and its bony socket

Periodontal membrane (= periodontal ligament) – the fibrous tissue which holds a tooth in its socket

Cranio-facial articulations – the joints of the face and the cranium (cranio-facial joints)

Cranio-mandibular joint – an alternative term for the temporo-mandibular joint

Masticatory apparatus – the various structures involved in mastication (chewing)

> Jaws, teeth, muscles of mastication, TMJ, tongue, lips, etc.

Stomatognathic system – the various structures of the mouth involved in eating, speaking, etc.

Classifications

a. Class 1:
Balanced position of upper and lower jaw

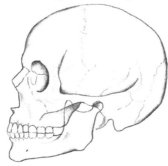

b. Class 2 Division 1:
Mandible retruded. Upper incisors protruding

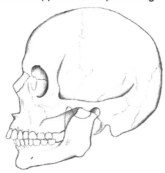

c. Class 2 Division 2:
Mandible retruded. Upper incisors retroclined

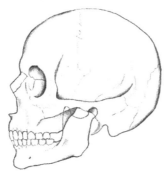

d. Class 3:
Mandible protruded

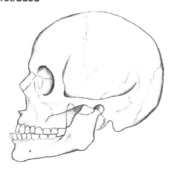

5.5   Classification of tooth and jaw alignment

Classification of jaw alignment

Within dentistry, there are several forms of classification for describing relative positions of teeth and jaw: dental classification, skeletal classification, functional classification, aesthetic classification, radiographic classification. Confusingly, several of these different classifications use the same terms (Class 1, Class 2, Class 3, etc.), although they are describing different forms of assessment, so it can be unclear which classification is being used. (There is also a separate military classification which also uses the same terms.) Different texts also use different terminology. The different classifications are also often mixed together. It therefore becomes impossible to provide a clear definitive explanation of the different classifications. The simplified summary given here follows the most commonly used form.

Alignment of the jaw and teeth is generally divided into three main classes, describing the relative position of the maxillae to the mandible – identified primarily through the relative position of the upper and lower molars (Figure 5.5):

- Class 1 – indicates a fundamentally healthy and balanced position of the upper and lower jaw.
- Class 2 – the mandible is set back (retruded) relative to the maxillae so that the upper jaw is set forward relative to the lower jaw.
- Class 3 – the mandible is set forward (protruded) relative to the maxillae so that the lower jaw (and teeth) protrudes in front of the upper jaw.

Class 2 is further subdivided into two divisions:

- Class 2 – Division 1 – the upper incisors are protruding forward (buck teeth). This occurs in approximately 34 per cent of the UK population (Figure 5.5b).
- Class 2 – Division 2 – the upper incisors are retroclined; in other words, angled back excessively towards the lower teeth (or at least too straight). This occurs in approximately 18 per cent of the UK population. It may arise because the maxillae are tilted forward and down (Figure 5.5c).
- Healthy upper teeth would be angled slightly forward at an angle of 25 degrees from the vertical.

Although Class 1 indicates a healthy and balanced position, this refers primarily to the alignment of the molars, specifically the 1st molar. Other teeth may be out of alignment, which may be described as a Class 1 Malocclusion (in other words, the jaws are aligned, but some teeth may be crooked, crowded or displaced). This is the case in a substantial proportion of the population.

Causes

Class 2 and Class 3 disturbances may arise as a result of various possible causes:

- birth compressions and trauma
- injuries, accidents and falls
- childhood habits – prolonged use of a dummy, thumb sucking, mouth breathing
- stress – clenching, grinding
- postural habits – uneven chewing, patterns reflected from elsewhere in the body
- congenital abnormalities
- growth and developmental abnormalities
- genetic influences
- iatrogenic causes – inappropriate extractions, etc.

For example, there could be maxillary or mandibular compression at birth, displacement of the maxillae or mandible through injury, or inadequate growth of the maxillae or mandible.

The maxillary arch may be too small, too narrow, compressed, or V-shaped instead of arched – this can entrap the mandible, holding it too far back and restricting its mobility (Class 2).

The mandible may be too small due to underdevelopment (Class 2) or too large (Class 3).

Imbalances of the mandible, or between the mandible and maxillae, may also adversely affect the temporo-mandibular joint.

Appliances

There are more than 200 different dental appliances currently in use – too many to describe in detail. They include bite plates, splints, braces, crowns, dentures, retainers and other devices commonly used in everyday dental practice. They also include more specialized appliances such as maxillary expansion devices, Advanced Lightwire Functionals (ALFs), bionators and twin blocks.

II

5

Chapter 6

A Practical Cranio-Sacral Approach to Dental and Jaw Issues

Cranio-sacral integration operates primarily by integrating the whole body–mind matrix, enhancing the body's natural resources, and allowing the body's inherent healing potential to address whatever needs to be addressed. This in itself will resolve many conditions, and reveal the source of disturbances on many levels. This applies to all circumstances, whether dealing with dental matters or any other health issues.

This process is enhanced through the informed awareness of the practitioner – his or her detailed knowledge and understanding of all the potentially relevant contributory factors and how they might manifest – thereby enabling specific identification of the relevant focal points or fulcrums revealed by the inherent treatment process.

In relation to dental issues, this informed awareness can be gained through a more detailed understanding of dental and orthodontic matters and also through specific exploration of the structures of the face, utilizing the information in previous and subsequent chapters of this book – including anatomical detail and contacts for the mandible, maxillae, palatine bones, vomer, nasal bones, zygomata and ethmoid, together with their associated muscles, fascia, nerve supply and blood supply.

By developing a more comprehensive informed awareness of dental issues, we can recognize them when they arise, identify more clearly which issues may specifically need dentistry or orthodontics as well as cranio-sacral integration, and refer for whole-person dentistry as necessary – or rest more securely in the knowledge that our cranio-sacral treatment is the appropriate way forward.

Cranio-sacral integration provides the least invasive, most comprehensive, and often the most profoundly transformative option. Where it is not possible to resolve issues completely, it will provide valuable preparation for any associated dental work that may be necessary.

Common scenarios

In cranio-sacral practice, various scenarios relating to dental issues commonly arise:

- Patients with dental or temporo-mandibular joint symptoms.

- Patients asking whether they should undergo extensive dental or orthodontic treatment that has been recommended.

- Parents asking whether their children should undergo extensive dental or orthodontic treatment that has been recommended.

- Patients with multiple non-dental symptoms, or recurrent symptoms, or who are not responding consistently to cranio-sacral treatment.

Approach

All of these scenarios can be effectively addressed through an appropriate informed approach based on the following principles.

Symptoms

- Recognize that dental and TMJ symptoms may be arising from anywhere in the body and from non-dental sources.

- Recognize that symptoms and dysfunctions anywhere in the body and general debilitation may come from a primary source in the teeth.

- Remain alert to all the possible symptoms that might be related to the teeth and jaw.

Diagnosis

- When a patient presents with dental or TMJ symptoms, evaluate thoroughly (based on the information below), establishing whether the cause is a primary dental source, or whether there are other non-dental factors that explain the condition, and consequently whether the source can be resolved through cranio-sacral integration or requires dental treatment.
- When a patient with non-dental symptoms is not responding consistently or symptoms are recurring, remember to consider the possibility of a dental source (since this is often neglected or missed).
- Maintain an awareness of this possibility with all patients, as a matter of course (through informed awareness of dental and orthodontic matters).

Application

- Observe patients with an awareness of dental issues, as a matter of course.
- Remain alert to all possibilities, including abscesses and cavitations.
- Where necessary, make a more detailed evaluation of dental matters (as elaborated below).

Symptoms associated with the teeth and jaw

Symptoms potentially indicating a dental disturbance (primary or compensatory) include:

Local symptoms

- Tooth pain, jaw pain, TMJ syndrome
- Clicking jaw, crepitus and other sounds in the temporo-mandibular joint
- Facial pain
- Pain in the muscles of mastication (the chewing muscles of the jaw)
- Teeth clenching, teeth grinding
- Limited opening of the jaw
- Jaw deviating on opening or closing
- Difficulty opening or closing the jaw
- Difficulty biting the teeth together, difficulty chewing

Symptoms within the cranium

- Headache, migraine
- Earache, recurrent ear infection, tinnitus, vertigo, hearing loss
- Sinus issues
- Catarrh, rhinitis
- Allergies and hypersensitivities
- Suboccipital tension

Symptoms in the rest of the body

- Throat tension, sore throat
- Larynx and voice symptoms
- Difficulty swallowing, swallowing repeatedly
- Coughing or clearing the throat repeatedly
- Recurrent tonsillitis and other infections
- Neck pain, shoulder pain
- Symptoms in the arms and hands – pain, numbness, weakness
- Back pain, low back pain, pelvic pain
- Knee pain
- Symptoms in the legs and feet – pain, numbness, weakness
- Ramifications throughout the body
- Persistent symptoms anywhere in the body
- Chain effects through the body
- Multiple symptoms
- Symptoms that cannot readily be explained
- Symptoms that are unresponsive to treatment
- Symptoms that recur despite apparently effective treatment

Systemic symptoms

- Weakness, numbness, lethargy
- Depression, anxiety, irritability, tension

II

6

- Mental disorientation
- Poor concentration
- Learning difficulties
- Persistent exhaustion
- Debilitation
- Feeling shut down, weighed down, walled in, blocked, compressed
- Attention deficit hyperactivity disorder (ADHD)
- Chronic fatigue

Clearly, any symptom or disturbance could arise from a primary dental source, so it is necessary to be alert to dental sources in every patient.

Diagnosis

Cranio-sacral integration will very often resolve a multitude of health issues, simply by applying general principles and allowing the inherent treatment process to take its course. Most patients will feel a general improvement in their overall health. However, it is not adequate for a practitioner simply to carry out whatever he or she is trained to do in the hope that this may resolve the issues and, if it is not effective, then refer them elsewhere – even though that may be common practice in many areas of medicine and therapy. It is preferable to make an accurate diagnosis from the start, to be alert to every possibility, to identify causative factors whatever their source, and thereby provide patients with the most appropriate treatment for their situation.

This can largely be enabled through effective application of standard procedures:

- A detailed case history – specifically including dental issues, dental history, orthodontics, and facial injuries, including during childhood.
- Accurate observation of the patient – including a detailed observation and assessment of the teeth and jaw (described below).

- Evaluation of the whole picture through the cranio-sacral process, including stress levels, trauma, birth patterns, whole-body imbalances arising from elsewhere in the body, and local imbalances within the maxillae, mandible, face or cranium that can be resolved through cranio-sacral integration.
- Where necessary, making a more detailed evaluation of dental matters (as elaborated below).
- Thereby establishing whether the source of the symptoms is a primary dental issue or is due to other identifiable factors.

Case history

Patients may not mention symptoms or issues relating to their teeth or temporo-mandibular joint, either because they have more immediate concerns, or because they occurred a long time ago, or because they may not think it is relevant. They might also think that dental issues are not the domain of a cranio-sacral therapist – so it is essential to ask patients specifically about their dental symptoms and history.

If their symptoms are not in the teeth and jaw, they are unlikely to consider or be aware of underlying dental imbalances as a possible cause for their non-dental symptoms elsewhere, but their dental history may still be crucial.

Children and teenagers in particular are often particularly unforthcoming, and may need more specific prompting and enquiry.

In every patient, it is necessary to include, as a matter of course, awareness of potential dental or jaw-related issues, current or previous – observing, asking about the case history, and evaluating through cranio-sacral palpation.

Whenever a primary dental cause appears to be a possibility – whether involving local symptoms, general debilitation, or apparent lack of lasting response to treatment – a more detailed evaluation of the teeth and jaw can be carried out.

A more detailed evaluation of the teeth and jaw

This is a comprehensive checklist. It will be followed by a more succinct summary for regular day-to-day application. In practice, much of this will become instinctive, particularly once it is familiar. The key is to make it a part of your thought process, your informed awareness, so that you will recognize relevant factors when they arise.

Questions to ask the patient

- What symptoms are they experiencing?
  - in their teeth
  - in their jaw
  - elsewhere.
- Are they currently undergoing any dental work?
  - What is the dentist's assessment and suggested approach?
- Do they have any persistent or recurrent tooth infection or inflammation?
- Do they grind or clench their teeth?
  - Might they do so without knowing?
  - Does their partner or dentist say that they grind their teeth?
- Do they feel that they are stressed, under pressure, or aware of stresses in their life?
  - Bear in mind that the underlying stress might be from childhood or early life or many years past, and may be such a familiar habit that the patient takes it for granted and is unaware of it. Many teeth-grinding habit patterns arise from childhood trauma.
- Do they experience any sounds when opening or closing the mouth, or when chewing?
  - Clicking, popping, crepitus (crackling).
- Do they experience, or have they experienced, any tinnitus?
- Do they wear bridges, braces or dentures?

Relevant factors in their history

- Have they experienced any injuries to their teeth, jaw, or face?
  - Recent or in the past, including childhood.
- Have they experienced any previous dentistry or orthodontic treatment?
  - Recent or in the past, including childhood.
- Have they experienced any previous persistent tooth infection or inflammation?
- Have they undergone any tooth extractions?
  - Wisdom teeth, molars or other teeth.
- Do they know what their birth was like?
  - In general – traumatic, long, difficult, interventions.
  - In particular, was it a back-to-back or a face presentation?
- Do they experience or have they in the past experienced any other symptoms relating to the mouth, nose, ears, breathing, swallowing, clenching, grinding?

Observation and examination

Observe the face both from the front (anterior view) and from the side (in profile).

From the front

- Observe whether the face and body are level and balanced:
  - the optic plane (eyes)
  - the maxillary plane
  - the mandibular plane
  - the otic plane (the ears) – possibly reflecting a temporal bone imbalance
  - the shoulders, pelvis, knees, feet.
- Observe any asymmetries in the face and jaw – bulges, twists, lop-sided, unbalanced.
- Observe whether the face, particularly the maxillae, appears squashed or medially compressed.
- Observe the overall facial expression and demeanour. Does it appear tight-lipped, held, compressed, squashed, withdrawn, protruded, strained, uncomfortable, open-mouthed?

II

6

From the side

- Are the maxillae compressed, distorted, too far posterior, or too far anterior?
- Is the mandible protruded or retruded, distorted or unbalanced?
- Observe the overall alignment and balance of the maxillae, mandible and face.

Inside the mouth

- Ask the patient to open their mouth and look for:
  - Extractions or missing teeth
  - Worn teeth or ground-down teeth
  - Crooked teeth
  - Crowded teeth
  - Overall balance of the teeth, jaw, mouth
  - Arch size and symmetry – maxillary and mandibular.
- In babies and children, check for tongue tie.

With the teeth closed

- Ask the patient to bare their teeth (retracting their lips) and observe for:
  - Arch size and symmetry – maxillary and mandibular
  - A compressed, distorted, or narrow maxillary arch
  - An uneven bite
  - Malocclusion
  - Teeth not meeting
  - Open bite
  - Overbite
  - Deep bite
  - Overjet
  - Crossbite
  - Underbite
  - Loss of vertical dimension – on one side or both

  - Bridges, braces, dentures, looking in particular to see if they cross significant sutures
    - › in the mandible – the midline sagittal suture
    - › in the maxillae
      - › the midline sagittal suture
      - › the pre-maxillary sutures (between the 2nd and 3rd tooth on each side).

Testing and measuring

Opening

Evaluate the degree of opening of the jaw (using a small ruler) (Figure 6.1).

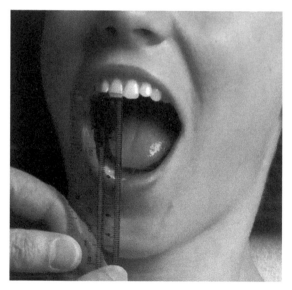

6.1 *Measuring maximum opening of the jaw*

A healthy adult jaw will open to between 48mm and 52mm, measured from the superior margin of the lower incisors to the inferior margin of the upper incisors. (In children, the measurement will vary according to their size.)

Restricted opening (less than 48mm) may indicate either a temporo-mandibular joint disturbance, or muscle spasm. Anything less than 21mm suggests an acute closed lock, in which the disc within the temporo-mandibular joint has moved out of position and become stuck, leaving the jaw locked.

Lateral movement

Ask the patient to move their mandible as far as possible from side to side. Note any imbalance between the two sides. Standard range of movement is 15mm to each side (Figure 6.2).

Alignment

With the teeth closed and lips drawn back, check that the centreline of the upper incisors is in line with the centreline of the lower incisors (Figure 6.3).

Ask the patient to bring their front teeth together gently, then to clench and relax repeatedly. Observe any shift in the mandible or the teeth as they clench – this may indicate an occlusal imbalance (the biting surface is not even).

Temporo-mandibular joint (TMJ)

Assess condylar position and balance:

- Ask the patient to open and close their mouth repeatedly.
- Observe from the front for:
  - deflection – the mandible shifts to one side on opening. This may indicate a displacement (dislocation) of the articular disc within the TMJ.
  - deviation – the mandible wobbles to one side and back to the centre again. This may indicate a self-reducing displacement (dislocation) of the articular disc, in which the disc displaces and clicks back into place, often with an audible click or clunk.

Place the pads of your middle fingers over the temporo-mandibular joints (in front of the ears) (Figure 6.4a):

- Ask the patient to open and close their mouth repeatedly.
- Feel for any imbalance.

Place your index or little fingers in the patient's ears, with the finger pads facing anteriorly to contact the mandibular condyles (Figure 6.4b):

- Ask the patient to open and close their mouth repeatedly.
- Feel for any imbalance (the condyle pressing against your finger more on one side).
- Notice any clicks or crepitus.

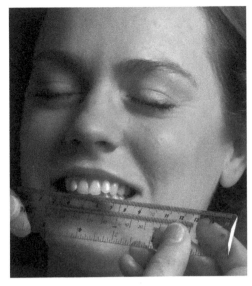

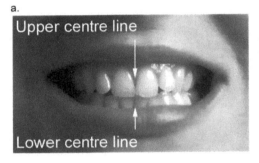

6.2   Assessing lateral movement of the mandible

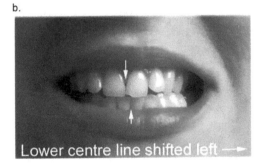

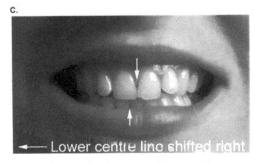

6.3   Checking the alignment of the centrelines

a.

b.

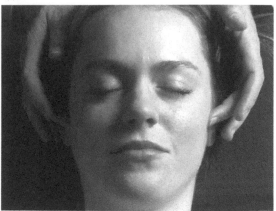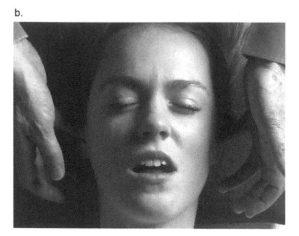

6.4   Assessing condylar position and balance within the TMJ

Hidden factors

Be alert to the possibility of any hidden factors, such as:

Abscesses

- Abscesses may sometimes not display any local symptoms.
- At other times they may be indicated by persistent tooth pain or inflammation.
- Check whether this possibility has been thoroughly investigated by a dentist.
- Abscesses may manifest as widespread symptoms such as headache, neck pain, exhaustion and general debilitation (easily mistaken for stress) without any tooth symptoms.

Cavitations (NICOs)

- Particular care needs to be taken to investigate this possibility where there are multiple debilitating symptoms such as those described above under abscesses – even when the patient has seen a dentist.

- They are difficult to identify because they may not be apparent on any standard tests including X-rays, and may therefore also be overlooked by dentists.

Babies and children

In babies and children, it is also relevant to look out for any indications of mouth breathing, difficulty latching on, difficulty in swallowing, chewing or yawning, persistent or recurrent ear infections, or tongue tie – along with standard indications such as head shape, face shape and any history of birth trauma. Ideally, between the ages of three and five, there will be a 1mm–2mm space between each tooth, in order to allow enough space for the adult teeth to come through. If any disturbances are identified, it is preferable to address them by the age of five, before the adult teeth start to erupt.

A succinct summary

It is not, of course, necessary to work methodically through this list with every patient. Once this information has become familiar, it should be possible to incorporate the principles into one's standard practice, and remain observant and alert to such matters. The approach can therefore be reduced to the following:

- Incorporate awareness of dental issues into your approach, knowing what to look out for.
- Ask specifically about dental issues and dental and facial history during case-history taking.
- Observe and evaluate your patient's face and teeth with awareness, as a matter of course.
- Be alert to hidden sources, such as abscesses, especially in patients suffering debilitation or whose condition is recurrent or unresponsive.
- Be prepared to carry out a more comprehensive check where this is indicated.

The *principal factors which might alert you to a possible primary dental source*, or which might merit a more comprehensive dental check, could be:

- symptoms involving the teeth, jaw or TMJ
- persistent or recurrent symptoms that are not responding consistently to cranio-sacral treatment
- widespread unexplained symptoms – headache, neck pain, tiredness, debilitation, etc. (easily mistaken for stress), which do not respond to treatment (typical of an abscess or cavitation)
- symptoms of feeling locked up, closed down, walled in
- factors in the case history – injuries to the face, dentistry, orthodontics

- observation of the patient – facial or dental asymmetries and disturbances
- cranio-sacral palpation and assessment.

The *principal factors which might lead you to refer a patient for whole-person dentistry or orthodontics* (assuming that there are persistent symptoms) include:

- suspected abscesses and cavitations
- bridges, braces or dentures which cross suture lines or which adversely affect cranio-sacral mobility
- loss of vertical dimension (once any stress factors and teeth grinding have been addressed)
- an unbalanced bite due to missing teeth
- malocclusions due to missing teeth, worn teeth, teeth growing out of position, open bite, deep bite
- an asymmetrical centreline at the incisors
- crowded teeth
- maxillary arch narrowing
- deeply ingrained maxillary and mandibular distortions, protrusions or retrusions
- restricted opening of the mouth
- temporo-mandibular disc displacements
- inappropriate previous dentistry.

Children (and parents) may of course wish to have teeth straightened for aesthetic reasons, which might be another reason for going to a dentist or orthodontist – always checking cranio-sacrally for any underlying reasons for the crooked or crowded teeth beforehand.

Cranio-sacral assessment and integration

As a cranio-sacral therapist, your main diagnostic and therapeutic tool is cranio-sacral palpation and the cranio-sacral process, so you will presumably have carried out a comprehensive cranio-sacral assessment and integration prior to identifying the need for a more specific dental and jaw assessment. Through this it should be possible to evaluate whether there are other (non-dental) factors which might explain the patient's symptoms.

Caroline's Story

Caroline had suffered persistent TMJ pain for years. It was mildly painful all the time, always painful when she chewed, and would often spread through the right side of her face and head. Two of her teeth, one on the left side and one on the right side, were also persistently painful. She also tended to grind her teeth.

She had been receiving regular dental treatment for over three years to try and resolve the symptoms, but without success. Her dentist had given her a bite plate which immediately threw her system into chaos with constant headaches, neck pain, mental confusion and emotional distress, and a locked-up feeling. She stopped using it after a few days. Her dentist persuaded her to try it again at least part-time, saying that she would need to put up with the symptoms for a while until her jaw and TMJ adjusted. But her symptoms were unbearable and she could not continue wearing it. Her dentist was also keen to embark on further substantial dental work to try and align her jaw, and retrain her jaw muscles.

Caroline's case history was long and complex. Among the list of various injuries, her story revealed certain particularly significant points. She had been hit by a car 23 years previously and her left hip had remained intermittently painful ever since. She had fallen on her right shoulder 12 years ago, and her neck and right shoulder were usually tight and painful, particularly when her hip was playing up. Her childhood had been stressful and she had learnt to be submissive, suppressing her feelings of anger and resentment in order to avoid trouble.

External observation of her face showed a well-balanced appearance. Looking inside her mouth revealed two missing teeth, one on each side, but this was not affecting her bite significantly, and otherwise she had a well-balanced set of teeth. The muscles around her jaw were tighter on the right-hand side.

Cranio-sacral palpation revealed a very clear whole-body twist, passing up from her left hip through the right shoulder into the right TMJ, with a corresponding torsion in the cranium, where the temporal bones were struggling to maintain balance within this whole-body twist, putting strain on her TMJ. The contraction in her right shoulder and neck was also pulling the right side of her head downwards, particularly affecting the temporal bone and TMJ. The suppressed anger was clearly palpable in the tight contracted quality of her system as a whole, and particularly in her solar plexus and heart centre.

She had brought her bite plate with her, even though she had not used it for a long time. We palpated her system with and without the bite plate in place, and her cranio-sacral system definitely did not like the bite plate, locking up immediately.

Addressing the hip injury and releasing the tension throughout her system reduced the whole-body twist substantially. After her first treatment, she reported that she felt more comfortable and balanced throughout her body and that her TMJ pain had disappeared. Working with the childhood trauma enabled significant changes in the overall quality of her system, and significantly reduced her teeth grinding.

These patterns were, however, deeply ingrained from childhood and from long-standing injuries, and regular consistent treatment was needed to maintain balance and integration. Initially the symptoms tended to creep back gradually. With each treatment, the improvement lasted longer, and she was soon spending most of her time feeling relatively comfortable. Circumstances prevented her from receiving as much treatment as she would have liked, so it was difficult to reach complete resolution. At times of stress or overexertion, the symptoms would start to return, and she would come back for further treatment.

She did not need any further dentistry, because the source of her TMJ and tooth pain was not in the teeth or jaw. Initially, when her TMJ symptoms tended to recur, she wondered (understandably) if there was something fundamentally wrong with her jaw that needed dental or orthodontic treatment. But it was clear from the evidence of the cranio-sacral system that her TMJ symptoms were not coming from her jaw and that further dentistry was not necessary.

Specific evaluation

For a more experienced therapist, a whole-person evaluation as in Caroline's story may arise spontaneously as an inevitable part of the cranio-sacral process. However, where the picture is not clear, or for less experienced practitioners, and particularly in cases of severe debilitation or persistent ill health where the patient is not responding readily to treatment, it may be helpful to give specific diagnostic consideration to each area:

- the overall quality of the system – stress, trauma, or shock held in the system
- whole-body balance
- the whole matrix
- the suboccipital region
- the neck – vertebral, muscular and neurological
- the throat
- the whole cranium – with particular attention to the occiput, sphenoid, temporal bones, occipitomastoid sutures and jugular foramina
- the whole face
- the mandible
- the maxillae, palatines, vomer
- the muscles of mastication – temporalis, masseter, medial pterygoid, lateral pterygoid
- individual teeth – quality, mobility, integration.

Evaluating removable appliances

In patients who are wearing removable dentures or bite plates, it is useful to palpate the cranio-sacral system both with and without the appliance in place where possible. Often, in patients who are suffering debilitating symptoms, the system may seize up or feel locked when the appliance is in place, indicating that the device is adversely affecting the system and needs to be adjusted or discarded.

Scanning

As cranio-sacral therapists, we have the added resource of being able to scan or survey the whole person and every aspect of the person while monitoring the cranio-sacral response.

Having engaged with the system, you can take your attention to each area, structure, or potential source of disturbance throughout the body, observing changes in quality, symmetry or motion as your attention moves from place to place – noting whether the cranio-sacral system closes down, becomes agitated, or reacts in any way to each enquiry.

Focal points and other responses will often arise spontaneously (without scanning systematically) as part of the usual cranio-sacral process, particularly when you maintain a broad perspective. For more precise and thorough diagnosis and identification of obscure hidden sources, you can survey more methodically through the body, asking questions of the system (or yourself) and noting the response at each area.

In this way you can explore the relevance to the patient's condition of every structure – the feet, ankles, knees, hips, pelvis, sacroiliac joints, coccyx, sacrum, each individual vertebral segment, the organs, the muscles, the diaphragms, the membranes, the individual bones and sutures of the cranium, the individual bones and sutures of the face, the mandible, each temporo-mandibular joint, each maxilla, each palatine bone, individual teeth, crowns, implants, dentures and other appliances. You can also explore the relevance of time fulcrums, toxicity, mercury and allergy, asking the system about abscesses, cavitations, or anything else of significance – and noting the response of the system to each enquiry.

Summary of approach

In summary, this approach consists of:

1. Cranio-sacral assessment and integration of the whole system
   - either resolving the issues completely
   - or identifying non-dental primary sources which are responsible for the patient's condition
   - or identifying a possible primary dental cause.

If a dental primary is suspected:

2. Undertake a detailed evaluation of the teeth, jaw and all related structures.

3. Address any stress and trauma factors as a priority
   - even if there is a dental primary, stress factors need to be addressed first, or in conjunction with any dentistry.
4. Refer if necessary for whole-person dentistry or orthodontics.
5. Maintain cranio-sacral integration in conjunction with any dentistry or orthodontics that may be necessary – before, during and after.

Further scenarios

Teeth grinding and reduced vertical dimension

Where bruxism has led to the teeth being ground down, or in any situation where there is a reduced vertical dimension, it is necessary to rebuild the teeth, but it is also essential to address any underlying stress that is causing the teeth-grinding habit.

A bite plate (on the lower jaw) may be beneficial to protect the teeth and to retrain the muscles, while cranio-sacral integration addresses the underlying causes – the stress and any cranio-sacral imbalances. Once the underlying stress has been addressed, dentistry may be necessary to build up the teeth and restore the vertical dimension, maintaining cranio-sacral integration in order to reintegrate the system both during and after dental treatment.

It is of course essential for the patient (and dentist) to acknowledge the need for addressing the stress and cranio-sacral imbalances, not just ploughing ahead with dentistry on its own and ignoring the underlying cause.

Patients with several teeth missing on one side or habitual chewing on one side

When patients are missing several teeth on one side, or have persistent pain on one side, they may tend to chew habitually on the opposite side. This invariably places unbalanced forces on the jaw and the temporo-mandibular joint and will often lead to TMJ pain, more widespread face, head and neck pain, and imbalances throughout the body.

Cranio-sacral integration will generally relieve the symptoms, but if the unbalanced forces are constantly being reintroduced and perpetuated, then the symptoms will recur. In such cases, it is essential to replace missing teeth, restore a balanced bite, and encourage the patient to do whatever is necessary to restore balanced, even chewing habits, in order to prevent recurrence of the symptoms.

Patients who have already undergone major dentistry or orthodontics

When patients have already undergone major orthodontic treatment, there are certain considerations to take into account.

If the orthodontic treatment has been carried out without any cranio-sacral integration, then it is likely that the orthodontic treatment has adapted the jaw to an unbalanced underlying structure, and that the underlying structure is still unbalanced.

If the patient subsequently receives cranio-sacral treatment which brings their underlying structure into balance, the orthodontics that have already been carried out may then be inappropriate and out of kilter with the newly balanced healthy underlying system. It is therefore necessary to consider whether it is appropriate to embark on cranio-sacral treatment, which may require the orthodontics to be re-done to fit the newly balanced structure.

This may initially appear to be a very difficult question, but although it may be a major decision and possibly a decision involving a significant financial cost for the patient, the options are relatively straightforward:

- If the patient is still suffering significant discomfort, then there is clearly a need for further treatment, so it is necessary to go ahead with cranio-sacral integration – with the understanding that it may render the orthodontics inappropriate – and for the patient then to proceed with any further adaptation of the orthodontics as necessary.
- If the patient is not suffering any symptoms (dental or systemic), then their system can be left well alone in its maladapted but comfortable state, even if it is not perfectly balanced.

The priority is to ensure that patients are aware before embarking on substantial cranio-sacral treatment that the realignment of their system may render their orthodontic treatment inappropriate, and the possible need to have the orthodontics re-done (probably at great expense).

The need for re-doing the orthodontics is only a possibility, not an inevitability, so it is not necessary to incur undue apprehension on this subject. The key issue is whether the patient is still suffering any symptoms.

Patients asking whether to proceed with major orthodontics

In cranio-sacral practice, it is common to encounter patients asking if they need the extensive dental or orthodontic treatment that has been recommended to them, or to their children.

With the information provided above, it is hoped that the cranio-sacral therapist will be able to make an accurate evaluation of the situation from a whole-person perspective and provide a well-informed opinion as to the appropriate way forward. However, patients are likely to believe their dentist or orthodontist – because it is logical for them to think that dentists and orthodontists know more about teeth and jaws than cranio-sacral therapists.

You cannot make a decision for them, but you can help them to make a well-informed decision for themselves, and this could be based on the following considerations:

- The majority of dentists and orthodontists view the situation only from a local perspective, without awareness of the whole person.
- Looking at the situation from a whole-person perspective, you can give them your own evaluation and recommendation.
- If you can identify the primary source of their issues, then the way forward will be clear – whether dental or cranio-sacral, or both.
- However, even if the way forward seems clear to you, it may not be so clear or convincing to the patient.

So the following suggestions might be appropriate:

- Encourage them to obtain more than one opinion.
- Encourage them to obtain an opinion from an experienced whole-person dentist, rather than only from a conventional dentist or orthodontist.
- Encourage them to obtain more than one opinion from a well-informed cranio-sacral therapist with experience of orthodontics, not just any cranial practitioner.
- If they are still in doubt, encourage them to follow the least invasive course of action first.
- If cranio-sacral treatment were to prove ineffective or inadequate, then they can always move on to orthodontics; whereas if they go ahead with major orthodontics, there is no way back, and no way to reverse it.
- Encourage an understanding of the value of a whole-person approach and whole-person integration as the basis for any decision.
- They may also wish to consider the relative expense (orthodontics often costs many thousands of pounds), although this consideration is ideally secondary to an accurate diagnosis.

If a primary dental cause is identified, and dentistry or orthodontics is considered necessary, or if they decide to go ahead with orthodontics anyway:

- Encourage them to see a whole-person orthodontist rather than a conventional orthodontist.
- Encourage them to maintain cranio-sacral integration before, during and after treatment, for the most effective results.

Referral

It has been suggested here that patients who need dentistry or orthodontics are referred to whole-person dentists, which is a very good idea in theory. The difficulty is that there are very few of them around.

There is a small number of excellent whole-person dentists and orthodontists, with variable degrees of awareness. Very few of them actually use cranio-sacral therapy themselves, but they may work in conjunction with cranial practitioners.

Unfortunately, geography and cost are likely to be the most significant factors in many people's decision.

The most valuable option is word of mouth, and even this is very variable, as different patients have very different experiences even from the same practitioner.

But it is helpful to encourage patients to make what personal contacts and enquiries they can, and to explore for themselves. For such a major issue, it is worth taking the time and trouble, and worth travelling long distances for the right practitioner.

Let us hope for a continuing increasing awareness of whole-person perspectives and cranio-sacral awareness among dentists, and an expanding population of cranio-sacrally-aware dentists – not just aware of it but actually using it themselves in their everyday practice. (At the College of Cranio-Sacral Therapy, we run regular courses for dentists and orthodontists, presented by whole-person dentists and cranio-sacral therapists.)

Conclusion

Through utilizing this approach with informed awareness, the vast majority of dental and TMJ issues will be resolved through effective cranio-sacral integration.

Chapter 7

Dentistry and the Cranio-Sacral System
Dr Granville Langly-Smith

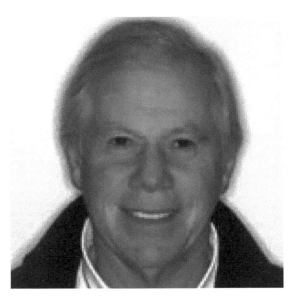

Dr Granville Langly-Smith

As an undergraduate, I found it an onerous task to study so many different textbooks. It was therefore with some relief that I noticed there was only one line in our Pathology and Oral Medicine book describing patients with temporo-mandibular joint (TMJ) disorders. It described these long-suffering souls as too difficult to treat as dentists, and stated that the patient should only be dealt with by a psychiatrist.

With that sort of background, I ignored the presence of TMJ dysfunction and all its accompanying symptoms for my first few years in practice. I rested easy in my conscience, as the textbook had definitely said that these patients should only be looked at on the psychiatrist's couch.

I travelled extensively in my early days after qualifying, and it was only after I settled down and had a family that I developed a stable practice and started to really get to know my patients. I began to see recurring symptoms in some people who exhibited clicking jaw joints, head, neck and back pain, and many other symptoms. Despite

what I had been taught as an undergraduate, I just knew that I did have a responsibility to try and help these patients. It was the start of my quest over almost a forty-year period to look for answers.

It soon became apparent to me that all these often complex problems could not be solved by dentistry alone. I started working with chiropractors and osteopaths and then studied cranio-sacral therapy to see how everything interrelated.

Dentists and cranio-sacral therapists who help patients with cranio-mandibular disorders often find that these patients have a long and often desperate history of pain and ever-increasing misery.

Susan's Story

Susan had a challenging start to her life. Her mother had a prolonged labour as Susan was in an awkward position when she was born. The obstetrician had to use a ventouse suction cup on the top of Susan's head to try and bring her out, but this had to be followed up by forceps to eventually bring her into the world. Susan's head was severely cone-shaped and she looked very battered and bruised when she was finally born.

As a baby she was fussy and frequently had colic. Her mother was very concerned as she failed to gain weight like other babies of her age. When she was an infant, she rejected nutrient-rich foods such as vegetables and high quality protein. When she went to kindergarten, she was always going to matron with earaches and headaches. Eventually she had an operation where grommets (tiny tubes) were placed in her ear drums to help drain the build-up of fluid and infection in her middle ear.

As Susan grew towards becoming a teenager, her headaches became worse and she developed a bucked tooth appearance, with a narrow upper palate and her upper front teeth sticking out, whilst her lower jaw was too far back. Her teeth were crowded, especially at the front. Her head craned forward and, quite early on, she started to develop a dowager's hump where her neck met her shoulders. Her mother was constantly admonishing her for her poor posture. She always seemed to have colds and flu, and she found it difficult to compete in sporting activities. Her self-esteem was very low and she was shy and retiring, finding it difficult to make friends. She was frequently teased for looking like 'Bugs Bunny'.

By twelve years of age, Susan's mother pointed out to her dentist that she was very concerned about Susan's appearance and her constant mouth breathing, which seemed to make her gums red and inflamed. Her dentist referred Susan to an orthodontist who recommended extractions of her first permanent premolar teeth in order to create space for the remaining crowded teeth. He explained that this would be followed by fixed braces to align the remaining teeth and to create a more aesthetic-looking smile.

Following this treatment, Susan was still getting headaches and these became even worse with the braces. She also had pain and clicking in her temporo-mandibular joints. Her headaches were now so debilitating that she was having to take time off school. She had also started her menstrual cycle, which was irregular, caused heavy bleeding and was very painful. Susan was told by the paediatrician that she would grow out of these symptoms as she matured through puberty. Her mother observed differently, however, because as time went on, she appeared to grow into them and there was no abating of her symptoms.

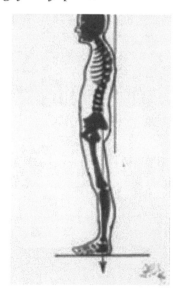

7.1   Postural alignment

Because her head was forward all the time, she complained of a stiff back and aching shoulders. Any athletic event at school was a nightmare for her. Although her teeth were now straight, her smile was not a full one and her lower jaw was still very far back, giving her a 'chinless wonder' appearance.

Susan left school and went on to university. Her family were hopeful that a new environment would help her and that all her symptoms would be a thing of the past. However, life's pressures increased, with home sickness and a heavy work load. Her head, neck and back pain became intolerable and her jaw was locking up, so that it no longer clicked, but she could not open her mouth very wide, as she used to be able to do. The muscles around her jaws and TMJs became constantly sore, and eating became exhausting. Susan started to lose even more weight. She was on various medications by now to control the muscle spasms and to treat her for her depressed state as she was finding it increasingly difficult to cope with life, let alone to form any meaningful relationships.

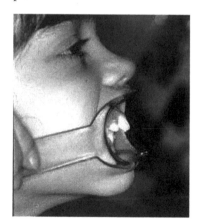

7.2   Susan's teeth

It was while Susan was at the dentist for her usual check-up that she was introduced to a new dentist at the practice. He commented on the fact that Susan could not open her jaw very wide and he asked her whether she ever had headaches. MRI studies indicated that both the articular discs in her temporo-mandibular joints were dislocated. Susan had been suffering for all those years with what early researchers termed 'Dental Distress Syndrome'. In fact, with the knowledge that we have today, it would be more accurate to describe it as the 'Cranio-sacral and Dental Distress Syndrome'.

Susan's story is not uncommon, and many patients that I have seen over my years in practice have similar stories, although they all differ as to timing and content. Why do these patients suffer so terribly and why are they often underdiagnosed, or not diagnosed at all?

Many of the reasons are due to the way we are trained. Doctors and dentists, especially the former, become specialized to the point that patients go to see the 'knee man' or the cardiologist or the urologist. In dentistry we have the orthodontist, the periodontist and the maxillofacial surgeon. Although all of us learnt anatomy as undergraduates and we know, as it says in the song, that 'the leg bone is connected to the ankle bone', somehow, due to specialization, the integrated whole is forgotten. Even in holistic medicine and dentistry, the body connections are often overlooked.

Fundamentally, the human body is made up of mind, body and spirit. For the body to function in a harmonious way, these components need to be in balance. Bodyworkers tend to be in tune with these concepts and to see the human body as a 'joined up' system. However, it has been my experience that, even with many holistic bodyworkers, what can often be missed is the dental component.

The teeth, the jaws and the cranio-sacral system

Our teeth are on the end of our upper and lower jaws – namely the *maxillae* and the *mandible*. Our jaws are part of our craniums (Figure 7.3).

The *maxillae* connect with 45 per cent of the cranial bones and are therefore highly influential. A misaligned maxilla can cause havoc with the fronto-sphenoidal complex and the facial bones. The maxillae are attached to the sphenoid through the vomer and the palatine bones and can therefore in fact be looked upon as an extension of the sphenoid and the *ventral* end of the spheno-basilar synchondrosis (SBS) (Figure 7.3a, b).

a.

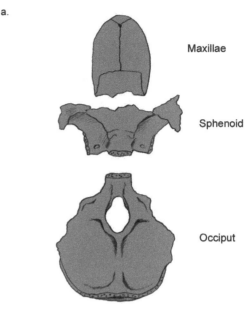

Maxillae

Sphenoid

Occiput

b.

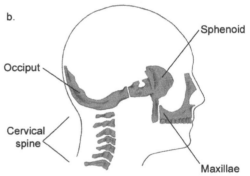

Sphenoid

Occiput

Cervical spine

Maxillae

c.

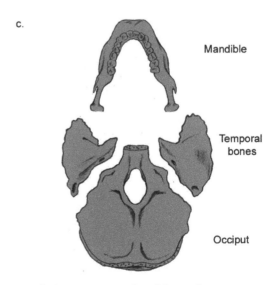

Mandible

Temporal bones

Occiput

7.3   The jaws are an extension of the cranium

II

7

The *mandible* has its articulations in the glenoid fossae of the temporal bones and functionally it is a major component of the temporal-occipital complex. A misaligned mandible will cause the temporal bones and the occiput to be out of alignment. As an extension of the temporal-occipital complex, it can also be regarded as the *caudal* end of the SBS via the temporal bones (Figure 7.3c).

Any discrepancy in the way that the jaws relate to each other is usually a reflection of what is happening at the spheno-basilar synchondrosis (as we shall examine shortly), or sometimes at the spheno-maxillary relationship.

How the bite impacts on the cranio-sacral system

Dr Dietricht Klinghardt is a remarkable, innovative doctor, who was awarded the physician of the year both in 2007 and 2011 from the Global Foundation of Integrative Medicine and the International Academy of Biological Dentistry and Medicine respectively. As a patient once remarked, 'There are doctors, and there are healers, and then there is Dietricht!'

I was chatting to Dietricht one day about the merits of cranio-sacral therapy. He turned to me and said, 'Cranio-sacral therapy is excellent, and this cranio-sacral treatment, if used correctly, can be good for a patient, especially the developing child. However, you are also an orthodontist, and cranio-sacral therapy combined with good dentistry can be nothing less than awesome!'

My personal experience of using cranio-sacral therapy with my orthodontic work has been simply amazing. The treatment seems to flow effortlessly, compared with how I used to work earlier in my career. Even the most challenging cases seem to unwind back towards nature's design. Children develop beautiful broad smiles on balanced postures and go out into the world healthy and confident.

I believe that both dentists and cranio-sacral therapists have the power to do so much good – but ignorance of the interconnectedness of these two disciplines can cause problems.

The crown that is too high

Many of us have experienced having a restoration done at the dentist and, because we are still numb from the local anaesthetic, we cannot ascertain whether the crown or filling is a little too high and in the bite too much.

Sometimes things can wear in, but it has been my experience that patients can start to exhibit symptoms elsewhere in their bodies if this state of affairs is left untreated. As the patient bites together, an excessive force will go into that tooth and there will be a transfer of that force into the bone of both the upper and lower jaws on that side. The mandible will be forced down and the maxilla will be forced up very slightly.

Because of the connections of the maxilla to the sphenoid through the palatine bones and the vomer, the sphenoid will respond by also moving. The spheno-mandibular ligament on that side will also influence the sphenoid and either a torsion or a sidebending-rotation can develop. The imbalance in dural tension will be reflected all the way down to the sacrum (Figure 7.4).

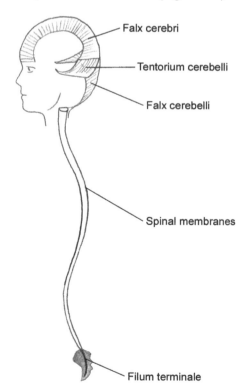

Falx cerebri

Tentorium cerebelli

Falx cerebelli

Spinal membranes

Filum terminale

7.4   Imbalances of the teeth may be reflected all the way down to the sacrum through the reciprocal tension membrane system

The situation can be likened to an 'ascending pattern' such as a stone in someone's shoe. If they were to walk around for long enough, the body would start compensating on that side, the pelvis would twist and tilt in an attempt to even itself out, and the sacrum would go into an asymmetrical pattern which would be reflected up through the dural membrane to the cranium. Eventually symptoms could develop as high up as in the head, neck and jaws. The history of events and diagnosis is critical in achieving effective treatment.

Dr Fonder and the Dental Distress Syndrome

I have had the great pleasure and privilege to have met and been taught by some very fine and forward-thinking clinicians. The grandfather of these researchers and the man who recognized 'Dental Distress' was Dr Aelred Fonder.

After the Second World War, Dr Fonder worked as a general dentist in a small town in Illinois, USA. He was a meticulous practitioner and did beautiful work reconstructing patients' occlusions, trying to save their teeth wherever possible. Because restorative techniques were not so advanced in those days, many patients were edentulous and Dr Fonder developed techniques to construct successful dentures in many of his patients.

Patients who had had their bites reconstructed started to comment at their follow-up appointments as to how they were experiencing improvements in their health, which seemed to coincide with their improved dental situation. At first, Dr Fonder just thought it was coincidence and put it down to the placebo effect from his 'excellent care'. However, as time went by, he examined his patients' records and a pattern emerged that could not be ignored. It seemed that an improvement in a patient's bite really did improve the patient's health. Their postures improved, skin rashes disappeared, headaches disappeared and ear problems and gynaecological problems all improved, as well as many other disorders.

Dr Fonder teamed up with Dr Hans Selye, who is now renowned as the world expert on stress. Dr Selye concluded that the body's adaptive mechanism can only cope so far when under prolonged stress, and that its ability to compensate eventually breaks down and homeostasis is threatened. Disease processes take over as the immune system is weakened and adrenaline and cortisol flood the blood stream. Dr Fonder and Dr Selye, with their research, concluded that imbalanced jaw relationships, poor vertical support and malocclusion of the teeth were a persistent source of stress on the body. They named these sources of stress the 'Dental Distress Syndrome'.

It has been my experience that treating these patients over many years has been a fascinating and most rewarding experience. It changes people's lives for the better and in many cases actually gives them their lives back. I believe that Dr Fonder was correct in his dental distress diagnosis. However, I believe that he was unaware that he was actually benefiting the cranio-sacral system. Even today, it is only a small proportion of dentists who know about cranio-sacral therapy and the involuntary respiratory mechanism. This is why teaching and spreading the word is so important, as both dentists and cranio-sacral therapists are in a position to do so much good and to help a great number of people.

George's Story

Almost twenty years ago a young boy of twelve was brought to me by his mother, as she was very concerned about his crowded teeth. She had been given an opinion already that involved extracting permanent dental units (adult teeth) in order to make room for his other permanent teeth.

The boy was called George and he not only had excessively crowded teeth but he was also a very sick boy, having a very serious condition known as neurofibromatosis. He was also asthmatic and suffered from eczema. He found it difficult to walk and run or to join in with sporting activities.

On examination, it was clear that George had very narrow upper and lower dental arches, combined with a collapsed deep bite which lacked vertical support. He was barrel-chested, with an unbalanced shoulder girdle, and an excessive lordotic curve in his lower back. His face was often puffy and his countenance was sad and listless. He was a mouth breather, the consequences of which are that the air is not cleaned by the vibrissae (nasal hairs) nor moistened and warmed by the membranes of the nose, resulting in poor assimilation of oxygen in the lungs.

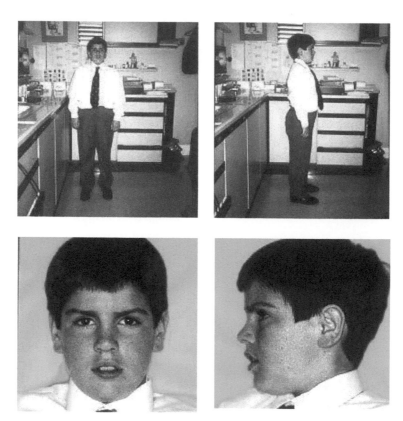

7.5   *George*

Both dental arches exhibited extreme crowding. The lower front teeth were so crowded that the teeth stood in front of one another instead of being side by side.

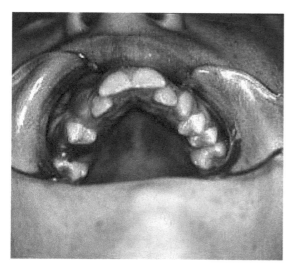

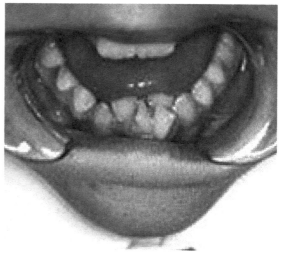

7.6   *(a) Narrow upper dental arch*   *(b) Narrow lower dental arch*

The bite relationship was totally collapsed into a deep bite – where the lower teeth are covered excessively by the upper teeth (Figure 7.7).

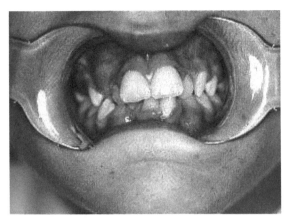

7.7   **Deep bite**

George had been given an orthodontic treatment plan, which involved extracting his two upper permanent first premolars and his two lower permanent central incisors. This was to be followed by fixed braces to align his teeth. From a purely dental perspective, carrying out this treatment plan could have improved the alignment and appearance of his teeth. However, from a cranio-sacral and overall health standpoint, a great opportunity would have been missed to transform his health and to help him achieve homeostasis and wellbeing.

The point here is that George was stuck in a cranio-sacral extension pattern. His sacrum was in extension and side-bent, and his whole body was internally rotated.

Both his jaws were internally rotated, making them narrow and causing the teeth to become crowded.

If the adult teeth had been removed and the teeth aligned in their existing underlying pattern of hyperextended jaws, head and body, then it would have left him in that disturbed extended situation, together with all its accompanying symptomatology. George was already having chiropractic treatment and phytobiophysics, which was helping to a degree, but there could be no proper breakthrough without attending to his cranium and his bite. Mainstream medication, according to his mother, made his symptoms worse.

Fortunately, George was a wonderful patient and I used appliances which encouraged his jaws and cranium to achieve a neutral pattern (Figure 7.8). These appliances, if used judicially and combined with cranio-sacral therapy, can achieve truly amazing results, especially in the young patient, where everything is more adaptable and flexible.

After six months of treatment, George had changed out of all recognition. He was moving properly and joining athletic activities at school. His academic work was improving and his mother said he was becoming such a pleasure to be with. All his symptoms of neurofibromatosis, asthma and eczema seemed to be improving dramatically.

As an orthodontist, I treat jaw relationships and malocclusion – not medical problems. However, I have seen so many apparently miraculous spin-offs when the jaws and occlusion are in harmonious balance. Dr Fonder was right in every way about the Dental Distress Syndrome.

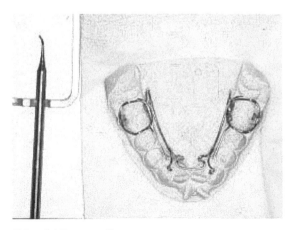

7.8   (a) Lower appliance

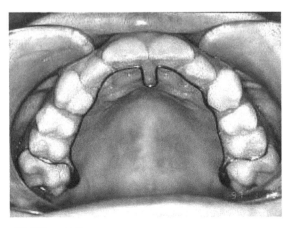

(b) Upper appliance

The light wire appliances shown in the pictures above do not move the teeth via the bone, but through a piezoelectric effect, which encourages bone growth and development. By using cranio-sacral therapy, the cranial sutures of the surrounding adnexa can be kept open and healthy, so that treatment proceeds quickly and with the minimum of discomfort. It has been my experience that the cranial rhythmic index is practically always enhanced significantly.

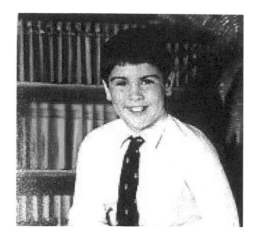 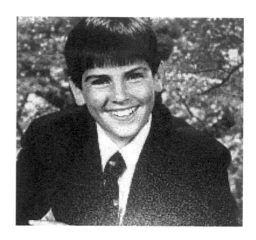

7.9   *(a) George before treatment*   *(b) After six months' treatment*

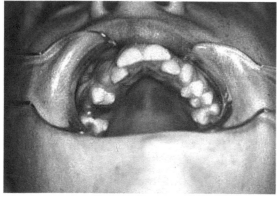 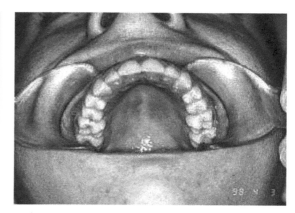

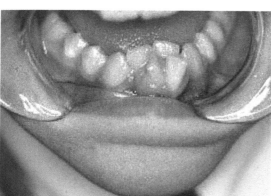 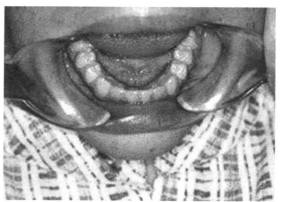

7.10   *(a) Upper arch before treatment*   *(b) Upper arch after treatment*
        (c) Lower arch before treatment   *(d) Lower arch after treatment*

At this point, after six months, it was clear to see the energy and the 'juices flowing' again, because the cranio-sacral imbalances had been addressed through normalizing the jaw relationships as well as using cranio-sacral therapy to rebalance the other body restrictions. George still required another eighteen months of orthodontic treatment to align all his teeth correctly with fixed braces. Note that the centre lines are now coincident in the 'after treatment' photograph (Figure 7.11b).

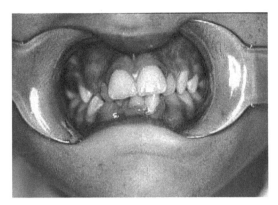

7.11 (a) Deep bite before treatment

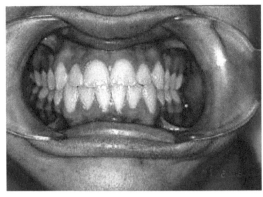

(b) Correct bite after treatment

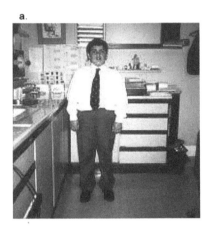

a.

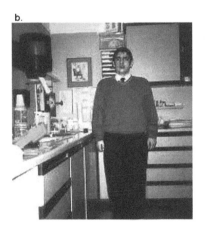

b.

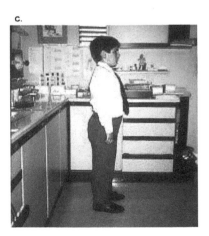

c.

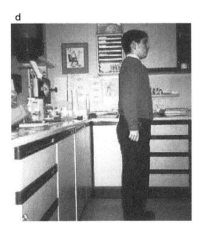

d

7.12 (a) Posture before treatment
(b) Posture after treatment

(c) Posture before treatment
(d) Posture after treatment

The development of the dental arches and the correction of the deep bite, combined with cranio-sacral therapy, all served to rebalance the cranio-sacral system. It is clear to see in the above posture photographs how the twisted shoulder girdle (up on the right-hand side) and the excessive lumbar lordosis have all improved.

The reason that George originally found it difficult to walk and to join in athletic activities was because his sacrum was in extension and jammed into a sidebending-rotation pattern which was driven, as a descending pattern, from the cranium. The severely crowded teeth and narrow extended dental arches were a manifestation of his general hyperextension habitus.

The key to treatment was to retain all his teeth and to use them as handles to redevelop and remodel the bony cranial complex. To have extracted permanent teeth and merely aligned his teeth to the underlying distortion would have kept him in a hyperextended and side-bent pattern for the rest of his life, with all the associated symptomatology.

There were amazing changes to George's health which coincided with his orthodontic and cranio-sacral therapy. His neurofibromatosis has not returned, and his asthma and eczema disappeared.

It is my belief that this treatment helps the body to rebalance itself towards homeostasis. As Dr Fonder found, once the traumatic occlusion and the source of dental distress is addressed, so many somatic disorders self-correct. Fonder was not so aware of the cranio-sacral system and so was treating everything from the dental and head end. Even doing this alone, he was achieving astonishing results, as he shows in his book *The Dental Physician*.[2] However, with all our present knowledge and experience with both holistic dentistry and cranio-sacral therapy, patients have the opportunity to achieve even greater improvements.

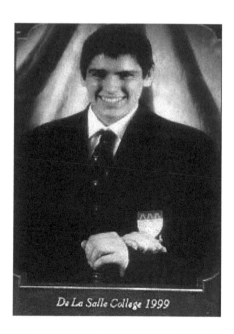

De La Salle College 1999

7.13 *There were amazing changes to George's health which coincided with his orthodontic and cranio-sacral therapy*

Cranial base distortions and malocclusion of the teeth – relationships between SBS (spheno-basilar synchondrosis) patterns and malocclusions

Hyperflexion (flexion at the SBS) (Figure 7.14)

Dental classification:

○ Class 2 Division 2

○ Deep overbite. Retroclined incisors

In hyperflexion cases (flexion patterns of the SBS):

• The hyperflexed maxillae and retroclined upper incisors trap the mandible.

• The mandible is pulled back and up, leading to TMJ dysfunction.

• The temporal bones are in external rotation and the occiput is in flexion.

• Frequently, the patient exhibits a kyphotic neck (military neck) with a loss of lordosis.

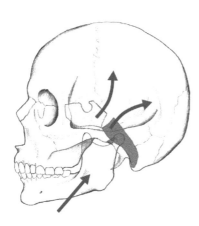

7.14 (a) Hyperflexion at the SBS.
Class 2 Division 2 malocclusion

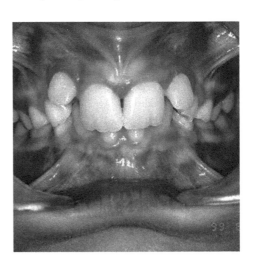

(b) Deep overbite; retroclined incisors

Inferior vertical strain (Figure 7.15)

Dental classification:

○ Class 2 Division 1

○ Large overjet and overbite

In inferior vertical strain cases:

• The sphenoid is in extension.

• Consequently, the maxillae are also in extension, leading to an elongated and narrow palate, often with a high vault.

• The occiput is in flexion, together with the temporal bones in external rotation.

• The mandible is therefore brought back and up into a retruded position, together with the externally rotated temporal bones.

• TMJ problems are common because of the compressed position of the mandible.

These patients also tend to be mouth breathers and have forward head postures (as in the case of Susan). Ear, nose and throat problems are very common, especially in the early developing years.

Figure 7.15b shows the excessive horizontal 'overjet' between the upper and lower incisors, with the lower incisors biting into the palate.

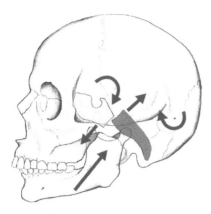

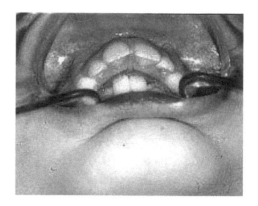

7.15 (a) Inferior vertical strain at the SBS. Class 2 Division 1 malocclusion

(b) Large overjet and overbite

Superior vertical strain (Figure 7.16)

Dental classification:

◦ Class 3

◦ Underbite

In superior vertical strain cases:

- The occiput is in extension, with the temporal bones in internal rotation, thrusting the mandible forwards, creating a 'reverse overbite' (underbite).

- The sphenoid, however, is in flexion, as are the maxillae – which are consequently shortened in the anteroposterior dimension.

- Because of this loss of length, it is common to see crowding in the upper dental arch, with teeth sometimes completely blocked out, especially the premolars.

- Because the mandible is pushed forward and the maxillae flexed back, the teeth end up in a crossbite anteriorly.

- Hyperlordosis of the neck, due to the extension pattern of the occiput, is a common feature giving rise to headaches and neck pain.

- Sometimes the mandible is abnormally large.

- TMJ problems are less common in these cases as the mandible is not being restricted in a backwards direction.

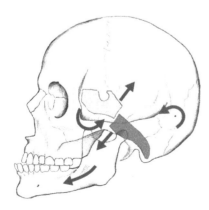

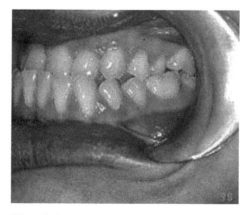

7.16 (a) Superior vertical strain at the SBS. Class 3 malocclusion

(b) Underbite

Lateral strain (lateral shift) (Figure 7.17)

Dental classification:

- Unilateral crowding
- Centre lines non-coincident

Lateral strain patterns are usually due to direct trauma, as often seen during the birth process or due to in-utero moulding.

In lateral strain cases:

- The occipital part of the SBS is strained (shifted) horizontally to one side, whilst the sphenoidal part is strained (shifted) to the opposite side in the same horizontal plane.
- The face often looks asymmetrical, with one side more open than the other.
- The eyes, maxillae and frontal bone follow the sphenoid, whilst the mandible follows the occiput (and temporals).
- The teeth do not fit together properly and a crossbite is a common feature.

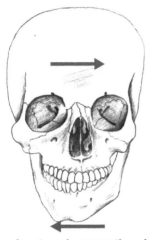 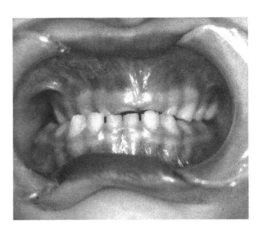

7.17   *Lateral strain at the SBS. Unilateral crowding and centre lines non-coincident. In this example, the maxillae and sphenoid are shifted to the left, and the mandible is shifted to the right*

Sidebending-rotation (side-bending) (Figures 7.18 and 7.19)

Dental classification:

- Class 1 molar relationship on one side
- Class 2 molar relationship on the other side

Sidebending with rotation at the SBS is one of the most complex of the cranial strain patterns and can have varying effects on the occlusion of the teeth, as well as often devastating symptoms – including headaches, neck-ache, back-ache, ear problems and loss of balance.

In sidebending-rotation cases:

- The head is shorter (compressed) on the side-bent side.
- The maxilla also often moves up on this side, but can slope down with the sphenoid.

- On the side-bent (compressed) side, the temporal bone is externally rotated, drawing the glenoid fossa posteriorly, along with the condyle of the mandible, causing a shift of the lower centre line (the line between the lower incisors) as the mandible swings across towards the side-bent side.
- Tightness of the muscles on the side-bent (compressed) side leads to a loss of vertical dimension on that side, causing the teeth to be crowded or in crossbite.
- TMJ dysfunction is common because of the asymmetry of the temporal bones (i.e. one being in external rotation and the other being in internal rotation) causing the TMJ sockets (glenoid fossae) to be out of alignment.
- The cervical spine has to adapt to the tilted occiput, as does the rest of the musculoskeletal system.

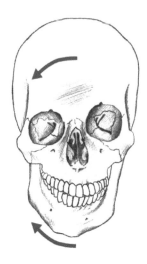

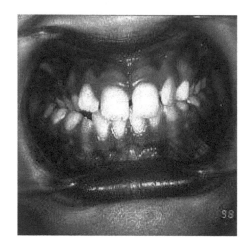

7.18   Sidebending-rotation to the right. Class 1 molar relationship on one side. Class 2 molar relationship on the other side

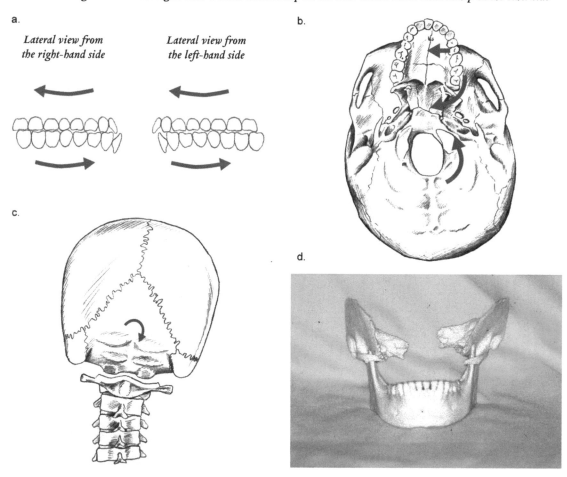

a.

*Lateral view from
the right-hand side*   *Lateral view from
the left-hand side*

b.

c.

d.

7.19   (a) Molar relationship with a left sidebending-rotation
(b) Sidebending-rotation – inferior view
(c) Sidebending-rotation – posterior view
(d) Internal and external rotation of the temporals with consequent shift of the mandible to the left. In this case, the
temporal bone on the right is internally rotated and the temporal bone on the left is externally rotated, so the mandible
swings to the left

Torsion (Figure 7.20)

Dental classification:

- Unilateral crossbite
- Centre line discrepancy

In torsion cases:

- Torsions occur around the anteroposterior axis of the cranium.
- At the SBS, the occiput twists one way round the AP (anterior–posterior) axis, whilst the sphenoid twists the other way.

- With a left torsion (as in Figure 7.20):
  - The sphenoid moves superiorly on the patient's left (high eye) while the occiput moves inferiorly on the left.
  - The left temporal bone moves into external rotation, along with the flexed occiput on the left side, drawing the glenoid fossa posteriorly, which causes the mandible to swing over to the left (the high eye side). The teeth consequently go into crossbite on this side in a large number of cases.

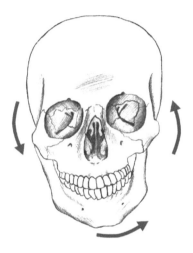

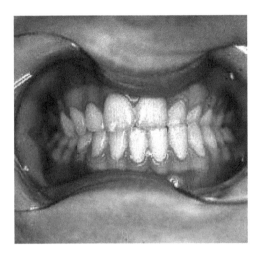

7.20   (a) Torsion at the SBS

(b) Unilateral crossbite. Centre line discrepancy

The cranio-sacral therapist and dentistry

There are various factors involving dentistry, awareness of which may be of value to the cranio-sacral therapist.

Cranio-sacral strain patterns

As I have stated previously, the teeth are on the end of the jaws and the jaws are part of the cranium. It would therefore not be unreasonable for the cranio-sacral therapist to observe the patient's bite and facial characteristics, in order to glean further diagnostic information. When I say observe the bite, I do not mean acting like a dentist, but merely asking the patient to bite together normally and to smile.

Observe the following:

1. Is the anterior bite relationship normal? Is there any tendency to a deep overbite or a large overjet, indicating a possible hyperflexion or inferior vertical strain pattern?

2. Is there a reverse overbite (underbite) anteriorly, as in a superior vertical strain?

3. Ask the patient to keep their teeth together and draw their lips back, so that you can see if there is a crossbite.

4. Are the jaws in line and are the upper and lower centre lines coincident?

5. Observe whether the teeth are crowded. Is one side worse than the other?

6. Are there any missing teeth? If so, approximately how many and where?

7. As well as looking at the teeth, examine the patient's facial features, assessing the three levels (triplanar analysis) – the eyes, the maxillae and the mandible. Is one eye higher, smaller or larger than the other? Are the ears level? Is one ear more flared than the other, hinting at external rotation of the temporal bone on that side and a tilted occiput? Look at the level of the maxillae relative to the otic plane (ears). Is the mandible centred or off to one side?

It can be helpful to match the patient's triplanar analysis to the cranial base patterns described above. What you see with the facial features and the bite relationship is likely to correlate with what you are feeling cranio-sacrally.

This does not need to be a detailed examination, but it can provide valuable information regarding the significance of the teeth and jaws in relation to any cranial patterns you might encounter. It can also help in identifying whether the patient may need referral to an orthodontist or general dentist. Many restrictions can be released with cranio-sacral therapy, but not if the bite is in crossbite or in a vertical strain pattern. Every time that patient bites together, they will perpetuate the same pattern and undo all your treatment.

Patients who have had recent dental procedures

As a therapist you may sometimes find that you are struggling to make headway and the patient keeps 'boomeranging' on you. This could be due to a primary dental/jaw cause. If so, it will be helpful to explore the following.

Recent extractions

Extractions can put abnormal forces into the cranium, thereby causing cranial disturbances. Finding out how and in which direction the extraction forces were applied can help in releasing the restricted area.

With the back teeth, the sphenoid is almost always involved. An upper extraction will cause a significant force through the maxilla, potentially affecting the sphenoid. A lower extraction on the mandible can affect the sphenoid through the spheno-mandibular ligament, the masticatory muscles and the fascia.

Sphenopetrous lesions are common in these situations.

Neuralgia and NICO lesions (Neuralgia Inducing Cavitational Osteonecrosis)

Patients will sometimes present with facial neuralgia, and again it is important to take a careful history before embarking on treatment, in order to distinguish the different possible causes.

Some neuralgias can be due to cranial strains, which may cause irritation of a cranial nerve, especially at the ganglion, as in trigeminal neuralgia.

One of the more unusual causes of neuralgia is from a NICO lesion (Neuralgia Inducing Cavitational Osteonecrosis). This can occur where a tooth has been extracted, sometimes many years previously, and the socket has never healed properly with new bone formation. Instead, there is a gelatinous substance in the socket which is acutely toxic, being full of potent bacteria and their poisonous breakdown products. Besides being a breeding ground for bacteria, this site may also become a dumping ground for heavy metals, especially mercury. There are dentists who can test for NICO lesions, though it is difficult to see them on X-ray. It is only after a NICO lesion is removed and the bone is cleaned up that the symptoms of neuralgia clear.

Wisdom teeth extraction sites are a common area for NICO lesions.

Since the advent of implants, it is possible for an implant to be inadvertently placed into a NICO lesion site with disastrous consequences, producing much pain and distress for the patient. The whole implant needs to be removed in these cases.

Sometimes, with so many complicated causes of neuralgia, it is easy to overlook pulpitis. When a tooth has an inflamed pulp, the pressure builds up in the confined pulp chamber and the tooth can become exquisitely painful, giving off all sorts of referred pain very similar to neuralgia.

Naturally in these cases the patient needs referring to their dentist.

Orthodontics

This is such a big subject that there is not space to cover everything here. However, as a cranio-sacral therapist, it is helpful to be aware of certain orthodontic procedures which may impinge on the primary respiratory mechanism and hence the health of the patient.

It is perfectly possible to treat even some of the most severe malocclusions with appropriate orthodontic appliances which do *not* adversely affect the cranio-sacral mechanism.

MAXILLAE

However, it is important to watch out for appliances, either removable or fixed, that bind the two halves of the maxillary complex together in a rigid way.

Similarly, certain appliances, especially rigid expansion screws, can cause asymmetry in the face if the upper maxillary arch is asymmetric, that is, one maxilla is in internal rotation and the other is in external rotation (as in Figure 7.21c). As the expansion screw is turned, the internal side will improve, whereas the external side will become more externally rotated and flared. This will have an adverse knock-on effect on the rest of the cranium.

The effects of inappropriate appliances are clearly demonstrated in the following item from a local newspaper cutting:

> A schoolgirl with an illness that baffled doctors began to recover rapidly after throwing out her dental brace, her family said. Stephanie Fender, 15, from Mount Pleasant, Swansea, was confined to bed for months, feeling sick and lethargic. Now she is recovering after her mother read of a similar case apparently triggered by a dental brace. Since then, Stephanie has started visiting a 'cranially aware dentist' who said the brace was blocking passages allowing vital fluid to circulate around her brain and body, causing disruption to her immune system. Her mother, Donna Fender, 31, said, 'She is now seeing a dental specialist in Bristol, who is going to fit a metal brace behind her teeth to push them out and unlock everything.'[3]

Figure 7.21a is an example of a bilaterally internally rotated maxilla. When the two halves are symmetrical, it is quite in order to use an expansion device to enlarge the palate to normal dimensions, thereby making space for the teeth. This usually has a beneficial effect on the cranio-sacral system (as in George's case).

a.
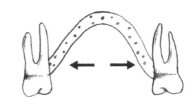

b.
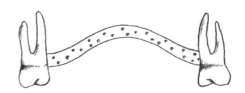

c.
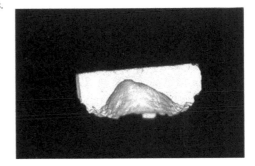

7.21 (a) Narrow gothic arch
(b) Wide maxillary arch
(c) When the palate is internally rotated on one side (left-hand side) and externally rotated on the other (right-hand side), it is not appropriate to use a central expansion device

Problems arise when the palate is internally rotated on one side (left-hand side) and externally rotated on the other (right-hand side) – as in the model in Figure 7.21c. It is not appropriate to use a central expansion device here as each side needs a different input, so this requires a more sophisticated form of treatment involving light wire appliances using asymmetric forces and light elastics

MANDIBLE

Any treatment which causes the mandible to be forced back and up, with a loss of vertical dimension, will result in possible TMJ dysfunction, and the neck is likely to go into a dysfunctional pattern. This compensatory pattern in the neck will be impossible to resolve satisfactorily whilst the bite is incorrect and unphysiologic for that patient.

The case of Jimmy (13 years old)

Jimmy had a narrow upper jaw, with his teeth crowded out of the arch. His mandible was retruded and he could only bite in a backward position because this was the only position of relative comfort.

In addition to having this very significant malocclusion, he had been diagnosed with 'petit mal' epilepsy, blanking out at times, though not totally collapsing. He had had various diagnostic scans including EEGs and MRIs which were inconclusive.

His mandible was not only retruded, but was also rotated back on one side more than the other.

It has been my experience that, with this sort of picture, the atlas is always involved, and in his case it was not only rotated back on one side, but was also canted down on the same side. This was probably affecting blood flow through the basilar artery.

I worked on opening up the upper dental arch with light wire appliances, so that there was space for his teeth, which I later aligned with fixed braces. Throughout these procedures, Jimmy had cranio-sacral therapy, with particular focus on the occiput–atlas relationship.

As the tissues of his neck released and the occiput–atlas relationship rebalanced and stabilized, so his mandible repositioned forward and centred itself under the now corrected maxillary arch. Everything now fitted together as nature designed and his symptoms never returned.

Bridge work

It must be remembered that the hard palate is made up of six sections (two maxillae, two premaxillae, two palatine bones) with sutures in between each section, as shown in Figure 7.22.

A bridge is an appliance for restoring a space which has resulted from losing a tooth. The teeth on either side of the space usually have crowns on them, and the replacement for the 'missing tooth' is joined to these crowns and is known as a pontic. This is skilful work requiring planning and meticulous support from the dental technician who constructs the bridgework.

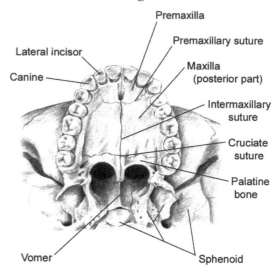

7.22   The hard palate is made up of six sections with sutures in between each section

A dentist carrying out this high-level work may be extremely adept at what he or she does dentally, but may not be aware that it is very important *not* to cross any of the sutures without incorporating some stress-breaking mechanism, so that there is still movement in the suture.

Locking up of any of these sutures, especially the midline suture, can have devastating effects on the health of the patient. I have had to cut an anterior bridge in the midline on quite a few patients before their cranio-sacral systems could rebalance and their health could recover. From my experience, some of the symptoms that can occur are:

- headaches, tightness in the head
- feeling stressed and irritable continuously
- neck pain, especially in the upper neck, with limited neck movement
- loss of balance, vertigo, hyperacusis and dizziness
- loss of hearing
- progressive chronic fatigue and generalized muscle weakness
- progressive paraesthesia and abnormal sensations in the arms and legs.

Implants

Implants have been around for a number of years. Initially, although many were successful, in a substantial number of cases the materials used failed to integrate with the bone, leading to infection and rejection. However, over the past twenty years or so, with the advent of titanium and zirconium oxide, the implant can in most cases integrate successfully with the bone, making a very strong base onto which the restorative work can be built. This has proved to be a very big leap forward for patients with missing teeth and poor dental support, especially in edentulous patients.

However, the same principles apply to patients undergoing implantology as with those undergoing bridge work with regard to the maxillary sutures. It is most important that the integrity of the sutures and the cranio-sacral mechanism is not violated.

As a cranio-sacral therapist, it is advisable to ask the patient questions regarding any restorative work, as it is rarely the case that the patient is aware of the aforementioned phenomena, and very often the well-meaning dentist is unaware as well.

In the early 1990s, I spent a great deal of time learning from various clinicians in the United States. I will never forget the expression on the face of a neurologically compromised patient who had been in a wheelchair for several years, when her anterior bridge was removed. Her completely dead and vacant expression became animated and she started to cry, as she realized that she had been released from her incarcerated existence. The bridge was modified with a stress-breaking device which allowed the two halves of the maxilla to move again and was then re-cemented. She continued with her chiropractic treatment and physical therapy, making a complete recovery – after all those years in a wheelchair.

Summary

Dentistry and cranio-sacral therapy can play a massive role in working together. No one person can treat everything, but by forming a team – especially in the treatment of young children who have malocclusions with a compromised cranial system and other such debilitating situations – dentists and cranio-sacral therapists, working cooperatively, can have remarkable results in helping those children (and adults) to develop normally and healthily into nature's design.

II

7

Chapter 8

Dentistry in the Context of Cranio-Sacral Therapy

Dr Wojciech Tarnowski

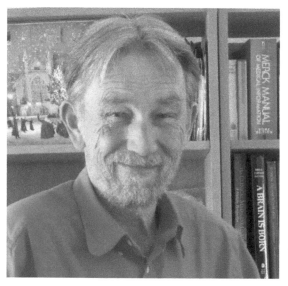

Dr Wojciech Tarnowski

Many years ago, Sally came to my surgery with an unusual dental problem. For about a year she had been receiving dental treatment which had totally failed, leaving her in pain and distress.

What was unusual about Sally was that the problem was only affecting one tooth, in an otherwise perfect mouth. There was no tooth displacement, no decay, no fillings, no gum disease, and no discoloration, except around the first molar on the lower right side, which was shattered, in a swollen, bleeding gum with pus.

Every clinically correct procedure that was done had failed. The story began with some tenderness in the tooth which her dentist had ground down to avoid pressure from the tooth above during clenching. This did not help. A micro-fracture was suspected – which does not usually show up on X-ray – and the tooth was root-canal treated and filled. The filling broke and

the tooth was restored with a gold crown, which fell off when the tooth broke in half. Sally was now on antibiotics and the remnants of the tooth were due to be extracted. She had come to me not so much in the hope of saving it, but more to try to find out what had happened.

At that time, a group of dentists was training with the Sutherland Society in cranial osteopathy and also participating in postgraduate programmes at the British School of Osteopathy. We were trying to apply the principles of whole-body mechanics to dental problems, so we tended to attract patients with unusual dental problems, such as Sally. With Sally, a visual examination revealed pelvic distortion with a history of trauma – a road traffic accident about a year before her jaw symptoms started, in which she was hit on her left hip by a motorcycle.

Unfortunately, appropriate cranial treatment came too late to prevent Sally from developing a full-blown osteomyelitis following the tooth extraction, necessitating admission to hospital for intravenous antibiotics and maxillofacial surgery. But her story certainly demonstrated to me that a tooth problem can arise from a hip injury, and opened my eyes to the need to explore the relationship between the 'Masticatory Apparatus' (where dentists work) and the whole body.

Dental training

The training of dentists in England takes just over four years, or at least it did when I qualified in the early 1960s. The first year was largely shared with medical students, although in the dissecting room our cutting up was confined to the head and a bit of neck, while they had the run of the rest of the body. Anyway, although we were aware that there was a body, we were not supposed to touch it. Dentists deal with the mouth and adjoining structures, doctors deal with the body.

Personal experience

Before going into general dental practice, I spent a hectic six months as a Resident Dental House Surgeon. If there had been any idea about not being able to survive without eight hours continuous sleep every night then that was very quickly banished. We were on call 24 hours a day 7 days a week, with two days off every three weeks, for three months. The duties were to look after the dental needs of all the in-patients at the main hospital during the day and to be on call at the casualty department for dental emergencies every night.

One incident in the early hours one morning brought home the potential practice of whole-body dentistry. A woman was brought into casualty with her jaw dislocated and jammed open. She was in severe pain as her jaw muscles were in spasm and so tight that it was impossible to put her jaw back. The procedure in such a case would be to give an inhalation anaesthetic to relax all the muscles of the body and so enable the dislocated jaw to be replaced. Unfortunately all the anaesthetists were busy with people involved in a road traffic accident and not available for some time. The muscle spasm was getting worse by the minute; there was only one thing to do. I placed my thumbs on both sides of the jaw and kicked her shin hard. As she yelled with pain and surprise – using the jaw-opening muscles which managed to overcome the spasm of the jaw-closing muscles for a moment – her jaw snapped back into place. Considering the look of relief on her face, I'm sure I was forgiven for the tender shin. This was a rather crude example of how one part of the body can affect another, and it left a deep mark on my memory and attitude over the years – much deeper, I hope, than my shoe on the lady's shin.

After leaving the hospital service, I went into general practice as an assistant. Still being full of surgical experience and expertise, most dental solutions were usually surgical. One day a patient arrived who had impacted lower wisdom teeth. Although they were not causing any problems, they were just ripe for surgical extraction. However, the young man was going away to America for two years, so he promised to come back when he returned, in order to have them removed. When he did come back, these teeth were fully erupted and in a perfectly healthy position – something that was considered impossible by the then current dental opinion, especially of surgeons. This was another little wake-up call to the possibility that current good dental practice might not always be the best solution for the benefit of the whole patient.

These were the days of experiment with all sorts of methods and drugs. I had joined the Society for the Advancement of Anaesthesia in Dentistry and the training was in the use of many intravenous and inhalation systems of sedation and anaesthesia. One of these was developed by the US army as a perfect battlefield anaesthetic. An injection anywhere on the body produced total loss of pain sensation for a few hours without loss of consciousness. However, it had an unfortunate side effect – it made the patient have death-like feelings. This particular drug was not a great success in dental practice, but I gather that it is now apparently used as a recreational drug.

There was not much regulation in those days and I worked for a dentist whose assessment of a patient's heart condition and suitability for sedation and anaesthesia was whether they could climb a steep flight of stairs to his surgery. It is amazing that there were no fatalities. All this seemed somewhat risky, and when I opened my own practice, I stayed with gas and air sedation, relaxation and a little hypnosis, in which some of us were lucky to be trained as undergraduates.

Looking deeper

Associating with these unusual people brought me in touch with like-minded dentists who were looking for something more than tackling endless dental disease, and looking rather to investigate its causes and how to integrate their dental training with the whole-body approach. The big breakthrough came in the late 1970s.

At this time there had been a rising wave of 'alternatives', especially in the USA, which started to spill into England and into Europe. I explored courses on all sorts of systems including

II

8

ayurveda, acupuncture, homoeopathy, yoga and transcendental meditation.

At one of these meetings I heard about a lady whose torus palatinus was reduced by cranial manipulation. A torus palatinus is a bony lump in the palate, and in my surgery days we used to remove these with a hammer and chisel in an operating theatre. I booked an appointment with a cranial osteopath and was so impressed with the experience that I decided to study cranial osteopathy.

Sutherland Society courses

The postgraduate department of the British School of Osteopathy was running courses in association with the Sutherland Society to train people in cranial work. As in America, they not only accepted osteopaths but also dentists, doctors and veterinarians. The courses were run under strict Sutherland Society rules and had to have a participant from the American Sutherland Society as an observer. In this way I was lucky enough to meet and work with some of Sutherland's direct pupils. They were the most experienced cranial osteopaths in the world and, although they shared a common system and training, they each expressed it in a completely individual way.

At these courses, the basic training was strictly controlled and guided to enable participants to feel the cranial mechanism. At the first course I attended, by the third day many of the participating osteopaths had not felt the cranial rhythm and walked out in disgust, but those of us who persisted were rewarded with our first experience of 'the Tide'.

The Sutherland System is very anatomy-based as a grounding tool, and I remember sitting with my hands on somebody's temporal bones trying to work out how on earth they could move, when my mind wandered off to the top of a red London bus that was passing the window – and suddenly my hands expanded into this glorious, peaceful rhythm. Once experienced, it cannot be forgotten, but it took me, working as a dentist, a great deal of practice to establish it on demand.

With cranial treatment, traumas healed

Working in general dental practice every day was not conducive to practising cranial osteopathy, but I decided to tune in to every single dental patient every time through the mandible. For a long time nothing happened, except that patients commented how relaxed and cared for they felt having their face held. Then one day I could instantly tune in to the cranial rhythm and assess its quality. This enabled me to monitor the effect that common dental procedures had on the cranial mechanism. I was appalled by what I discovered.

For example, once, it was necessary to remove a misplaced upper wisdom tooth which was causing lacerations to the cheek. With local anaesthetic, the extraction was very quick and painless, but on checking the cranial system, I found that it was in a profound state of shock. It took a good few minutes to dissipate the shock and re-establish the rhythm.

After this, I monitored all dental procedures and attempted to dissipate the aftershock. I soon realized that, with cranial treatment, traumas healed up much more quickly, and with no post-operative complications. This also applied to infections and inflammations and even pericoronitis.

Pericoronitis is an inflammation of the gum surrounding partially erupted wisdom teeth, which is not only uncomfortable but can lead to serious infection. The usual treatment is a week of antibiotics, hot salt water mouthwashes and, usually, eventual extraction. With cranial treatment, I found that a pericoronitis tended to resolve in about two days with no antibiotics. It was even possible sometimes to resolve pain of unknown origin which could otherwise, in conventional dentistry, have resulted in a great deal of unnecessary and unsuccessful dental treatment.

Practising cranially – as a dentist

It should be remembered that at this time my cranial work was carried out within the context of dentistry – with the intention of making dental work more successful or solving dental problems – and it was all carried out from the head and jaw. Dentistry is a self-governing profession in England and is regulated mainly by dentists on the basic assumption that 'dentists do what dentists normally do'. So I considered it potentially risky to treat anything but dental, or at least oral, problems – and certainly not from anywhere but the head and neck (as a few dentists found to their cost). In time, I managed to develop a system that I was comfortable with, which encompassed both diagnosis and treatment, and which was powerful and discreet.

Direct pupils of Sutherland

After the first Sutherland course – where I was the only dentist – more dentists joined the courses. We trained with the Sutherland Society for over a decade, meeting and working with the American observers who came to oversee the courses. They were mostly direct pupils of Sutherland such as Rollin Becker, Anne Wales, Alan Becker, Robert Fulford and John Harakal, who each expressed the Tide in their own unique way.

The Postgraduate Department of the British School of Osteopathy at that time organized courses with members of every medical profession, including many complementary and alternative therapies. As dentists, we were quite actively involved, giving courses on dental topics and in turn receiving private tuition from the tutors. This was suddenly disbanded at the beginning of the 1990s as the osteopaths sought self-regulation by statute. Now the osteopathic profession no longer trains non-osteopaths in England – and cranio-sacral therapy, which had by then already been around for several years, flourished all the more.

The cranio-sacral rhythm stopped

About that time, one of the tutors who specially liked to train dentists asked me to see her husband who had been fitted with a metal partial denture and was reacting to it adversely for no apparent reason. Having some experience of dowsing, it occurred to me that the cranial rhythm might work in a similar way. I checked the husband dentally and cranially and, sure enough, the cranial rhythm altered with the metal denture in the mouth, even though it fitted perfectly. Then, using the cranio-sacral rhythm as a 'dowsing' tool, I asked the system if the man was reacting to the metal content of the denture and the rhythm suddenly stopped dead. The tutor, who was monitoring the rhythm at the feet, looked up with surprise and said 'it stopped'. This was the first time that I had independent confirmation that this phenomenon could be detected by other experienced practitioners, so I went through it again – and again I got the response 'it stopped'. This senior tutor could not acknowledge that this was possible, but I had the confirmation I needed, and I still use this 'Indicator Pulse' today, although in a more refined way.

We each have to find our own way of working with the Tide, and although over the years I was fortunate enough to meet and work with many talented people, some left a more lasting impression than others. The two American osteopaths who were the greatest inspiration for me were Robert Fulford (Figure 8.1a, b) and Rollin Becker (Figure 8.2). For me, Fulford was 'the Prana Man', and Becker was 'the Fulcrum Man', because they said that is how they worked.

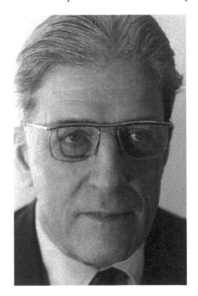

8.1   (a) Dr Robert Fulford D.O.

When I first saw Robert Fulford he apologized for feeling somewhat tired, but explained that when he had got off his flight from the States, a distraught young osteopath had asked him to treat his brain-damaged baby. He held the baby in a Still Point for three hours. We only discovered afterwards what a Fulford Still Point was. We had all been taught to practise the 'feather touch' – which was difficult enough if you had been originally trained as a dentist – and here Dr Fulford clamped your head in a vice-like grip and held on. At some point or other his hands would spring apart as if by themselves, and that was it – treatment over.

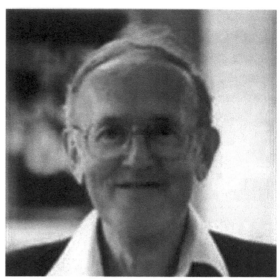

8.2   *Dr Rollin Becker D.O.*

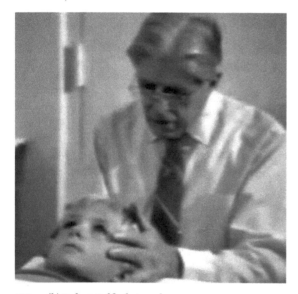

8.1   *(b) Robert Fulford at work*

Robert Fulford worked with universal prana, or rather universal prana worked through him. The prana did the work and decided when his hands should stop the contact. This at first seemed too good to be true, but I soon discovered from personal experience both as a patient and a practitioner that it works. However, it needs a certain type of personality to use this system all the time. Robert Fulford was a rock-solid, steady man who could sit for three hours holding a baby in his vice grip, but for me it was necessary to adapt his system to my own personality and feather-light way of working.

It is very difficult to describe what it was about Rollin Becker that left such a deep impression. Like all Sutherland's students, he was deeply grounded in anatomy and physiology, but his basic philosophy was that of the Fulcrum. It is an axiom that there can be no movement without a relative Still Point, and Rollin Becker called that the Fulcrum.

It took me many years to understand that this process is so completely natural that it goes on by itself, whether we are aware of it or not – but only when we know about it do we have any chance of utilizing it or having any control over it.

Invasion

Why would we want to utilize or have any control over such a process? One of the most important lessons, if not *the* most important lesson, I learnt during training in cranial osteopathy was how not to 'invade' the patient and how not to be 'invaded' by them.

On Sutherland Society training courses, it was rightly assumed that after a week of work and experiment, often with inexperienced hands, it would be necessary in the final session for the students to be 'put together' by their tutor, and I was duly checked and balanced by my tutor. On that particular occasion I felt quite odd for a number of weeks, but did not think anything of it, until, some months later, I was asked to assess dentally a patient of that particular tutor. When I tuned in to this patient, I experienced the same feeling that I had after the course and suddenly realized that this particular osteopath was probably invading his patients.

On a subsequent course I was fortunate enough to encounter a tutor who spent a whole day teaching non-invasion. The answer of course lies in maintaining a constant awareness of the Fulcrum, which is not as easy as it sounds. It is almost a meditative state, and without constant practice the mind can slip away all too easily. Also, as well as preventing invasion, resting in a Fulcrum can avoid the use of the practitioner's own energy in treatment. It is a sure sign that, if the practitioner experiences any fatigue after treatment, a form of invasion has taken place and the results may not be beneficial. This is how Bob Fulford worked – he utilized only Universal Energy, which filled him and the patient so that both benefited as it flowed through to earth.

TMJ

During the 1980s, within cutting-edge dentistry, the focus was on the temporo-mandibular joint (TMJ). Anatomically it is a lever, so it can also be considered to have a fulcrum. It was the centre of research and practice of aware dental practitioners. It could be affected by many specialities within dentistry, and the results of treatment were often quite spectacular in curing not only migraines but also all manner of pains and dysfunction all around the body.

Conventional Western dentistry often considered the TMJ to be the province of general (non-dental) surgery and did not specifically train dental students to treat its dysfunction. I remember during my surgery days assisting with injecting some poor man's TMJs with sclerosing solution to immobilize them as a means of ameliorating his pain! However, among dentists the awareness started to dawn that working in the mouth might have an effect on the whole head and even the whole body.

Moffett's Orders

The question arises, 'What is so special about the TMJ?' In the early 1990s, I came across the work of Benjamin Moffett, an anatomist who

was professor of orthodontics at the University of Washington. His aim was to show that dealing with the TMJ should be a speciality of dentistry, rather than general surgery. To this end he devised a system of 'Four Orders of Cranio-facial Articulations'; in other words, four types of joint through which forces are distributed within the head:[1]

- First Order Articulations are the occlusal joints, where the lower teeth meet the upper teeth. This is where most force is generated.
- Second Order Articulations are the gomphoses or periodontal membranes which suspend each tooth in its socket.
- Third Order Articulations are the cranio-mandibular joints, that is, the temporo-mandibular joints (but he also includes the maxillofacial sutures).
- Fourth Order Articulations are the cranial sutures.

Moffett proposed that all these four orders are interdependent, and that working on one order would therefore influence all the others. So dentists working on teeth would be affecting the other three orders – and vice versa. Therefore, what conventional dentists do – drilling, filling, extracting and replacing teeth, and even orthodontics – will have an effect on the other orders, that is, periodontal, TMJ and cranial, for better or worse. However, he emphasized that Order One is the only one that has no natural cellular repair mechanism and is affected only by wear, disease and dentistry.

Most dentists work with Orders One and Two, working with the occlusal articulations and periodontal disturbances, without awareness of the other orders. Some work with Order Three, incorporating an awareness of the TMJ. Very few work with Order Four – that is, with awareness of the effect that they may have on the cranial articulations, and consequently on the whole body, through the vestibular system (as we will see shortly).

If the TMJs are in balance, the whole body will tend to self-heal

During the 1980s and 1990s, while most dentists in the world kept their patients' mouths pain- and disease-free, and kept them smiling and chewing, with plastic, porcelain and gold, a small but enthusiastic minority spread the gospel of the TMJ. The basic premise was that if the TMJs were kept in a good functioning position, then the whole body would tend to become more balanced, less painful, more energetic and would tend to self-heal. This was the world of the Third Order dentist. Third Order dentistry covered many approaches, from the coarsest surgical replacement to the finest orthodontics. I met many Third Order dentists and went on many courses in Britain and America – but the people who made the biggest impact on the way I work were the Fourth Order workers, and they were by no means all dentists, or even therapists.

When visiting Aelred Fonder in Illinois, author of *The Dental Physician*[2] and *The Dental Distress Syndrome*,[3] I was introduced to many concepts such as Hans Selye's Stress and the General Adaptive Syndrome,[4] Whatmore and Kohli's Physiopathology and Dysponesis,[5] and others such as Weston Price's work on nutrition, *Nutrition and Physical Degeneration*.[6]

One of the most interesting concepts for me was the Quadrant Theorem of Casey Guzay.[7] The importance of the position of the odontoid peg (dens) is well documented, especially in literature concerning whiplash injuries, yet here we have an indication that the position of the dens would have an implication on the position of the mandible and the position of the mandible on the position of the dens. This is highly significant considering the anatomical position of the dens with its relationship to the spinal cord. After all, fracture or displacement of the dens can mean instant death.

Examining the anatomy of the TMJs, it may be noticed that they are designed for adaptation – in order to keep the mandible functioning as well as possible in all situations. This is not really surprising considering the importance of the mandible. Normal life would be impossible without a mandible, as it is essential for functions such as chewing, swallowing, speech and even keeping an open airway for breathing. Yet people with severely compromised dentitions and TMJs can still do these things with greater or lesser degrees of efficiency.

So in what possible ways can an efficient masticatory mechanism have an influence on pain and health in the whole body?

The vestibular system

In the petrous portion of each of the two temporal bones lies the vestibular system of the body. For all intents and purposes its connections function as the homeostatic system of the body, balancing, coordinating and repairing, internally and in action. This is the 'Operating System' of the body (in computer terminology) and it will try to perform its function automatically, however severely compromised.

This may be the point where cranio-sacral therapy, dentistry and many other therapies come together – where treatment consists of removing obstacles to the full functioning of the vestibular system in its role of maintaining the homeostatic function of the body.

A few years ago, by chance, I found an article by Dr Richard Belli titled 'A Brief Discussion of Cranial Manipulation and Visceral and Somatic Response'.[8] In this article, he suggests that some, if not all, therapeutic and physiological responses to cranial manipulation are brought about through the vestibular system. He also suggests that the vestibular system cannot function properly unless the two 'vestibular apparatuses' are in correct juxtaposition to one another.

There are, of course, two vestibular apparatuses, one on each side of the head. Each side is designed to detect movement, acceleration and deceleration in three dimensions. There are connections on both sides to the hearing system, the optical system, the cerebellum, the reticular system, the brainstem and the hypothalamus.

Normalization – acquired habitual patterns

This system, when working properly, enables us to perform complex multiple tasks automatically. So what can happen when things are altered by wear, disease or trauma? We carry on anyway, but not very efficiently, until the mind considers it can no longer cope, the prana is shut off, and the body disintegrates. However, until then it has coping strategies, and probably the most insidious of these is normalization – the formation of a habit where a pathological pattern is considered normal and therefore works automatically.

For example, when people talk or eat with a damaged dentition or other dysponetic Orders, the mandible will acquire habitual pattern generators which will prioritize talking and eating over the balance of the temporal bones.

The mandible plays a crucial role in the relationship of the temporal bones because of its functions. It is not separate either from the head or from the rest of the body, but because of the way we use it to chew, swallow or speak, or even breathe, habitual automatic patterns are learned. Take as an example trauma to the hip, where the body has to adapt by twisting, in order to function. The whole body compensates around the twist and the temporal bones move out of balance. The mandible then functions out of balance as well, putting extra stress on the teeth, more on one side than the other, as a result of which the teeth may then wear or break. The chewing function then adapts, eventually changing the anatomy, and the situation becomes habitually 'normal'. The hip may eventually heal – but the effect is perpetuated in the body through the chewing mechanism.

Such habitual patterns are cumulative and can lead to complex adaptation throughout the body unless rectified. Quite often, cranial adjustments do not hold, or compensation occurs rather than resolution. Very often it is useful to balance the chewing mechanism using a removable, adjustable plastic overlay called a splint, in order to stabilize the temporal bones and thus facilitate many therapies and therapeutic responses.

Every therapy works, but only to the extent that it is able to relieve stress on the homeostatic system, and those therapies that appear to be most effective are the ones that have a more direct influence on the vestibular system.

How I work

Over the years I have tried all the systems that I have encountered, but I only use them when there is a specific indication for their use. Every person is unique, and the most effective treatment would be specific to them.

I use the Indicator Pulse every time, in the same order, with every patient, and I notate it using a code. This sets a base where it is relatively easy to spot any changes and deviations in the habitual pattern. However, there are many ways of doing this, and during teaching or training I find that students have different aptitudes, so I try not to impose my system but try to encourage their own natural ability or inclination to achieve their own way of working.

My basic attitude is that human bodies are by and large able to heal themselves if enabled to do so. In essence, treatment consists of removing obstacles on energetic, subtle levels and allowing the causal level to manifest – but leaving it to the patient's system to decide whether to clear it or not. From past experience I have found that it is potentially disruptive to release deep emotions for the patient. I let them decide for themselves when they are ready and I provide support.

With the patient lying down, to obviate as much as possible the influence of gravity, and working from the head, I initiate connection with the patient and mentally ask for acknowledgement and permission to proceed. I then check the quality of the cranial rhythm at the temporal bones and upper cervical vertebrae and then check the quality of the chakras and the amount of energy available to the whole system. All this takes just a few seconds and provides an overview of the general functioning of the body.

I then check the adaptability of the vestibular system by putting cotton wool rolls (a dentist thing) between the teeth on both sides of the mouth, and then on each side of the mouth separately, to check if the cranial rhythm changes. If it is perceivable and does change then I conclude that the vestibular system is compromised somewhere. Before going on to scan for ascending and descending patterns or any dysponetic signals, I allow the temporal bones to come into balance by the simple procedure of asking the patient to hold a cotton wool roll between their front teeth in the midline, while I monitor through the mandible. In this position, the pulse always disappears and goes through a Still Point for varying amounts of time. Often it is a few minutes, but with a seriously compromised system it can take much longer. The system spontaneously goes through a series of unwinds and readjustments until it is completed, and finishes with a strong even pulse which lasts for 33 seconds.

II

8

I have never really found out why it lasts for 33 seconds, but very occasionally I find it lasting a few seconds longer. In such cases, the only common factor is that these people have at some time or other been on anti-depressant drugs. I can only surmise that the beat has to do with the polypeptide circulation.[9]

Ascending and descending patterns

Ascending and descending patterns are a convenient way of describing the effect that cranio-facial joints have on the body, and the rest of the body has on the cranio-facial joints. Accumulated trauma seems to leave affected joints unable to contribute accurate information back to the vestibular system. This leaves a distorted body image, and movement takes place without taking these joints into account, leading to physical body distortion and its many consequences.

J.P. Meersseman, a chiropractor, was recently the fitness supervisor for AC Milan, a very successful European football club. His system of assessing ascending and descending patterns enabled him to detect an injury-prone player, affecting the transfer decisions of multi-million-euro players.

Scanning

After the temporal bones, and therefore the vestibular system, come into balance as much as they can, I mentally scan the four 'Orders of Craniofacial Joints' and the major joints of the rest of the body, starting with the feet. The procedure is that when I hold a joint in mind and the Indicator Pulse stops, this implies that the area indicated is dysponetic (functionally disturbed).

Dysponesis is a physiopathological state where various organs and systems of the body are no longer fully coordinated with the homeostatic system of the body.

When I mention a 'dysponetic point' I mean a point or joint that is no longer recognized by the vestibular system as being part of the whole-body image and so the body as a whole automatically functions as if that joint or point was not there and compensation takes place. For example, very often a stressed joint breaks down because it has to bear an excessive load due to compensation for a cause elsewhere, so that when it is treated it eventually breaks down again because the real cause has not been addressed. A good case in point is a hip replacement operation.

Over the years, with experience, it became clear to me that some dysponetic joints were much more significant than others.

Lock Foot

The most significant and also the most neglected is Lock Foot. In the 1990s a very enthusiastic dentist from Oslo named Kjell Bjørner attended many holistic dental seminars in Britain, emphasizing the importance of what he called 'Lock Foot' in relation to the difficulty of stabilizing the chewing mechanism, because of instability in the pelvic girdle. He used to go around with an enormous set of calipers containing a spirit level which, when placed on the iliac crests of a standing person, demonstrated their unevenness. He would then lie the person down and manipulate their feet, then stand them up and demonstrate with his gadget that the iliac crests were now even.

I was very sceptical about the whole thing, especially when he said that he was not able to clear my Lock Foot. However, some time later during a futile attempt to stabilize a patient's splint, it occurred to me to check for Lock Foot with the Indicator Pulse. Sure enough it showed up but, much to my surprise, there was not one lock but two in the same foot. When these were cleared, the lower jaw stabilized and remained stable.

It was like having a new toy to play with. At that time, we were building up deciduous molars in children, after a research project by one of our colleagues showed that this helped to eliminate glue ear and improve hearing. A friend brought her six-year-old daughter, who had not been able to speak properly and was withdrawn and uncommunicative, to have the build-ups done, to see if that would help her. But it soon became obvious, as she curled up in the corner of the waiting room, that we would not be able to get anywhere near her mouth without a great deal of trauma. A quick check revealed that she had a Lock Foot and, when that was released, within half an hour this depressed child was wandering around smiling and hugging everyone. From that time, I check every patient, every time, for Lock Foot; and as Kjell Bjørner said, it only needs to be released once, like a switch being turned off. (His book is published in Norwegian.[10])

Most people that I see have a Lock Foot pattern, but not everybody; and nobody that I have talked to about it seems to know what could possibly cause it, but there are reasons to suspect that it is a product of Western civilization. Over the years there have been many examples of profound energy changes, especially in young people, after Lock Foot release. A typical example was a teenage girl who was undergoing orthodontic treatment and suffering headaches and mental fog. Releasing a Lock Foot, along with some cranial treatment, soon got rid of the headaches without the need to remove the orthodontic appliances; and we subsequently received a statement from the orthodontist reporting on how rapidly the treatment was progressing. Once orthodontic treatment has begun, it is rarely necessary to discontinue it in order to alleviate side effects, since releasing ascending patterns is often enough.

Coccyx

Another dysponetic area I always check for is coccyx damage. Some years ago, a medical doctor in the Midlands specializing in the treatment of patients diagnosed with multiple sclerosis discovered that, when he put a wooden spatula in their mouth and got them to bite on it, they suddenly recovered their muscular strength and movement – but not every time and not for long. We had a holistic dental study group in that area at the time and my wife and I became involved in investigating his patients. My wife is a physiotherapist and Alexander Technique teacher and, since I was a dentist, she is much better at body work than I will ever be. She would check the patient's lower spine while I monitored at the cranium. I remember clearly with a particular patient resting my hands gently on the temporal bones while my wife had her hand at the base of the spine. Suddenly my left arm went into spasm and a few moments later the spasm disappeared. So I asked my wife where she had her hand and she said 'on the coccyx', so of course I asked her to put it back again, and as she did so the spasm

came back. We investigated all the patients using scanning, trauma history and touch over a period of a few weeks and discovered that every one of the forty patients diagnosed with MS had coccyx damage.

We had no way of treating coccyx damage at that time, but I often mentioned this finding at various courses and meetings, and one day an osteopath approached me at a conference and said that he had checked all the clients at his practice who were diagnosed with MS and discovered that nineteen out of twenty had coccyx damage. People rarely remember their coccyx damage, and not everyone with coccyx damage has MS symptoms, but we found it very difficult to successfully treat the coccyx dysponeses. After some experimentation, I found homeopathic Hypericum to be the most effective treatment, but since a few years ago, when I ran out of the actual remedy, I find thought-form homeopathy works just as well.

Odontoid peg

The next dysponetic area I always check is the odontoid peg. This is usually associated with whiplash injury and in most cases is very difficult to eliminate, especially if it has been there for some time. Its position is such that any displacement and dysponesis can lead to bizarre whole-body symptoms through its effect on the vestibular system.

The odontoid is in such a delicate area that although the dysponesis can be switched off – in other words, connected to the vestibular system successfully – when recognized and targeted, it is very unstable and keeps reappearing. With habitual use, the area does not appear to remain stable enough for the muscles and ligaments supporting it to heal. So far, the best results we tend to get are from multidisciplinary care – elimination of any ascending patterns (especially Lock Foot and coccyx) and cranio-sacral therapy, followed by construction of a dental splint on quadrant theorem principles and simultaneous Alexander lessons to re-pattern faulty use of the body and posture. One thing is for sure – treatment is quite complicated and there is no one system that will apply to every patient.

Hormonal, visceral, pathological

I then make a general scan, using the Indicator Pulse, of the hormonal system, the organs, any significant pathology and cancer states, and anything else that the vestibular system would like to tell me about. All this I notate in a shorthand code which anybody can make up for themselves, but it has to be flexible enough to account for many variations, and meaningful enough to make sensible comparisons.

Whole-body picture

After finishing the scan I have a whole-body picture, on the energetic level, of all the areas that the vestibular system wants me to address. Treatment can be carried out physically or mentally. I prefer to use two hands to move energy between them, but the most reliable method for me is to have an assistant who can put their hand or hands at the dysponetic spot, while I monitor at the head. This of course comes from my days working as a dentist. The Indicator Pulse is very accurate at indicating the precise spot where the touch needs to be.

This is not quite the same as Upledger's 'Inner Physician', as this is a notation system, so that when I go through the same procedure next time, there is a direct written comparison. With every session there are usually fewer and fewer dysponetic areas, until just a small number are left, which are often on a different level and are more of a core problem.

Various individual patterns can emerge. One important one is what I call the 'Double Whammy'. These are dysponetic points that affect ascending and descending patterns at the same time, so that when one is dealt with the other will bring it back. They both have to be addressed simultaneously. It is very rare that there are more than two points, but if this does occur and if there are not that many hands available, I tend to use the mental stacking technique.

Although I keep to this routine as a grounding method, there is huge variation from one person to another and in the symptoms that they present, so occasionally I do contact the Inner Physician for advice and try to follow instructions. That is how early cancer indicators can be switched off.

To sum up

When working with human beings, it is necessary to start with the whole person. Specialists often forget the effect that their speciality has on the larger whole, because there are other specialists who specialize in dealing with the side effects. This can be especially true for dentistry.

When any one part of the human body changes for whatever reason, it can be quite obvious (to those who look) that the whole body changes automatically to adapt. These adaptations are almost completely automatic and difficult to predict because there are so many variables – often including emotional levels – and they are often accepted as normal.

Much has been written about many aspects of the vestibular system, but not much from the point of view of dentistry and how treating the TMJ in fact works on the level of the whole body.

Similarly, much has been written and taught on the subtle aspects of cranio-sacral therapy, but not much on its association with the automatic control system of the body – the vestibular system.

The knowledge that such a system exists and how it works can bring together under one umbrella many different therapies and treatments.

It may be some time before dentistry in the context of cranio-sacral therapy is recognized and practised widely, so in the meantime let us consider a few questions regarding dentistry that may commonly arise among cranio-sacral therapists.

Q1. When would it be necessary to refer patients to a dentist?

When there are primary disturbances in the occlusion, periodontium or TMJ that require dental stabilization to help balance the vestibular system.

However, there are of course occasions when chronic toothache is not of dental origin and referral to a dentist would only perpetuate the problem, as most dentists always feel that they have to do something.

Q2. How to advise patients whether to have dentistry?

It is not so much a case of whether to have dentistry or not, but rather what type of dentistry to have.

Apart from acute states it would be sensible to advise patients, especially those with many dysponetic areas, not to have too much dentistry done at once, to have as little non-reversible work done as possible, and not to have permanent restorations done initially. With cranio-sacral treatment, all the Orders change and adjustments to dental work are often necessary.

There are also different qualities of dental work and different materials used. It is almost impossible to assess the quality of dental work, except within a few limited parameters, and even then dentists will disagree. I have seen really bad dentistry which has lasted for forty years and excellent dentistry which has failed within days.

As far as materials go, the controversy lies mainly with the use of amalgam, which is primarily a mixture of mercury and silver. It is cheap and easy to use, but concerns have been raised about the leakage of mercury vapour and its toxic effects on the nervous system. By and large it would be best avoided. Removal of old amalgam fillings should be undertaken with great care and precautions, so as not to inhale the aerosol produced by the removal process. One further issue is allergy to certain metals, notably silver. If you can't wear silver rings, you should not have amalgam fillings.

Q3. How to resolve the after-effects of dental treatment?

Even in modern times, dental treatment can be quite traumatic. Having the mouth open for long periods of time to its full extent can pull muscles and stretch ligaments, especially round the TMJ, and especially if combined with an arched back and head bent back.

Cranio-sacral therapy can be very helpful in resolving dental trauma and enabling more rapid and effective healing. Fascial unwinding can be beneficial after any visit to the dentist, to resolve stresses and strains in the muscles and fascia of an overarched neck and elsewhere.

If the patient has no access to a therapist, it could be useful to lie down for a few minutes in 'semi-supine' holding something firm but not hard between their front teeth. This allows the mandible to gently stimulate the vestibular system through the temporal bones, to balance itself, remove stress, and return the system to a healing equilibrium.

This would not really be adequate after an extraction. When a tooth is extracted, three structures can be traumatized – the nerve, the bone, and the periodontal membrane. The periodontal membrane has a histological structure very close to that of a cranial suture – so much so, that some practitioners consider the teeth to be cranial bones and treat them as such. It would be very valuable for the patient to have a treatment with a cranio-sacral therapist as soon as possible after an extraction, thereby almost certainly helping to avoid a healing complication and infection, which often go together.

Q4. How to prepare patients for dentistry and orthodontics?

Without doubt, it is very valuable for a patient to receive good quality cranio-sacral therapy before dentistry, in order to eliminate their ascending patterns and free up their cranial sutures.

Any dentistry and orthodontics will affect the descending patterns and challenge any ascending patterns to react. Without cranio-sacral therapy, instead of the body adapting smoothly to change, the system could lock up, not only precipitating pain but also interfering with the dentistry and slowing down orthodontic treatment. When working smoothly, following appropriate cranio-sacral therapy, the body will adapt and remain in dynamic equilibrium, and use energy efficiently. This can help to minimize any adverse effects of dentistry.

Each person is individual, but it is always worthwhile checking for Lock Foot, coccyx and spinal dysponeses. Certainly in my experience, the most rewarding and the easiest to switch off is the Lock Foot.

Q5. What are the limitations of conventional dentistry?

Dentists are trained in all the skills of Order One and Order Two dentistry, sometimes in Order Three (mainly on postgraduate courses) and almost never in Order Four. They know how to extract teeth and replace them both by fixed or removable appliances such as bridges and dentures. They repair broken or decayed teeth with various metals, plastics and ceramics. They remove dental nerves and replace them with various materials and chemicals. They even instruct you how to brush and floss your teeth and not to eat too much sugar in the hope of preventing dental disease.

A well-functioning vestibular system is fully capable, through homeostasis, of protecting the mouth against dental disease as has often been experienced. However, if dentists are not fully aware of the effect their excellent work has on the rest of the body or the effect that the body has on the masticatory system, there can be problems sooner or later.

For example, when someone loses an upper front tooth through an accident, it is usual to replace it with a bridge, which to avoid the destruction of healthy tooth tissue is glued to healthy teeth on both sides of the gap. A high failure rate was soon noticed where one side of the bridge tended to come away because nobody had acknowledged the movement between the maxillary bones at the midline suture. Many patients would also experience severe symptoms of various kinds while the fixed bridge was in place, because the bridge was restricting movement of the intermaxillary suture, preventing fluent cranio-sacral motion.

In orthodontics, the practice of extracting teeth and then moving the remaining teeth to align the dental arches often has the result of locking the mandible, affecting the cranial bones and playing havoc with the vestibular system. There are of course many other examples of how an awareness of the interconnectedness of the various levels would not only avoid unnecessary dentistry but also enhance the wellbeing of the whole person.

Q6. Does stress cause TMJ problems?

Hans Selye, who coined the word 'stress' in the 1930s, spent many years researching what he called the General Adaptive Syndrome and its effects.[11] He said that humans (and animals) cannot function efficiently without eustress (good stress), but when the system is overwhelmed (distress) then pain and dysfunction occur on many levels. The General Adaptive Syndrome describes the body's struggle to remain viable in a situation where increased effort brings a diminishing effect. Clenching and grinding is a common experience when the body is trying to steady the vestibular system.

TMJs are particularly relevant because of their close relationship with the temporal bones and the core of the vestibular system. The way to relieve TMJ problems is to relieve the excessive stress on the body. This can be done through a great many different therapies and on many different levels, from nutrition to meditation, which is why there are so many valuable therapies available.

Practitioners are highly skilled in their specialities, so every therapy will work no matter what it is. However, some therapies are more effective than others. Cranio-sacral therapy, with a little help from appropriate dentistry and an awareness of how the vestibular system works, has the potential for being the most effective holistic therapy of all by restoring homeostasis.

Part III

Essentials of Cranio-Sacral Integration

Chapter 9

Essentials of Cranio-Sacral Integration

Higgs boson

In 2013 Professor Peter Higgs received the Nobel prize for a concept he first proposed in 1964 and for which the experimental proof was finally provided at the CERN laboratory in Switzerland in 2012. Professor Higgs postulated that there is an invisible field pervading the whole universe.

Within quantum physics it has now been established that there is a universal field, a unifying matrix within which everything exists and interacts – every galaxy, star, planet, solid object, living being, molecule, atom, subatomic particle – a field from which particles take their mass.

In the quantum model of cranio-sacral integration, we also perceive a universal field or matrix, within which life on earth has come into being, and each one of us exists as an individual matrix within this wider matrix. We are formed embryologically, developed, maintained and sustained by the biodynamic forces within that field, and every cell, atom and subatomic particle within our body is an integral part of that wider field.

Overview

- In order to understand cranio-sacral integration, we need to think on a quantum level. The body is not just skin and bones, muscles and fluids. All of these structures are composed of cells, of molecules, of atoms, of subatomic particles, in constant motion and interaction.

- The body is a coherent living matrix, an integrated cohesive mass of particles and waves bound together by nuclear forces, existing within the wider matrix of the universal field around us and the biodynamic forces within that fluidic field (Figure 9.1).

- These forces of nature determine the natural process of growth, development, health, healing, balance and integration, from embryonic development and throughout life, providing the body with an inherent ability to heal itself.

- These forces are expressed within the body as rhythmic motion.

- By engaging with these forces we can enhance their potential for healing and integration.

- In order to engage with these subtle forces and rhythms, we need to establish our own profoundly therapeutic practitioner presence – a calm, quiet meditative presence, simply being there in stillness.

- In order to enable the patient's optimum responsiveness, it is helpful to establish a settled, grounded and receptive state in the patient.

- Through establishing appropriate levels of light contact, spacious attention and profound tissue awareness, we can engage with the subtle quantum levels of being which constitute the matrix.

- This can be experienced as a fluidic field surrounding and incorporating the body.

- Within this field, subtle impressions of quality, symmetry and motion will become apparent.

- Disturbance to health will manifest as variations in quality, symmetry and motion, thereby revealing the source of any dysfunction.

- The therapeutic process is guided by the inherent forces within the matrix – the inherent treatment process – the body's natural tendency to heal itself.

- This process can be enhanced by the practitioner's therapeutic presence and informed awareness.

- By settling into profound stillness, we can connect with deeper levels of consciousness.

- Through this profound stillness we can engage with the most profound levels of being.

- This can lead us to the deepest levels of healing.

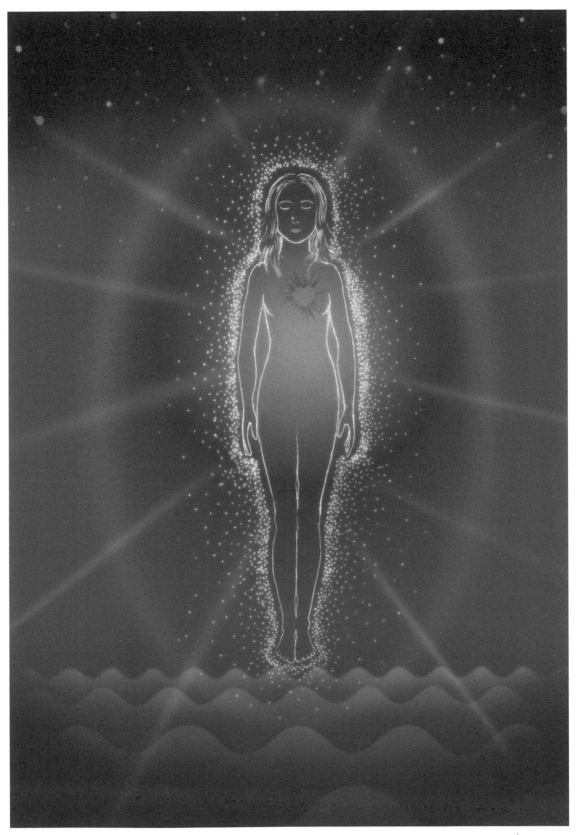

9.1   *The body is a coherent living matrix, existing within the wider matrix of the universal field around us and the biodynamic forces within that fluidic field*

Further elaboration

The therapeutic process

The body has the ability to heal and reintegrate itself through its own inherent treatment process.

Cranio-sacral integration involves engaging with and enhancing this natural inherent treatment process. Cranio-sacral integration is not specifically treating conditions; it is engaging with the whole person, reintegrating the fundamental matrix, establishing underlying health and vitality through which the body itself can resolve symptoms, conditions and their underlying causes, encouraging overall integration of structure and function.

Integrated approach

Cranio-sacral integration brings together the various approaches to cranio-sacral therapy – biodynamic, biomechanical, and other aspects – to create a broad-spectrum approach that can respond more comprehensively to each patient according to their individual needs.

The fundamental approach is biodynamic. In other words, it engages with the system and allows the inherent treatment process to take its course through the dynamic fluidic forces of nature expressed within the energetic matrix – rather than imposing forces on the body.

Within this context there is scope for more specific biomechanical stimuli and the use of other resources in response to the body's demands and individual needs.

The cranio-sacral system

The cranio-sacral system is the individual matrix – not just the anatomical structures which make up the physical body, but the whole energetic matrix or fluidic field within and around the body, within which the body forms, develops, exists and functions – incorporating the whole person and their response to the environment within which they are living, the whole body–mind complex within the context of their life.

Anatomy and physiology

Detailed knowledge of anatomy and physiology is fundamental to cranio-sacral integration. The physical body is the aspect of the matrix through which we experience day-to-day life, the physical medium through which life is expressed. Informed anatomical knowledge enables the practitioner to connect more effectively to the body through their attention and to become aware of significant fulcrums, tracing patterns of imbalance to their source, or surveying through the body for focal points of disturbance. The practitioner's informed awareness plays a significant part in the therapeutic response.

Membranes

The central nervous system (CNS) is enveloped in a triple membrane (the meninges), the three layers consisting of pia mater (inner layer), arachnoid mater (middle layer) and dura mater (outer layer), forming a reciprocal tension membrane system extending from the cranium to the sacrum (Figure 9.2). Within the cranium, the intracranial membranes form infoldings of membrane – the falx cerebri, the falx cerebelli and the tentorium cerebelli – which partially subdivide the cranium (Figure 9.3). The whole reciprocal tension membrane system including the intracranial membranes plays a significant part in maintaining the integrity of the system.

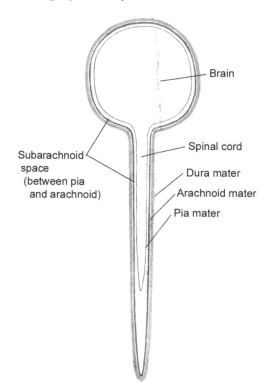

9.2   A triple layered membrane system

III

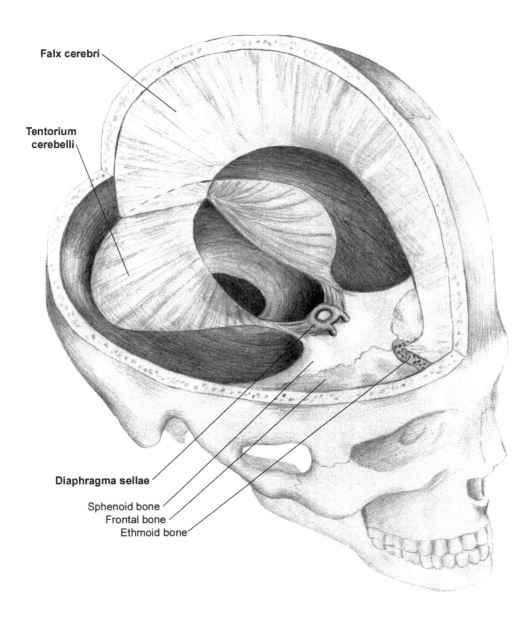

Falx cerebri

**Tentorium
cerebelli**

Diaphragma sellae

Sphenoid bone
Frontal bone
Ethmoid bone

9.3   The intracranial membranes – oblique view

Cerebrospinal fluid

Cerebrospinal fluid is contained within the membranes, bathing and protecting the brain and spinal cord. Cerebrospinal fluid is formed from arterial blood, circulates within the ventricular system (deep inside the brain and spinal cord) and in the subarachnoid space (the space surrounding the brain and spinal cord, between the pia mater and the arachnoid mater) and drains into the venous blood. It is continuously renewed, and provides oxygenation, nutrition and removal of waste products from the central nervous system (Figure 9.4).

Fascia

Fascia forms an interconnected sheath emanating from the membrane system to envelop every structure in the body – bones, muscles, organs, blood vessels, nerves – from the top of the head to the tips of the toes, providing structural continuity and interconnection throughout the body.

Rhythmic motion

The acknowledgement of cranio-sacral motion and engagement with this rhythmic motion is a feature which is distinctive to cranial therapies. This rhythmic motion has been shown on film to exist within a wide range of living matter, including humans. Within the cranial field, three principal rhythms are identified – the cranio-sacral rhythm, the middle tide and the long tide. Although these rhythms have identifiable rates, they are more meaningfully perceived as states of being, the longer rhythms reflecting deeper states of being and consequent deeper levels of healing. In engaging with these rhythms, the practitioner may, from time to time, perceive shifts to a deeper level. At the deepest level lies a state of being which is beyond rhythmic motion, a state of dynamic stillness where the deepest healing occurs.

Treatment process

An individual's state of health is the accumulation of everything that has happened to them. The role of cranio-sacral integration is to reintegrate and re-establish the underlying health which has been distorted and depleted by this accumulation. The essential function of treatment is to provide the therapeutic space within which the system can express and release its accumulated traumas, tensions and restrictions, thereby enabling the restoration of underlying mobility, integrity, health and vitality.

This is enabled by establishing the therapeutic presence within which engagement with the cranio-sacral system can develop, and allowing the spontaneous evolution of the inherent treatment process in accordance with the fundamental principles of cranio-sacral integration:

- *engagement*
- *allowing* the system to express itself
- *following* wherever the system may lead
- until the system draws to points of *stillness*
- leading in due course to *release*
- followed by *reorganization* throughout the system

– until it settles to a balanced *neutral* state, within a new-found freedom from previous restriction, with a more expansive quality, a greater degree of symmetry, and an enhanced expression of rhythmic motion or vitality.

The points of stillness (Still Points) are significant moments of therapeutic effect.

Cranio-sacral integration requires the development of a high degree of sensitivity. Through this sensitivity, the therapist can engage with subtle levels of being. The patient's whole life story is held in their system, ready to be read. Whatever their circumstances, condition, or symptoms, the cranio-sacral process simply involves engaging with the system on this subtle level and allowing the system to reveal its story. Through subtle variations in quality, symmetry and motion, the body will reveal whatever is relevant – injury, trauma, restriction, blockage, shock, disease, tension, emotion – thereby allowing the source of disturbance to be identified, allowing it to be expressed, to rise to the surface, to be released and resolved through the body's natural, inherent potential for healing and balance.

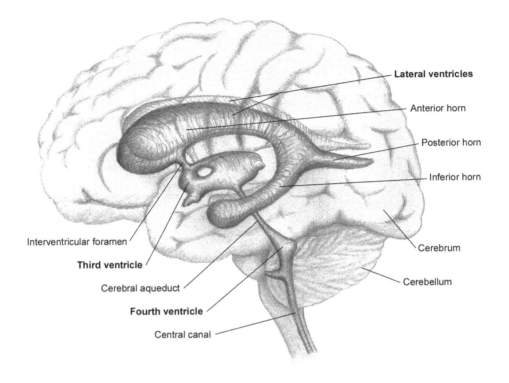

Lateral ventricles

Anterior horn

Posterior horn

Inferior horn

Cerebrum

Cerebellum

Interventricular foramen

Third ventricle

Cerebral aqueduct

Fourth ventricle

Central canal

III

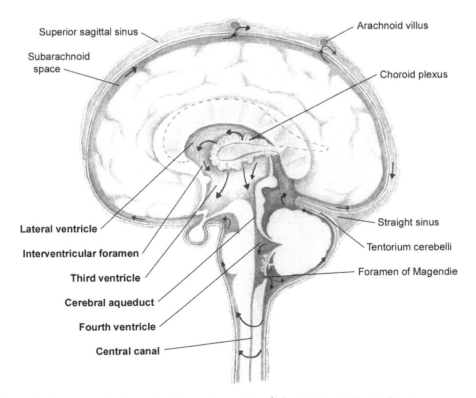

Superior sagittal sinus

Subarachnoid space

Arachnoid villus

Choroid plexus

Lateral ventricle

Interventricular foramen

Third ventricle

Cerebral aqueduct

Fourth ventricle

Central canal

Straight sinus

Tentorium cerebelli

Foramen of Magendie

9.4 The ventricular system and sub-arachnoid space: above – lateral view; below – mid-sagittal section

The treatment process therefore consists of:

- establishing a therapeutic space
- engaging with the subtle forces within the matrix
- allowing those therapeutic forces to be expressed
- enhancing the body's natural inherent potential to release, heal, and reintegrate.

The inherent healing potential is enhanced simply by the fact that the practitioner is engaging with it, while maintaining a spacious therapeutic presence and informed awareness, thereby allowing the system to express itself and reach resolution.

This could be compared to a psychotherapy session with a traumatized patient, in which the therapist interacts with the patient very gently, allows the patient time, space and freedom to express himself or herself without imposing any confining methodology, and through this process of self-expression the patient gains enhanced clarity and resolution of limiting issues.

Shock and trauma

Shock and trauma accumulate in the tissues, the cells, the matrix, the energy field, the mind and the heart, as the body's natural reaction to the injuries and stresses of everyday life. They wear us down and prevent us from functioning effectively, both mentally and physiologically. They are the underlying cause for the majority of health disturbances. Release of shock and trauma is fundamental to cranio-sacral integration, as a means of establishing a basis of healthy function. Nothing else engages with shock and trauma in this way. Their release is essential to health and healing.

Therapeutic presence

The cranio-sacral system and its expression are subtle. They are not likely to be noticed through casual superficial observation. In order to engage with the system, the practitioner needs to develop an appropriate state of stillness, spaciousness and peacefulness – a *therapeutic presence* – through which he or she will be more receptive to the subtleties of the cranio-sacral process.

Engagement with the subtle expressions of the cranio-sacral system is essential to the process. Cranio-sacral integration is not a matter of applying techniques on a mechanical superficial level, but an interaction – an interaction enabled and affected by various factors:

- an appropriate presence on the part of the practitioner
- establishing a suitably receptive state in the patient
- establishing *subtle levels of physical contact*, so light that the hands may not be touching the body at all
- establishing an *appropriate level of attention*, with a wide spacious perception
- developing an *awareness of different levels of tissue* structure – from the more solid physical structures of bone and membrane, through a more fluidic experience of the cranio-sacral system, to engagement with the quantum level of subatomic particles and pure energy.

The usual level of physical contact in cranio-sacral integration is extremely gentle, so light that it may not be touching the body at all – not holding, not gripping, simply being there in softness, stillness and spaciousness, engaging with the matrix or energy field rather than with the anatomical tissues.

The movement of energy within and around the body has a fluidic quality, as if the hands were immersed in warm fluidity, and is therefore described as a *fluidic field*.

Through engagement, the practitioner will become aware of quality, symmetry and motion – the individual characteristics of the person, any imbalances or asymmetries, movement in many different forms (vibration, pulsation, rocking, swirling, etc.) including rhythmic motion. These are the guiding elements which will enable the practitioner to make a comprehensive diagnosis and enable appropriate response and treatment.

The cranio-sacral process (inherent treatment process) is stimulated and enhanced by the therapeutic presence of the practitioner and by allowing the natural tendencies of the body to be expressed.

It may also be helpful in appropriate circumstances to respond to the body's demands with subtle levels of physical stimulus, including containment, traction, Still Point induction or fascial unwinding – in which the cranio-sacral process is expressed more visibly and physically – or through energy drives – in which the body's inherent energy is encouraged more specifically towards focal points of disturbance.

Responses

The most common response to cranio-sacral treatment is a profound sense of ease and relaxation as the whole person, body and mind, comes into a more integrated state of health. There may be different responses according to the nature and state of the individual – sleepy, tired, refreshed, stimulated. Vestiges of old injuries may arise as they are brought to the surface in order to be released and resolved, and in the same way past emotions and distant memories may arise in conjunction with the release of associated traumas and tensions in the tissues, as 'tissue memory'.

Time fulcrums

A specific age or time in a patient's life may be particularly significant to their history and progress. Engaging with such time fulcrums through the cranio-sacral process can enable profound responses. This may arise spontaneously or deliberately.

Suitable for all ages

Cranio-sacral integration is suitable for anyone, whatever their age or state, newborn to elderly, and whatever their condition – acute pain, chronic ill health, or simply maintaining wellbeing. Cranio-sacral integration is concerned with enhancing underlying vitality – and can therefore be of benefit to anyone. The process of overall integration and establishing underlying health will tend to eliminate symptoms and underlying causes whatever the situation.

Quality

Each person is different, and this will always be reflected in the quality of their system. Quality in cranio-sacral integration indicates the characteristics of the cranio-sacral system. Everything that happens throughout life is reflected in the cranio-sacral system as changes in quality, so the whole life story is there to be read, through the various qualities and multiple layers of quality encountered.

Emotional centres

Cranio-sacral integration recognizes the major part played by emotions in our health. Emotions are held in all parts of the body. They are particularly held in certain key areas known as the emotional centres – heart centre, solar plexus centre, pelvic centre, subocciput. Release of these emotional centres, where necessary, is a crucial component in settling and grounding the patient, and in enabling access to deeper levels. It is also profoundly therapeutic in itself, and is a vital element in the therapeutic process.

Integrated treatment framework

A feature of cranio-sacral integration is the integrated nature of a treatment session. This flexible framework consists of four stages:

- establishing initial engagement
- settling and grounding
- core treatment
- completion.

There are significant benefits to this approach, in terms of clearer perception of the whole picture, greater stability for the patient, increased responsiveness, more efficient progress, minimizing unwanted side effects, a greater degree of cohesion, more effective results, and more complete overall integration.

Every treatment session, whatever the symptoms or condition, is best carried out with a comprehensive understanding of the whole picture.

In every patient, it is essential to establish a powerful underlying level of health and vitality, since this is fundamental to the body's ability to resolve local factors.

Local disturbances can only be addressed effectively within the context of that overall perspective.

III

Every treatment needs to involve integration of the cranio-sacral system as a whole, since this is fundamental to overall health and vitality.

Working with the face

Any treatment of the face therefore needs to be carried out as an integral part of treatment of the whole person.

It is essential to address underlying disturbances throughout the body as necessary:

- because balance and integration of the core is always fundamental to overall health and vitality, whatever the patient's condition or symptoms

- in order to establish a stable and firm foundation upon which to carry out any facial work

- because imbalances elsewhere may be the underlying cause of disturbance in the face

- so that imbalances within the face can be seen within the context of the whole picture, thereby helping to recognize whether facial imbalances are primary patterns originating in the face, or secondary to patterns arising from elsewhere.

In working with the face, each contact is intended to be utilized within this integrated context. Each contact will need to be approached with an extremely light delicate touch, waiting in stillness, allowing the gradual emergence of engagement, allowing the evolution of the inherent treatment process, and following to resolution and completion, the whole process being integrated within the context of the overall perspective.

Chapter 10

Working with the Face – An Integral Part of the Body

As we have seen, working with the face can be relevant to many common conditions, both local and systemic. For some people, the key to their overall health may lie in the face, whether through a restricted palatine bone, an unbalanced vomer, a cranial nerve compression, an injury to the face that has affected their mechanical balance, or subtle disturbances affecting their personality.

The face is an integral part of the whole system, with many crucial connections and interactions with the rest of the body. It can be affected by facial injuries, dentistry, stress, structural imbalances from elsewhere, birth trauma, intrauterine compression, and many other sources.

Site of expression

The face is also our principal site of expression – whether smiling, laughing, frowning, crying, expressing surprise or joy, disapproval or distaste – and consequently our faces express our personalities, our nature, our upbringing, our feelings, our emotions. Our faces have been moulded by our experience of life and they reflect our very being (Figure 10.1).

Engaging personality

So when we work with the face, we can, on one level, contact the various structures that comprise it, and address infection, congestion, pain and local discomfort; but we can also engage with the whole personality that underlies the face, with all its profound intricacies and emotions. Through the face, we can feel everything about the person. We can engage with the deepest levels of their being.

The degree to which we engage with those deeper levels will depend on our awareness of these connections and the extent to which we view the face and treat the face within the context of the whole picture.

Relevant for every patient

Working with the face may be more specifically indicated for certain conditions, but it can also be relevant for any situation. Whatever the circumstances – local symptoms or widespread debilitation, evident facial involvement or not – we need to include the face in our assessment of every patient, and incorporate an awareness of the whole person in our assessment of the face.

Always incorporated into the whole

In the following chapters, we will be describing many contacts for the face, each of which may be useful in different circumstances. However, these are not techniques for 'fixing' the face. They are processes which might be incorporated into an overall treatment process, within a comprehensive understanding of the whole picture. The guiding principle is always overall whole-person integration in order to enable fluent function, rather than mechanical release of a particular structure or restriction.

Working within the essential principles of cranio-sacral integration

It is therefore always preferable and more profoundly effective to treat the face (and everything else) within the context of the essential principles of cranio-sacral integration:

III

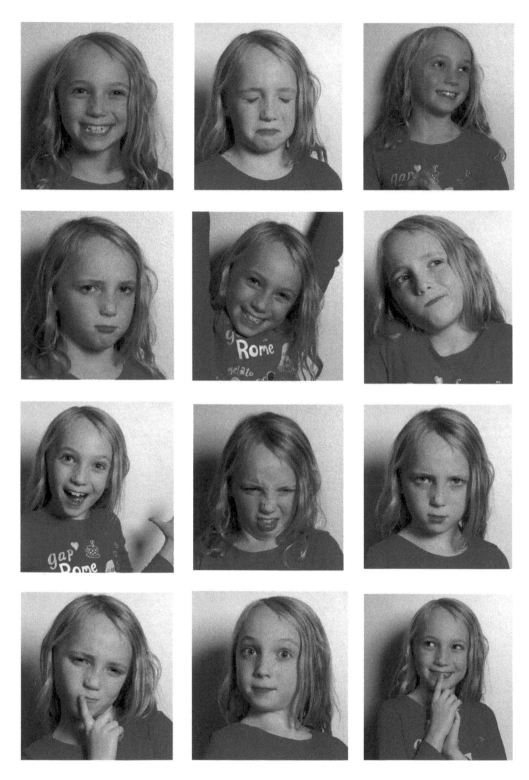

10.1   *The face is our principal site of expression – whether smiling, laughing, frowning, crying, expressing surprise or joy, disapproval or distaste. Our faces reflect our very being*

- Each treatment will involve an evaluation of the whole person (not mere local assessment).
- This will include evaluating and addressing psycho-emotional factors.
- Each treatment will involve integration of the person as a whole (not merely treating the symptom or condition).
- This can be enabled primarily by treating within the context of an *integrated treatment framework*:
  - settling, grounding, and opening up the system
  - balancing the core
  - establishing a powerful underlying vitality
  - allowing the *inherent treatment process* to take its course
  - bringing every treatment to a satisfactory and complete resolution.
- Within this context, various contacts for the face may be included, as appropriate.

- The level of physical contact is extremely light – simply being there in stillness, softness and spaciousness. (*Many of these contacts for the face require an extremely delicate and sensitive touch, and should only be used by those with sufficient training and experience in the exceptional gentleness, softness and delicacy of cranio-sacral integration.*)
- With each contact, the treatment process consists of:
  - establishing a therapeutic practitioner presence – calm, quiet, still
  - taking up a light, gentle contact
  - waiting for engagement to evolve
  - allowing the system to express itself
  - allowing the inherent treatment process to take its course
  - following to points of stillness, release and resolution
  - reintegrating within the system as a whole
  - bringing the session to an appropriate completion.

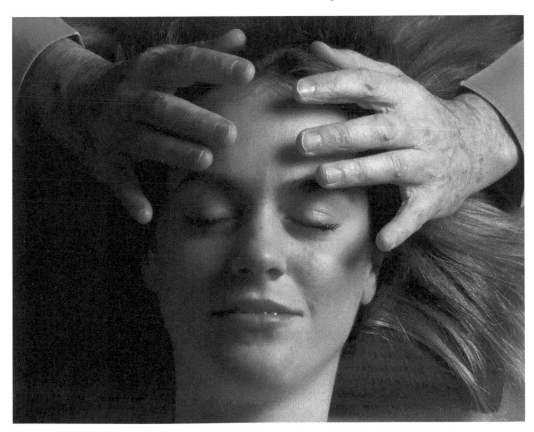

10.2   The level of physical contact is extremely light – simply being there in stillness, softness and spaciousness

Chapter 11

Anatomy of the Face

The bones of the face (Figures 11.1, 11.2 and 11.3)

The skull can be divided terminologically into two divisions:

- the *cranium* (also known as the neuro-cranium)
- the *face* (also known as the viscero-cranium).

The *cranium* consists of the bones which form the *cranial vault* and *cranial base*, housing and containing the brain. These are:

- the frontal bone
- two parietal bones
- the occipital bone
- two temporal bones
- the sphenoid bone.

The *face* consists of those bones attached to the anterior aspect of the cranium, but not directly forming a part of the cranium. The true bones of the face differ from the bones of the cranium in that they do not have direct attachment to the membrane system. The bones of the face are:

- two maxillae (maxillary bones)
- two palatine bones
- the vomer
- two nasal bones
- two zygomata (zygomatic bones)
- two lacrimal bones
- two inferior nasal conchae
- the ethmoid.

The *ethmoid* acts as a bridge between the cranium and the face. It moves functionally with the facial bones, but unlike true facial bones it has direct attachment to the dural membrane – like cranial bones – via the falx cerebri.

The mandible

Anatomically speaking, the mandible is not considered to be part of the face, but for practical purposes it belongs here with the rest of the face.

The ossicles

Within each middle ear, there are three tiny bones: the malleus, incus and stapes.

Internal structures

As well as those bones and portions of bones visible externally in Figures 11.1 and 11.2, there are certain bones or parts of bones which are only visible internally (Figure 11.3), or on a disarticulated skull. These include:

- the horizontal portions of the maxillae
  - which project internally to form the anterior two thirds of the hard palate
- the palatine bones
  - the horizontal portions forming the posterior third of the hard palate
  - the vertical portions forming the posterior part of the lateral walls of the nasal cavity
- the vomer
  - which forms the inferior part of the nasal septum (partly visible through the nose)
  - passing from the superior surface of the hard palate at the intermaxillary suture
  - up to the rostrum on the inferior surface of the sphenoid body
- the ethmoid
  - a delicate and complex box-like structure, composed of wafer-thin bone
  - located between the eyes, behind the nose, above the palate, in front of the sphenoid body.

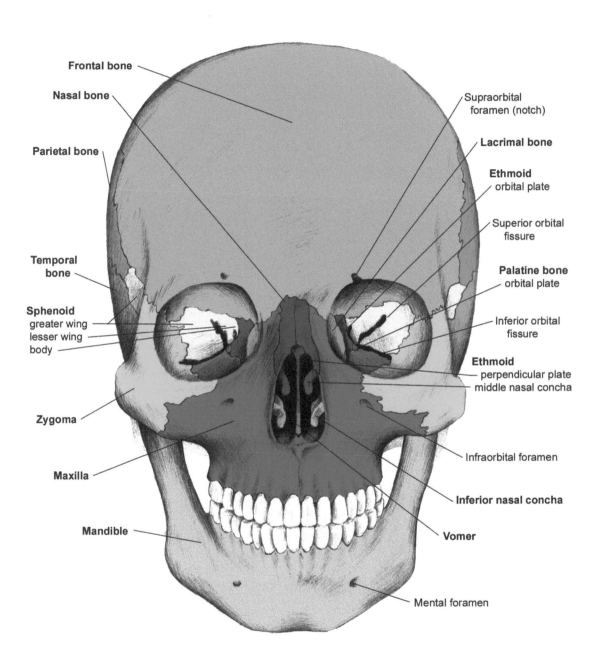

Frontal bone

Nasal bone

Parietal bone

Temporal bone

Sphenoid
greater wing
lesser wing
body

Zygoma

Maxilla

Mandible

Supraorbital foramen (notch)

Lacrimal bone

Ethmoid
orbital plate

Superior orbital fissure

Palatine bone
orbital plate

Inferior orbital fissure

Ethmoid
perpendicular plate
middle nasal concha

Infraorbital foramen

Inferior nasal concha

Vomer

Mental foramen

III

11.1   The face – anterior view

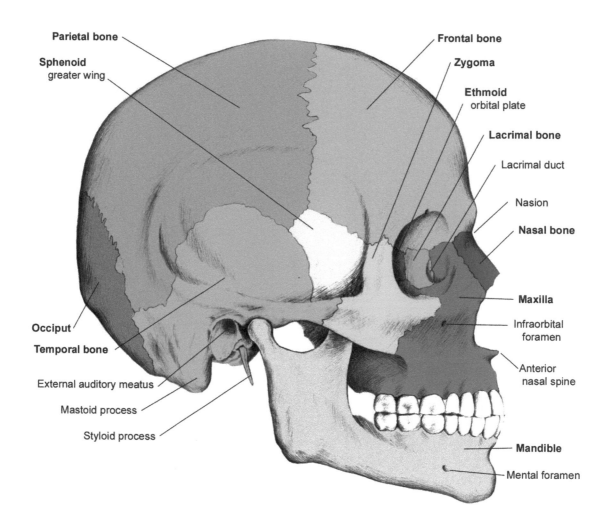

11.2   The face and cranium – lateral view

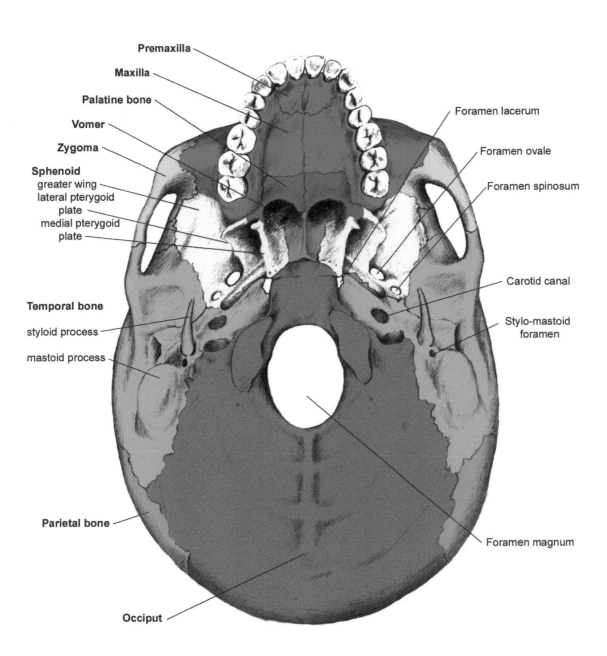

Premaxilla

Maxilla

Palatine bone

Vomer

Zygoma

Sphenoid
greater wing
lateral pterygoid
plate
medial pterygoid
plate

Temporal bone

styloid process

mastoid process

Parietal bone

Occiput

Foramen lacerum

Foramen ovale

Foramen spinosum

Carotid canal

Stylo-mastoid
foramen

Foramen magnum

III

11.3   The face and cranium – inferior view

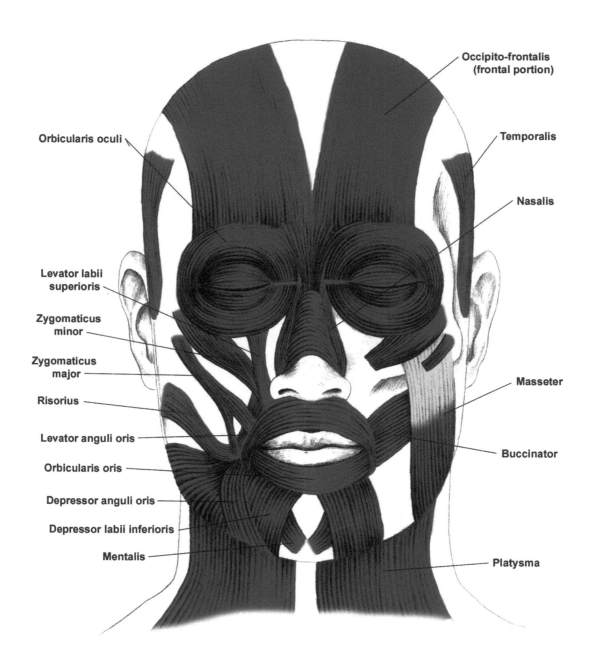

Occipito-frontalis
(frontal portion)

Temporalis

Nasalis

Orbicularis oculi

Masseter

Levator labii
superioris

Zygomaticus
minor

Zygomaticus
major

Risorius

Buccinator

Levator anguli oris

Orbicularis oris

Depressor anguli oris

Depressor labii inferioris

Mentalis

Platysma

11.4 Muscles of the face

The muscles of the face

The muscles of the face (Figure 11.4) are numerous, intricate and often overlapping. They enable the many movements of the face involved in talking, eating, smiling, laughing, frowning, scowling and the many other variations of facial expression.

Reflecting emotional tensions

In working cranio-sacrally with the face, patterns of tension and restriction within the muscles and their enveloping fascia will inevitably arise – reflecting injury and emotional tensions, often including lifetime habits of holding particular facial expressions. Working with the facial muscles can therefore engage with profound emotional levels.

Facial expressions set in childhood

Facial expressions may be set in childhood and maintained as deeply ingrained patterns of holding in the muscles of the face, moulding and establishing our facial features, reflecting the nature of our childhood experience and our underlying emotional state, reflecting fear, anxiety, suppression, recalcitrance, scowling, resentment, timidity, pursed lips, tight-lipped, a polite smile, and so on. Of course facial features may also reflect a childhood that was happy, joyful, carefree and relaxed – but these emotions are less likely to have imposed patterns of tension and restriction in the muscles of the face.

Injury

Patterns of injury will also be reflected in the muscles and fascia of the face, contributing to tensions, asymmetries, facial pain and neuralgia. The release of such patterns can help to restore symmetry and comfort. This is particularly relevant following facial injury, where substantial overall reintegration of the soft tissues of the face (as well as the underlying structure) can be very beneficial.

Memories

As physical patterns emerge in response to cranio-sacral engagement, releasing the effects of injury, they may be accompanied by memories associated with the incident, along with the underlying emotions – perhaps bringing up memories of childhood circumstances, and potentially changing the facial demeanour.

Paralysis and neuralgia

The muscles of the face may be subject to Bell's palsy (in which one side of the face is affected by flaccid paralysis) or trigeminal neuralgia. Both of these are conditions involving cranial nerves and will be dealt with more fully under the relevant chapters on cranial nerves, but working with the muscles of the face can also be relevant in such conditions, in conjunction with addressing any restrictions to the affected nerves.

Working with the muscles of the face

Working with the muscles and fascia of the face may be specifically indicated by the condition or symptoms involved, and is also something that may arise spontaneously in response to individual needs. It will primarily involve the usual process of cranio-sacral integration, engaging with the system through a light contact on the muscles of the face, and allowing the system to express itself through whatever pulls, twists or asymmetries may manifest, reaching points of stillness, leading to the release and reorganization of the patterns of restriction within the tissues, allowing the face to settle into a more comfortable, symmetrical, peaceful and serene state.

Fascial unwinding

The response may occur on a very subtle level, without any external movement, or it may evolve into a more visibly active process of fascial unwinding, with the soft tissues of the face sometimes moving into extreme positions and extreme facial distortions of expression, reflecting the effects of injury or deep emotional holding.

(*Note on terminology:* Note the distinction between the words *facial* (referring to the face) and *fascial* (referring to the fascia).)

Force vectors

Individual muscles may prove relevant, and awareness of the individual muscular structures as shown in Figure 11.4 can be helpful. However, more often the responses will be in the soft tissues as a whole, incorporating many muscles simultaneously and following force vectors or patterns of tension and restriction which transcend individual structures, in order to address the patterns in the face as a whole. This may arise in response to any facial contact.

In the following chapters, various contacts for the face will be described, and further individual contacts may also be improvised in order to address particular injuries or focal points of restriction. One particularly appropriate contact for assessing and addressing the muscles of the face (and the underlying structures) is the *general face contact*.

Chapter 12

General Face Contact

Deep engagement

The general face contact is a beautiful way to engage with the whole person. Just as one might tune in at the feet, or at the sphenoid, in the same way one can tune in at the face and evaluate the qualities, responses and impressions throughout the system as a whole, as expressed through this particular connection at the face.

It can also be a very pleasant experience from the patient's perspective. Patients often find it a particularly engaging contact which connects profoundly with their inner being.

Within the context of an overall treatment session, there will be many times when it is relevant to take up contact on the face, in order to engage with the various underlying structures – whether due to local symptoms, or in order to assess the state of the face, or because the practitioner is drawn to the face through the cranio-sacral process, or as a highly effective means of engaging with the system as a whole.

Specific focus

The general face contact also has more specific possibilities. It can be helpful in more clearly identifying primary patterns arising in the face, mouth, teeth and jaw. It can enable more specific focus on the individual structures of the face – the maxillae, the palatines, the vomer, the orbits, the teeth, the muscles of mastication, the temporo-mandibular joints, the maxillary sinuses – or whatever else might come to our attention as we rest there in deep engagement with the system.

Surveying

These specific focal points may come to our attention spontaneously. Alternatively, we could survey more specifically through the whole structure of the face, in order to identify specific fulcrums. As always, practising the process of surveying methodically helps to develop the anatomical knowledge and the informed awareness which, through experience, will enable these impressions to arise in our consciousness more spontaneously and intuitively.

Wider perspective

Our awareness will not of course be limited to the face. Through the face, we can pick up patterns and fulcrums throughout the body – either by allowing our whole-body awareness to expand out into the surrounding matrix, or by surveying methodically through the body – in order to gain a broad and comprehensive perspective on the whole system. We can notice how patterns in the face may be reflected elsewhere in the body, and identify whether the primary source is in the face, or whether the state of the face is secondary to a primary source elsewhere.

Contact

In order to take up a general face contact which will be comfortable for the patient and for the practitioner, and which also provides a comprehensive connection with the various components of the face, you could take up the following position (Figure 12.1):

- With your forearms or elbows resting on the couch for support, allow your hands to settle gently through the energy field to alight softly but comprehensively onto the face – hands and fingers spreading across the whole face. Your index fingers can rest on the cheeks, close to (but not touching) the nostrils, your middle fingers resting close to (but not touching) the corners of the mouth, your ring fingers extending down to the mandible, your thumbs resting on the forehead above the eyes.

  Take care not to invade or contact sensitive areas such as the lips, nostrils, eyes, eyebrows or eyelids.

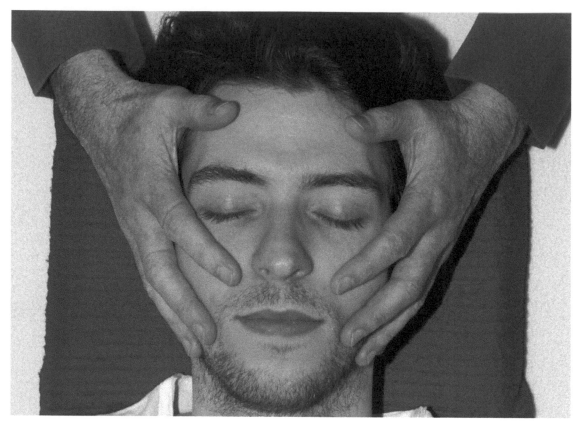

12.1   General face contact – anterior view. Take care not to invade or contact sensitive areas such as the lips, nostrils, eyes, eyebrows or eyelids

Don't be tentative

There can be a tendency to be tentative in contacting the face, thinking perhaps that it is such a sensitive area that we should not let our hands rest on it at all, perhaps holding your hands in some degree of tension. Tentativeness and hesitancy are not helpful features in any cranio-sacral treatment and will be transmitted into the patient and into the treatment process. Be sure to allow your hands (and your whole body) to relax totally – but not too rapidly – alighting as gently as a butterfly, then very gradually, almost imperceptibly, sinking into the contact, settling softly on to the face, the hands gradually letting go completely, the weight of your arms supported through your elbows on the couch.

Once you have settled into the contact, check again that you are letting go completely throughout your shoulders, arms, forearms and hands. Check with the patient that the contact is comfortable (not weighing too heavily onto their face). Encourage them to let you know if at any time any contact feels uncomfortable. (Comfort and relaxation in the patient are very beneficial in enabling the most effective therapeutic response to the cranio-sacral process.)

As you settle into the contact, allow engagement to evolve and allow awareness of the interaction to develop, becoming aware of local impressions and of whole-body patterns. Allow your hands to float fluently within the fluidic movements which you encounter.

Responses

Each face is of course individual. There might be a multitude of movements which gradually settle. There might be obvious focal points within the face – sites of injury, restriction or congestion – towards which your attention is drawn. The whole face may wish to unwind. You might be drawn to whole-body patterns and focal points elsewhere in the system. You might feel tensions in the face gradually relaxing and releasing – perhaps letting go of the face that the patient presents to the world – the face and the whole system settling into a more balanced easeful state. You might feel that, through this face contact, you are engaging with the patient's whole expression of themselves and their feelings, their underlying nature, their emotional being. You might feel the whole system engaging with the inherent treatment process and you can simply allow it to take its course.

Allow the picture of the whole person to emerge, aware simultaneously of the patterns reflected through the face and the patterns reflected through the whole body, all becoming one unified interaction. Within that perspective, explore the different qualities and impressions that will enable you (and the inherent treatment process) to identify the principal focal points within the context of the whole matrix.

You could evaluate whether the patterns you are experiencing are primary patterns arising from the face and affecting the rest of the body, or patterns arising from elsewhere affecting the face. This will be enabled primarily through exploring the relative quality in each area and through the responses that arise when your attention rests on a particular fulcrum.

You could identify focal points in the face which could benefit from a more specific focus of attention, or a particular change of hand contact, or which might be the primary source of a patient's overall state of health.

You might wish to stay at the face throughout the session, allowing the inherent treatment process to follow its course, observing the responses throughout the system, acknowledging moments of stillness and release, feeling the system as a whole settling into greater stillness, balance and integration – or it might be appropriate simply to make a brief assessment through the face and move on to other contacts.

Unwinding

Extensive unwinding of the face may particularly arise where there has been significant trauma to the face, tracing the profound effects of that trauma, not only through the face, but also deeper into the cranium and the whole body. Such journeys of unwinding may also arise in response to significant emotional tension held into the face, often enabling the patient to connect with those emotions, and with the events or circumstances which have led to that emotional holding. This in turn can lead to profound release of trauma and its associated emotions.

This may involve recent traumas or past traumas, including childhood injuries, dental treatment, and facial habit patterns developed during childhood with their associated emotional implications. This may occur on a visibly active (fascial unwinding) level, or within the subtle energetic matrix. Either way it is likely to involve and make profound connections with the whole of the system (as long as the practitioner is aware of and open to that possibility).

Spaciousness

At times, the system may require a more spacious contact, with the energy field expanding – sometimes immediately, sometimes gradually. A severely traumatized face might demand a more spacious contact from the start, with the energy field pushing your hands away until they reach a comfortable non-imposing distance. At other times, the matrix may expand more gently, in response to release of tensions and restrictions within the face, with the energy field softly expanding out to establish a new level of engagement, as if your hands were floating on a fluidic field of energy. At other times, your hands might be drawn into a firmer contact, perhaps engaging with traumatic forces imposed on the face by an injury.

As always, the practitioner needs to remain alert to the ever-changing demands of the system, in order to establish the appropriate level of physical contact from moment to moment, with the hands perhaps floating off the body until you encounter the edge of the field, wherever that may be. Wide spacious contacts often engage with profound levels of being and engage with the whole system more comprehensively – but they need to arise from genuine and full engagement, not from simply choosing to place the hands away from the body.

Maintaining contact

The general face contact can be maintained for a substantial length of time, and may constitute the predominant part of a complete treatment. This might be particularly relevant with a patient who has a primary facial injury which has created significant ramifications throughout the body–mind – perhaps from being hit in the face during a fight, perhaps from being thrown against the windscreen in a car crash, perhaps from major dentistry or orthodontics. As always, it is essential to consider the whole person, understanding that a blow to the face may have ramifications through the cranium, the subocciput, the neck and the overall body structure, as well as emotional repercussions.

It can also be a very effective contact in less traumatic circumstances. It might, for example, be relevant for a patient with sinusitis. Addressing sinusitis is likely to involve various other considerations such as the overall drainage of the face and cranium, the immune system, and the autonomic nerve supply – all of which may benefit from a variety of different contacts from subsequent chapters, as appropriate to the individual circumstances.

Overall fluent function

Facial treatment can enable the release of bony, muscular and fascial restrictions which may be contributing to nasal congestion, sinusitis, earache, hearing loss, facial pain, Bell's palsy, trigeminal neuralgia, and many other symptoms. Once again, however, relief of such symptoms is brought about primarily through an emphasis on the overall integration of the face and body into a more balanced state of fluent function, rather than through excessive focus on a particular restriction or structure.

Facial habit patterns

Facial expressions are instilled in our facial muscles from an early age – the persistently screaming colicky baby and the happy peaceful contented baby are already setting the patterns for their subsequent facial appearance. A constantly frowning, bitter, resentful personality may establish those expressions in the facial muscles. The happy smiling child or adult will establish a different appearance. Every individual will develop a different facial demeanour in accordance with their emotional state and personality. As you work with the face, those patterns established from early childhood and throughout life may be contacted, potentially engaging with the deep underlying emotional patterns that created those expressions and with deeply ingrained memories of those times of life.

Allowing the face to express itself and release its patterns of tension and trauma can bring about profound changes, as the patient lets go of the emotions that are contained within and expressed through the facial muscles. It can enable profound physical connections with past dental or facial trauma, or birth patterns, or other structural associations between the face and the rest of the body. It can bring a sense of deep relaxation.

Moving on

Having worked with the general face contact in whatever way is appropriate, assessing the overall picture and identifying any focal points of restriction, it may be appropriate to move on to more specific contacts on individual areas of the face – the mandible, the maxillae, the palatines, the vomer, the nasal bones, the zygomata – or elsewhere in the body, in accordance with the needs of the patient.

Part IV

The Mouth

Chapter 13

The Mandible

Introduction

The mandible is a particularly significant bone. It is crucial to our overall health, with potential repercussions anywhere and everywhere, as we have seen in the dentistry section of this book. We use our mandible much of the time – to eat, speak, yawn, and express ourselves. It is one of the most common sites of stress – as indicated by the prevalence of teeth grinding and temporo-mandibular joint discomfort – and is an area particularly susceptible to injury and trauma.

The mandible receives attachment from sixteen different muscles (more than any other bone apart from the scapula). It has direct associations with the throat through the various suprahyoid muscles. It is strongly influenced by the muscles of mastication (chewing muscles) which frequently impose unbalanced tensions. It is intimately involved in TMJ syndrome. It has significant connections to the emotional state.

Disturbances of the mandible may arise due to birth trauma, growth and developmental issues, habit patterns, stress, dentistry, structural strain from imbalances elsewhere (for example, disturbances to the temporal bones which may in turn be arising from anywhere else in the body), strains via the muscles of the throat, neck and jaw, or through the teeth (whether developmental or iatrogenic), or direct injury from being punched in the mouth, from sports injuries, from a car accident, or from a fall. It is of course an integral component of the whole body.

When we engage with the mandible, we are not merely concerned with the jaw and local symptoms. We are engaging with the whole person through the fulcrum of the mandible. At times, we might be engaging with the mandible in order to address local issues relating to the teeth, jaw or temporo-mandibular joint. We might be working with it to address tinnitus, earache or headaches. We could be addressing imbalances in the mandible which are affecting the rest of the system. We might check the mandible for dental primaries, or simply to explore whatever it may be expressing. We might be working with stress, teeth grinding, and profound deeply ingrained emotional patterns. So we can work with the mandible because it is symptomatic, because it is the underlying factor for issues elsewhere, to check its state, or as a means of integrating the whole person.

Anatomy

The mandible (from the Latin *mandere*, to chew) or lower jaw (Figure 13.1) consists of:

- the *body* of the mandible – forming the horizontal portion of the bone
- two *rami* – one ramus (*ramus* is Latin for branch) on each side, projecting up vertically from the posterior end of the body up to the *temporo-mandibular joints*, where the mandible articulates with the temporal bones.

The two *angles of the jaw* are the clearly palpable bony prominences at the inferior posterior corners of the mandible, where the body and the ramus meet on each side.

The *alveolar process* runs along the superior surface of the body of the mandible and contains the *lower teeth*. (*Alveolus* is Latin for a socket or cavity, and refers to the sockets for the teeth.)

The *submandibular glands*, one on each side, are located on the medial surface of the body of the mandible, close to the angle of the jaw, with a *submandibular ganglion* immediately above each gland.

Each ramus divides superiorly to form:

- a *condyle* (posteriorly) – which articulates with the *mandibular fossa* (glenoid fossa) of the temporal bone on each side, forming the temporo-mandibular joint
- a *coronoid* process (anteriorly) – for the attachment of muscles of mastication.

Anterior:

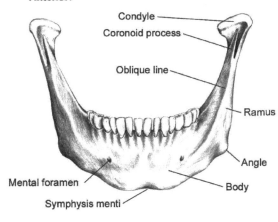

Condyle
Coronoid process
Oblique line
Ramus
Angle
Mental foramen
Symphysis menti
Body

Posterior:

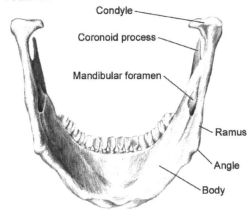

Condyle
Coronoid process
Mandibular foramen
Ramus
Angle
Body

Oblique:

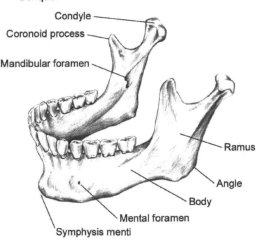

Condyle
Coronoid process
Mandibular foramen
Ramus
Angle
Body
Mental foramen
Symphysis menti

13.1   The mandible

Cranio-sacral motion

As the temporal bones flare forward and out into external rotation, the condyles, rami and body of the mandible follow them, moving forward and out during the expansion phase (flexion phase) of cranio-sacral motion, coming back and in during the contraction phase (extension phase). The mandible forms embryologically as two separate bones, meeting anteriorly at the symphysis menti. It continues to express cranio-sacral motion throughout life as if it were hingeing around the symphysis menti, externally rotating during the expansion phase of motion, internally rotating during the contraction phase.

Symptoms

Symptoms associated with the mandible may be local, such as jaw pain, temporo-mandibular joint dysfunction, persistent toothache and teeth grinding, but may also include a wide variety of symptoms and repercussions throughout the body, from ear infections and migraine to back pain, learning difficulties and general debilitation. The balance of the mandible is crucial to the balance of the whole person.

Many patients may have undergone substantial dentistry or orthodontics before they turn to cranio-sacral integration, but such cases are likely to have been viewed locally, and will probably not have included any effective approach to stress, or any awareness of whole-body connections.

The need, in all cases, is to view the situation within the context of the whole person, identifying the source of any disturbance accurately and integrating the whole body accordingly. The majority of cases will be responsive to cranio-sacral integration, often enabling the resolution of temporo-mandibular joint disturbances, tooth and jaw pain, headaches, earaches, and a multitude of different circumstances affecting any part of the body, but it is also necessary to be alert to the possibility of dental primaries and refer if necessary, and to sources of disturbance that may benefit from a different contact or approach.

IV

13

Deeper repercussions of trauma

The mandible, by virtue of its position, is an area which is particularly susceptible to direct trauma. In addressing direct trauma to the mandible, it is relevant to take into account not only the immediate local effects but also the potentially far-reaching consequences of such trauma, whether it be a blow, a fall or dental trauma. These consequences may be imprinted into the body on many different levels – mechanical, muscular, emotional, energetic.

Mechanical

A blow to the jaw may cause local bruising, a fractured jaw or a displacement of the jaw, but may also have more widespread effects. The force of the impact is likely to be reflected up into the temporo-mandibular joint, potentially leading to temporo-mandibular joint dysfunction. This may in turn create imbalance in the temporal bones with consequent ramifications to the other bones of the cranium or into the tentorium cerebelli and consequently down through the whole reciprocal tension membrane system to the sacrum and coccyx.

A blow to the face is also likely to push the whole head into backward bending, creating strain and trauma at the base of the cranium, at the occiput–atlas joint and in the suboccipital region, with consequent repercussions through the neck and vertebral column, potentially leading to back pain, and resultant mechanical imbalances throughout the whole body.

Muscular

These mechanical disturbances may also lead to stresses and strains in the muscles passing from the mandible to the throat (the suprahyoid muscles), in the muscles of mastication (temporalis, masseter and the medial and lateral pterygoid muscles), in the many suboccipital muscles, in the sterno-cleido-mastoid muscles, or in the various postural muscles of the neck and spine. All of these repercussions may become deeply ingrained into the system (particularly if the injury has been left untreated for some time), creating imbalance, restriction and resistance which can have profound effects on the system as a whole.

Emotional

In addition, any physical trauma is inevitably accompanied by emotional repercussions – major or minor, conscious or unconscious – particularly when it is accompanied by fear (which might arise from a serious accident) or anger (at being hit or attacked during a fight). These emotional consequences can also become deeply established in the individual's system on physical, mental and emotional levels, maintaining and perpetuating the physical imbalances, and potentially inducing far-reaching and long-term consequences in the emotional state, the personality, and therefore on the whole underlying vitality and health of the patient.

These effects can also become deeply ingrained in a mutually perpetuating cycle of interaction – the physical injury perpetuating the emotional reaction, the emotional reaction perpetuating the physical tension and imbalance. Such situations, where physical and psycho-emotional factors are inextricably intertwined, may be unresponsive to physical therapy and unresponsive to psychological therapies, but may be particularly responsive to cranio-sacral integration which, more than other therapies, engages with the combined effects of trauma as a unified totality.

Energetic

The force of the impact and the various effects of trauma may become energetically locked into the system, not only in the gross anatomical structures, but also in the energy field, and in the whole matrix. It is therefore also essential to maintain a spacious perception of the whole energetic matrix.

Approach

So we need to work with an awareness of the whole person – the mechanical structure, levels of stress (current stresses, past trauma, childhood patterning), the history (in relation to the jaw and the whole person), the underlying health and vitality.

Within our spacious awareness of all the various potential levels of trauma, we can connect with the whole-body patterns, tracing the forces from their source (the point of impact, in this case the mandible) throughout their pathway including both physical and emotional fulcrums, identifying and engaging with the points of stillness that arise and allowing the inherent treatment process to take its course.

Through this, we can enable overall integration of the system around the fulcrum of the mandible.

Contact

In order to take up contact on the mandible, bring the hands gently through the energy field towards the sides of the head. Let the heels of the hands come to rest softly onto the sides of the head around the temporal area (with whatever level of contact is indicated by the energy field). Let the fingers come to rest lightly under the inferior surface of the body of the mandible, the ring fingers close to the angle of the jaw, the rest of the fingers spreading forward towards the symphysis menti (Figure 13.2).

Having taken up contact, follow the usual principles of cranio-sacral integration, settling into engagement, simply being there in stillness, softness and spaciousness, allowing the inherent treatment process to evolve in its own way according to the needs of the patient. Be receptive to whatever impressions may arise, in terms of quality, symmetry and motion, or anything

a.

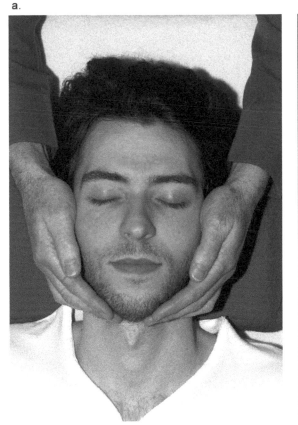

b.

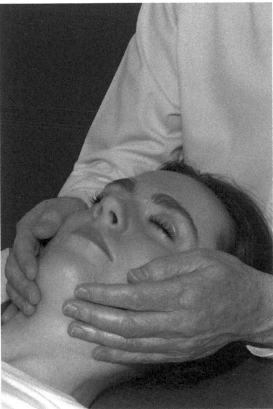

13.2   (a) Mandibular contact – anterior view; let the fingers come to rest lightly under the inferior surface of the body of the mandible
(b) Mandibular contact – oblique view

else that may come to your awareness. Let your attention expand to encompass the whole matrix, aware of whole-body patterns as well as local factors within that wider overall picture, sensing the interactive relationships between all the different components, seeing how they fit together to form the whole picture, and allowing the treatment process to develop through that awareness.

The mandible may unwind along its own intricate multi-directional journey, it may rock from side to side, it may draw up towards the temporo-mandibular joint on one side, or express many different variations of movement. As always, you can allow it to express itself. Allow it to find its own way to whatever focal points or fulcrums it may need to discover, reaching points of stillness, and eventual points of release, each release leading to a greater degree of balance throughout the whole system, and enabling a shift to a deeper level.

Through this continuing evolution, the system will gradually address whatever it needs to address, each release revealing the next layer, progressing steadily deeper into the history of the patient's process, gradually becoming more settled, gradually enabling deeper and more complete integration.

Informed awareness

It is the nature of the cranio-sacral process that much of this may happen spontaneously with or without your conscious awareness, as you maintain your steady fulcrum of therapeutic engagement (simply being there in stillness). However, your informed awareness can help the inherent treatment process to be more focused and effective, and your awareness of the evolving patterns and fulcrums may sometimes be crucial to the effective resolution of the therapeutic process. Through your informed awareness, you might be aware of various more-specific responses in the mandible.

You might encounter a sense of compression, drawing the mandible superiorly towards the temporal bones and temporo-mandibular joints, reflecting a tightly clenched jaw or an upward blow to the mandible, and as you allow the system to draw into that compressive pattern, this may enable the tensions to soften and release

(along with their repercussions throughout the body) and help the patient to release the associated emotional patterns underlying their teeth clenching.

You might feel the mandible shifting to one side, and as you allow this pattern to be expressed, this may engage more fully with an injury which imposed that lateral force on the jaw many years ago, perhaps emerging as a vivid picture of the incident and bringing up memories of the incident for the patient, as the jaw and the forces held there are allowed to release.

You might identify a sense of contraction pulling the mandible up into the temporo-mandibular joint on one side, drawing into a resistant temporal bone, with restriction at the occipitomastoid suture and associated tension in the tentorium with reflections down through all the transverse diaphragms to an unbalanced pelvis and a restricted sacroiliac joint – and as you acknowledge and engage with this pattern, so the whole system may release and resolve in response to your informed awareness.

As the system settles into an increasingly balanced state and deeper engagement, subtle patterns from deep within the system may arise, reveal themselves, and resolve, enabling a more complete integration of the whole system at increasingly profound levels. The degree to which we engage with deeper connections within the system will be dependent on the extent to which we maintain an awareness of the whole person.

Surveying

Experienced therapists are likely to find the overall picture of the patient and the significant fulcrums within the patient arising spontaneously, within the context of the practitioner's broad perspective and informed awareness. Less experienced therapists can develop this ability by surveying the body more methodically, until the process becomes more natural and spontaneous. You might therefore choose to survey the rest of the body more systematically, seeing what arises when you scan more thoroughly through the system, identifying previously unnoticed impressions and focal points.

You could take your attention on a journey from the mandible through the temporo-mandibular joints, the muscles of mastication, the temporal bones, the tentorium, the other transverse diaphragms – the subocciput, thoracic inlet, thoracic diaphragm, pelvic diaphragm – acknowledging the emotional associations with these structures at the heart centre, solar plexus and pelvic centre, through the throat and neck, the trunk and spine, the pelvis, legs and feet, observing any responses at the mandible or in the system as a whole, as your attention reaches different areas.

Your survey can also include not only the mechanical structures of the body but also any factor potentially relevant to the patient – the viscera, the endocrine organs, the emotional centres, toxicity, mercury, allergens – monitoring the response of the system to each enquiry. As always we are engaging with the whole system through a particular fulcrum.

Stimulus

It may be enough simply to stay with the system, in deep engagement, allowing the inherent treatment process to progress in its own way to whatever conclusion it may reach. At other times it may be helpful to ask questions of the system and to offer options to the system in order to explore further possibilities and perhaps reveal previously hidden patterns.

Compressive patterns

The mandible is often compressed or contracted superiorly towards and into the temporo-mandibular joint, whether as a result of a blow to the jaw, or prolonged clenching of the jaw. Consequently, as mentioned above, the mandible may at times draw spontaneously into compression, and may invite you to follow into that compression as a means of engaging with underlying patterns, perhaps engaging with deeply ingrained compressive forces held within the tissues and the matrix for many years. This may arise spontaneously.

Alternatively, if it does not arise spontaneously, you could ask yourself whether a compressive pattern is present, exploring whether the mandible wants to draw superiorly into compression, observing closely to see if any hint of compression becomes apparent, noticing how the mandible and the system respond to this enquiry, and allowing the response.

This process of 'asking' is sometimes described as 'asking the system'. What you are actually doing is asking yourself whether you can feel any forces which you have not previously noticed, any subtle sense of the mandible wanting to compress superiorly – asking through your fingers. It is an enquiry expressed through your fingers, rather than a physical force.

As with surveying and other cranio-sacral skills, the more you practise this process, the more likely it becomes that the impressions will arise spontaneously and that you will notice these forces instinctively.

Containment

At times, the mandible may remain persistently unsettled, or unengaged. At such times, having allowed adequate time for spontaneous expression, you could again offer the mandible the possibility of compression, introducing a very subtle level of containment. This can enable the system to come into focus, to engage more readily with forces held within the body, and thereby enable the therapeutic process to proceed more readily.

In order to offer this possibility, maintaining the same contact, you can offer through your fingers under the mandible the option of compression, inviting the mandible to compress superiorly towards the temporo-mandibular joints, allowing any responses, aware of the responses throughout the system. This stimulus is a thought rather than a physical force, an invitation rather than an imposition. Only the lightest of contacts is needed to engage the cranio-sacral system. Once engaged, the system is likely to continue along its own journey, revealing and addressing imbalances and fulcrums as appropriate, as it moves towards progressively deeper levels.

The body has powerful self-healing potential, and the inherent treatment process can lead the way to the most profound therapeutic responses. But the body also has protective mechanisms which can obstruct its own self-healing mechanisms. Offering options such as a very subtle compression or a gentle element of containment can help the body to make clearer decisions about its own needs – rather than shying away from its own self-healing processes – thereby enabling the therapeutic process to progress more readily

Decompression

Another option is to offer the mandible the option of decompression, inferiorly away from the temporo-mandibular joints. This can act as an alternative option to which the body may respond more readily, or which may be more appropriate to the body's needs. It can also be a useful sequitur to the compressive option. Having unlocked the deeply ingrained forces of contraction through the compressive stimulus, the decompressive option can help the body to open up and release the many years of tension held within the muscles of mastication, the temporo-mandibular joints, the tissues, the matrix, and the associated patterns throughout the body.

In order to offer a decompressive stimulus, keeping the heels of your hands in the same position over the temporal area, curl your fingers so that the tips of your fingers are resting lightly on the sides of the body of the mandible. Allow your fingers to settle and re-engage. With this contact, invite the mandible to decompress inferiorly (away from the temporo-mandibular joint) – as if the tips of your fingers were very gently trying to uncurl (Figure 13.3).

Working with the mandible does not have to include these options of compression and decompression. A great deal of profound therapeutic effect can be enabled simply through being there in stillness and deep engagement. But these options will often prove highly effective in enabling the system to engage more profoundly and in gaining access to patterns that are not arising spontaneously.

a.

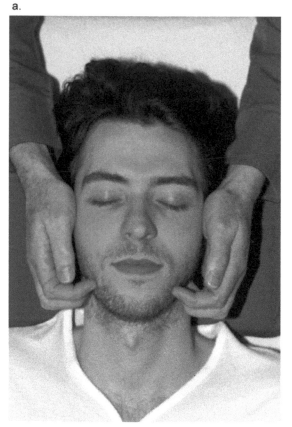

b.

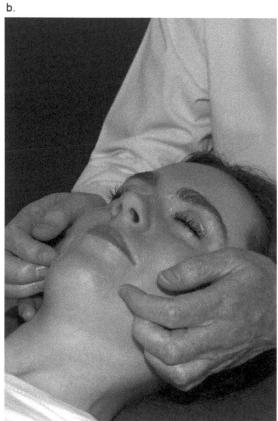

13.3 (a) Mandibular decompression – anterior view; curl your fingers so that the tips of your fingers are resting lightly on the sides of the body of the mandible
(b) Mandibular decompression – oblique view

Completion

You might work with the mandible at great length, or briefly, depending on the responses of the system and the relevance of that particular contact. Profound balancing and integration of the whole person can be enabled through the mandible and this may be all that is necessary. In the context of the overall treatment, it may also be appropriate to move on to other contacts in accordance with the needs of the patient.

When the inherent treatment process has reached its natural resolution and the system has settled once more into a balanced neutral state, with rhythmic motion expressed freely and expansively, you can allow the process to come to a conclusion and move on to whatever may be appropriate within the context of the overall integrated treatment.

IV

13

Chapter 14

The Muscles of Mastication

The muscles of mastication are often given insufficient attention, despite the fact that we use them constantly, that they are often held in an excessive degree of tension, and that they play a pivotal role in many disturbances, including the now familiar list of TMJ issues, jaw pain, tooth pain, worn teeth, earaches, congestion, hearing loss, tinnitus, headaches, migraine, neck pain and suboccipital tension, with inevitable widespread repercussions throughout the whole system.

They are the muscles through which we move the jaw and they are therefore in action much of the time. They are involved in chewing (mastication) and in teeth clenching and teeth grinding (bruxism). Even within dentistry and temporo-mandibular joint treatment, they are often neglected – and yet their role is crucial.

Dentist John Laughlin reports:

> In clinical practice, I have never found a patient with TMJ dysfunction who did not have problems with either one or both of the pterygoid muscles.[1]

Laughlin goes on to say that, in his dental practice, he uses medial pterygoid release before and after 90 per cent of all dental procedures.

John Upledger recommends assessment and treatment of the pterygoid muscles in every TMJ patient:[2]

> The TMJ is a frequent focus of difficulty when the medial pterygoid muscles are in a state of hypertonus.

> Our clinical experience indicates that contractile hypertonus of the lateral pterygoids is frequently involved in dysfunction of the TMJs.

Lateral pterygoids are a frequent cause of recurrent cranio-sacral and TMJ problems.

The muscles

The muscles of mastication comprise four pairs of muscles:

- the temporalis muscles
- the masseter muscles
- the medial pterygoid muscles
- the lateral pterygoid muscles.

Bony attachments – overview

All four muscles attach to the mandible:

- temporalis also attaches to the temporal bone, parietal bone, frontal bone, and sphenoid
- masseter attaches to the zygoma, and the temporal bone
- the medial and lateral pterygoid muscles both attach to the lateral pterygoid process of the sphenoid, the medial pterygoid also having a small attachment to the palatine bone and the maxilla.

Innervation

All four muscles are innervated by the motor branch of the trigeminal nerve (Cr V) travelling with the mandibular division of the trigeminal nerve, which passes down through the base of the cranium via the foramen ovale before branching out to the various muscles.

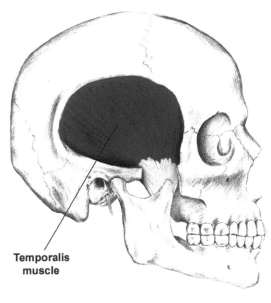

**Temporalis
muscle**

14.1   Temporalis muscle

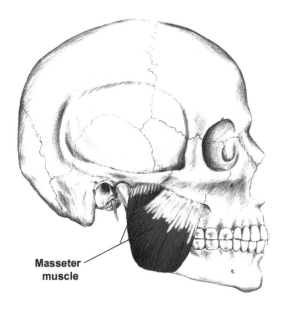

**Masseter
muscle**

14.2   Masseter muscle

Anatomy

Temporalis muscles

The temporalis muscles are the largest of the four pairs of muscles, with an extensive origin spreading around the temporal fossa on the lateral surface of the cranium on each side, attaching to the parietal bones, temporal bones, frontal bone and the greater wing of the sphenoid. They pass down medial to the zygomatic arch and attach onto the medial surface of the mandible at the coronoid process and ramus (Figure 14.1).

Their action is to raise the mandible and draw it posteriorly, closing the mouth, and clenching the teeth. They are therefore involved in chewing and talking and many other activities involving the mouth.

They can readily be palpated by placing the tips of your fingers on the sides of your head around the temporal area bilaterally and clenching and unclenching your jaw repeatedly.

Masseter muscles

The masseter muscles are the strongest muscles in the body in terms of strength per fibre,[3] as exemplified by the clamping jaws of a crocodile. However, once the jaw is closed, a crocodile, like other animals, has very little strength with which to open the jaws since jaw-opening muscles are few and weak.

The masseter muscles originate from the zygomatic arch – both the zygoma itself and the zygomatic process of the temporal bone. They pass down to insert onto the lateral surface of the ramus of the mandible, their attachment extending down almost to the angle of the jaw (Figure 14.2).

Their action is to raise the mandible, draw it anteriorly, close the mouth and clench the teeth. They are therefore also involved in chewing and talking and the many other activities involving the mouth.

They can readily be palpated by placing the tips of your fingers on the sides of your face below the zygomatic arch bilaterally and clenching and unclenching your jaw repeatedly.

Medial pterygoid muscles

The medial pterygoid muscles each have two heads (Figures 14.3 and 14.5). The larger head originates from the medial surface of the lateral pterygoid plates of the sphenoid; the smaller head originates from the palatine bone and the maxilla. Both heads pass inferiorly and laterally to attach to the medial surface of the ramus of the mandible on each side, their attachment extending from the angle of the jaw upward along the ramus as far as the mandibular foramen.

Their principal action is to raise the jaw and close the mouth, with minor contributions to sideways movement and protrusion of the jaw.

IV

14

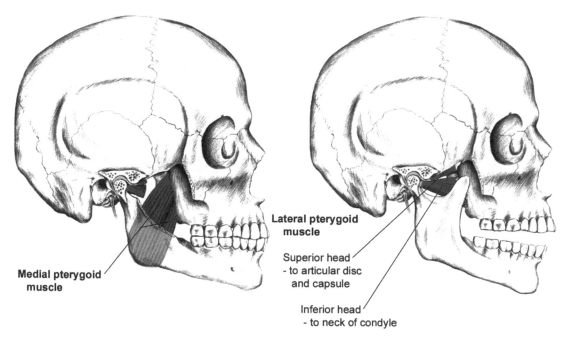

Lateral pterygoid muscle

Superior head
- to articular disc
and capsule

Inferior head
- to neck of condyle

Medial pterygoid muscle

14.3   The medial pterygoid muscles each have two heads

14.4   The lateral pterygoid muscles also each consist of two heads

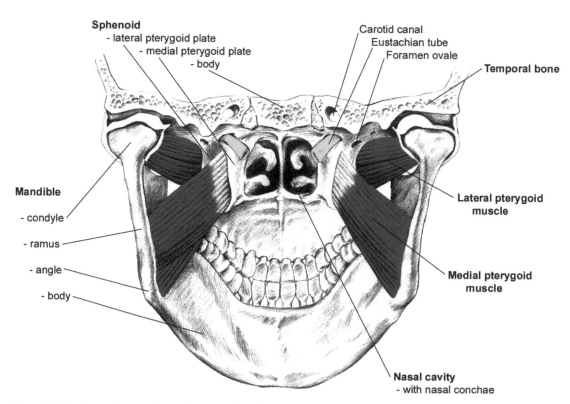

Sphenoid
- lateral pterygoid plate
- medial pterygoid plate
- body

Carotid canal
Eustachian tube
Foramen ovale

Temporal bone

Mandible

- condyle

- ramus

- angle

- body

Lateral pterygoid muscle

Medial pterygoid muscle

Nasal cavity
- with nasal conchae

14.5   Medial and lateral pterygoid muscles – posterior view

Lateral pterygoid muscles

The lateral pterygoid muscles also each consist of two heads, the inferior head originating from the lateral surface of the lateral pterygoid plates of the sphenoid, the superior head originating from the proximal portion of the greater wing of the sphenoid (Figures 14.4 and 14.5).

The inferior head passes out laterally to insert onto the neck of the mandible just below the condyle. The superior head inserts into the articular capsule of the temporo-mandibular joint and gives off fibres which penetrate into the temporo-mandibular joint and attach to the articular disc within the joint, thereby enabling the muscle to draw the disc and capsule forward during mouth opening. (The disc is drawn back into place by elastic tissue behind the disc during mouth closing.) It is this attachment to the articular disc within the joint that renders the lateral pterygoid muscles so significant in TMJ disturbances.

The lateral pterygoid muscles may also sometimes insert into the malleus within each middle ear, with potential consequences for hearing.[4]

The principal function of the lateral pterygoid muscles is to draw the mandibular condyle forward and out of the mandibular fossa along the articular eminence during mouth opening and jaw protrusion. They also contribute to lateral movement and, unlike any of the other muscles of mastication, also play a part in lowering the jaw (together with various suprahyoid muscles of the throat).

The lateral pterygoids are therefore involved in opening and closing the mouth, protruding the jaw, moving it from side to side, and the various movements of chewing, as well as drawing the articular disc and capsule forward during mouth opening.

Disturbances of the lateral pterygoids are often missed:

> Lateral pterygoid hypertonus is often overshadowed by other lesion patterns and is difficult to discover until many layers of adaptive lesion patterns have been removed.[5]

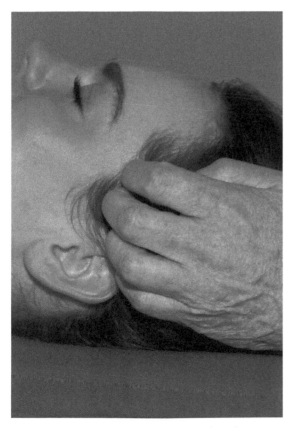

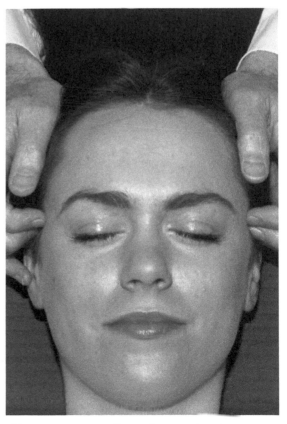

14.6 (a) Contact for temporalis muscles – lateral view　　*(b) Contact for temporalis muscles – anterior view*

Contacts

Temporalis muscles (Figure 14.6)

Contact can be taken up by resting the heels of the hands gently on the sides of the head in the parietal area, with the tips of the curled fingers resting onto the body of the muscle within the temporal fossa. Alternatively, the straight fingers can rest gently onto the muscle.

Their location, the extent of their attachment, their tone and their balance can readily be identified and assessed by asking the patient to clench and release their jaw a few times, whereupon the muscles can be felt contracting and relaxing.

Having established contact, their quality, symmetry and relative tension can be evaluated and addressed as you settle into stillness and engagement and allow the inherent treatment process to take its course with an awareness of not only the muscles themselves, but also the connections and repercussions throughout the body, both physical and emotional.

Masseter muscles (Figure 14.7)

Contact can be taken up in a similar manner to the temporalis contact, but with the hands positioned further down the sides of the head, so that the fingers are resting on the body of the masseter muscle below the zygomatic arch. Their location, and the state of the muscles, can again readily be identified and assessed in the same way as the temporalis muscles, asking the patient to clench and release their jaw a few times. Having established contact, their condition and response can also be evaluated and addressed as for the temporalis muscles, settling into stillness and engagement and allowing the inherent treatment process to take its course.

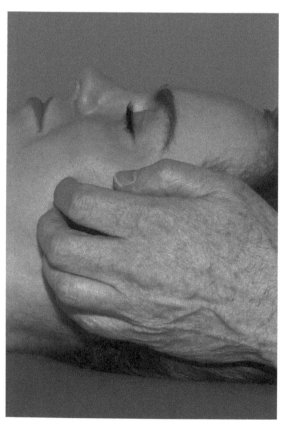

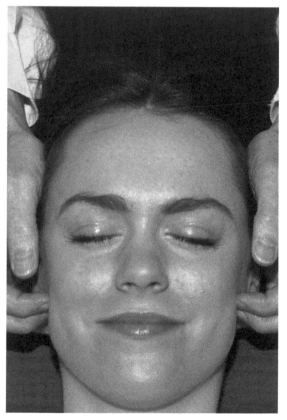

14.7 (a) Contact for masseter muscles – lateral view

(b) Contact for masseter muscles – anterior view

Medial pterygoid muscles
(Figures 14.8 and 14.9)

The medial pterygoid muscles can be contacted by curling your fingers deeply under the medial surface of the angle of the jaw, where the muscles have their insertion. Resting the hands gently on the sides of the head in the temporal area, the fingers can be curled up into position. In order to gain direct contact with the muscles, it is necessary for the fingers to curl some distance up within the inner surface of the mandible. There will often be tightness and tenderness here, perhaps more evident on one side than the other, but despite any tenderness, a deep penetrating contact is often the most effective means of release, particularly for the long-held deeply ingrained tension patterns which are common here.

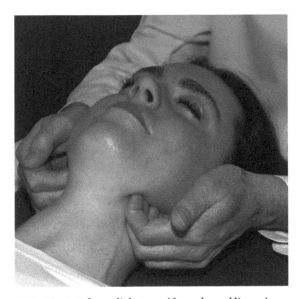

14.8   Contact for medial pterygoid muscles – oblique view

Deep contacts can be very beneficial and will be perfectly acceptable to the body, but they need to be approached very gradually. Whenever using a deeper firmer contact anywhere in the body, it is essential to start with a very light contact and to deepen very slowly. Allow the fingers to sink gently through the superficial tissues, penetrating gradually deeper and deeper. As always, the ramifications through the whole system need to be maintained in your awareness at all times.

Patients can also work on their own medial pterygoid muscles, inserting their thumbs up along the inner (medial) surface of the angle of the jaw on each side, with the fingers resting on the lateral surface of the ramus, and allowing their thumbs to sink in gradually deeper and deeper (encouraging the patient to settle into softness, stillness and relaxation rather than actively massaging the muscles).

Patients with contracted muscles of mastication, who grind their teeth, can also readily massage their own masseter muscles, their temporalis muscles, and their jaw and temporal area generally, to help release tension and to raise their awareness of the tension they hold in those muscles. They can also learn to relax their jaw and change their jaw-clenching habit pattern. It can also be very beneficial to raise their awareness of these muscles and their tendency to hold tension in the body through mindfulness training.

When one medial pterygoid muscle is found to be a particular focus, it can be helpful, while maintaining the deep contact with the affected muscle, to take up contact with the other hand over the opposite pole of the cranium, allowing and monitoring the responses between your hands, throughout the cranium and beyond.

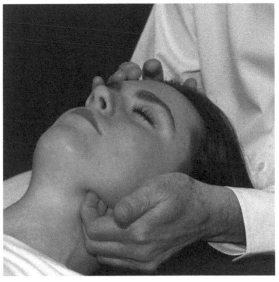

14.9   Contact for engaging with one medial pterygoid muscle unilaterally

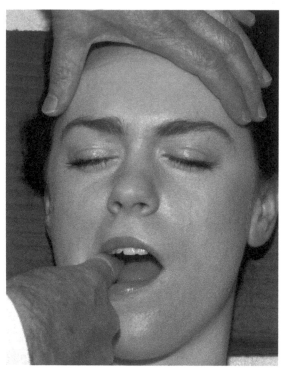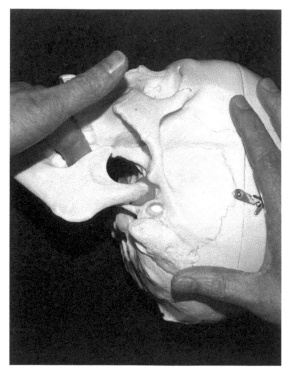

14.10 Intraoral contact for medial pterygoid muscle

a.

b.

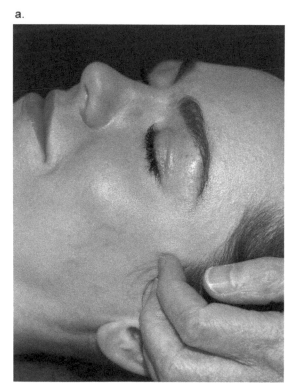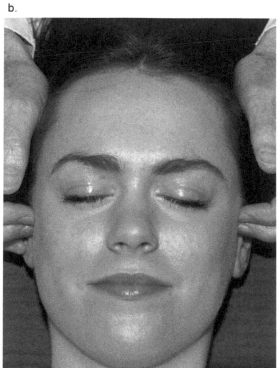

14.11 (a) External contact for lateral pterygoid muscles – lateral view
(b) External contact for lateral pterygoid muscles – anterior view

a.

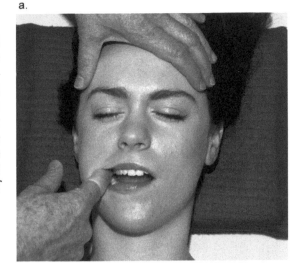

Intraoral contact (Figure 14.10)

The medial pterygoid muscle can also be contacted intraorally. Stand at the side of the head – on the opposite side from the muscle to be addressed – and with one hand resting over the spheno-frontal area of the cranial vault, invite the patient to open their mouth and run the index finger of your other hand down inside the medial surface of the mandible on the far side, as far down towards the angle of the jaw as possible. The medial pterygoid muscle can then be contacted through the pad of your finger.

Lateral pterygoid muscles

Indirect contact (Figure 14.11)

The lateral pterygoid muscles are not directly accessible externally but may be contacted indirectly through a bilateral external contact with the fingers of each hand resting gently over the TMJs (into which they insert), extending your attention through the TMJs into the lateral pterygoid muscles and their attachments. Energy drives directed towards the affected area can be usefully employed through this contact.

b.

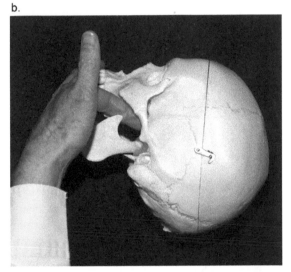

Intraoral contact (Figure 14.12)

The lateral pterygoid muscles can also be contacted intraorally. Stand at the side of the head, on the same side as the muscle to be addressed. With one hand over the spheno-frontal area, ask the patient to open their mouth and insert the index finger of your other hand – with the pad facing superiorly – medial to the mandible but lateral to the maxilla, posterior to the upper molar teeth, as far up towards the TMJ as possible, on the near side. The pad of the finger will then be resting on the lateral pterygoid muscle, close to its insertion into the neck of the condyle and into the temporo-mandibular joint. (Figure 14.12c shows an alternative contact for the lateral pterygoid muscle.)

c.

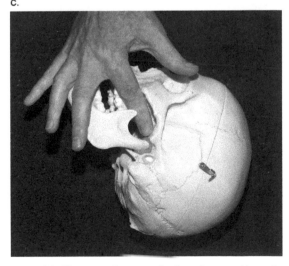

*14.12 (a), (b) Intraoral contacts for lateral pterygoid muscle
(c) Alternative contact for lateral pterygoid muscle*

IV

14

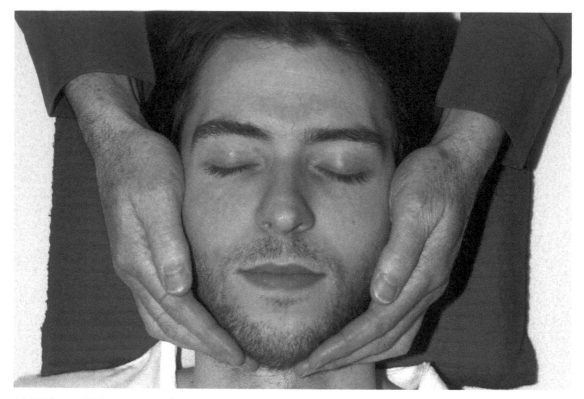

14.13 The mandibular contact can be the most effective means of addressing the overall balance and integration of the muscles of mastication

Mandibular contact (Figure 14.13)

Perhaps the most valuable contact for addressing the muscles of mastication is the mandibular contact (described in Chapter 13). The various individual contacts described above can each be useful and relevant at different times. However, all four muscles attach to the mandible, and consequently a contact on the mandible can provide a means of engaging with all four muscles simultaneously and can often be the most effective way to address the overall balance and integration of their function, monitoring the responses, identifying the various pulls and imbalances exerted on the mandible by the various muscles individually or together. Allow your attention to be drawn to any focal points whether in the muscles themselves, the surrounding tissues, or in the matrix as a whole, projecting your attention through the various muscles in order to survey the area and identify specific focal points, and engaging with the local area within the wider context of the whole person through a widening of perception to engage with the whole body and the whole matrix.

Tension

Tension in the muscles of mastication is often accompanied by tension in the suboccipital region with all its potential consequences on arterial supply to the brain, venous drainage from the brain, sympathetic nerve supply to the head, and compression of the vagus nerve – with repercussions on the heart, lungs and other organs, and on the many other vital structures passing through this region.

The tensions associated with teeth clenching and teeth grinding are likely to have significant psycho-emotional associations, and in working with the muscles of mastication this needs to be taken into account and addressed appropriately. The underlying emotional factors may reflect current stresses and pressures, but will often also relate to long-held deeply ingrained emotional patterns arising from childhood.

The emotional source of the tensions may also be explored and identified through the case history, through dialogue with the patient, through time fulcrums, through the quality of tissue tension, and through the nature of the response to treatment.

Tensions in the muscles of mastication may also often lead to restricted drainage of the middle ear through the Eustachian tube – which passes along the base of the skull at the spheno-temporal suture – thereby contributing to earache and ear infections. The ears may also be affected by the lateral pterygoid muscle, which has variable attachments to the malleus within the middle ear.

Physical causes

As well as psycho-emotional tensions, the muscles of mastication may be disturbed by physical traumas, including direct injury to the mandible and other associated bones of the face and cranium, and by dentistry. The effects of such injuries – including the usual list of headaches, jaw pain, ear infections, and so on – may develop insidiously, perhaps some time after the original injury. The connection between the injury and the symptoms may therefore pass unrecognized and much inappropriate treatment may be sought before the true source is identified.

It is necessary to give consideration to these muscles as a matter of course in every patient, and it is particularly relevant to investigate them in any case of jaw or temporo-mandibular joint dysfunction.

IV

14

Chapter 15

The Temporo-Mandibular Joint (TMJ)

When suffering from TMJ or jaw pain, most people will understandably go to a dentist or orthodontist, and a great deal of dentistry and orthodontics is carried out in an attempt to resolve such issues.

Whilst there are undoubtedly some TMJ disturbances which do need dental and orthodontic treatment, for a great many cases this may not be the appropriate approach. As one experienced dentist reports:

> Less than 10 per cent of patients with temporo-mandibular joint symptoms have actual TMJ dysfunction.[1]

Upledger states:[2]

> TMJ syndrome is usually a symptom not a cause. Ninety per cent of cases are not primary temporo-mandibular joint disturbances. They are usually a result of cranio-sacral system dysfunction, or stress.
>
> A minority require occlusal work – i.e. mandibular splints and vertical bite dimension.
>
> To treat only the TMJ dysfunction is to invite eventual failure of treatment. The joint is part of a whole person. Its dysfunction usually signifies that something else is wrong.
>
> It is clear that, in the future, the significance of the cranio-sacral system in the diagnosis and treatment of TMJ syndrome will be more fully appreciated by the dental profession.

In addressing TMJ disturbances, we need to take into account stress, trauma, psycho-emotional factors, teeth grinding, balance and integration of local structures – mandible, maxillae, muscles of mastication, temporal bones, cranium – and integration of the whole person.

We also need to be alert to the small percentage of cases where there is a primary TMJ disturbance which requires dental or orthodontic treatment.

As always, addressing stress factors where appropriate (through cranio-sacral integration) needs to be the first priority, since it is the most common cause, and because there is little point in doing anything else without addressing this fundamental factor. This includes not just current stresses and conscious stresses, but also, more significantly, deeply ingrained patterns from the past. Unfortunately, although stress is the most probable underlying cause, it is often the factor that is least likely to be addressed, and patients will often undergo extensive and unnecessary dental and orthodontic treatment in order to avoid this conclusion, or before eventually coming to this realization.

Anatomy

The temporo-mandibular joints are synovial joints, enveloped in a synovial capsule; they are the only synovial joints in the head, since they are the only freely mobile joints in the head. Each temporo-mandibular joint is formed between the condyle of the mandible fitting into the socket of the mandibular fossa (glenoid fossa) of the temporal bone.

Each temporo-mandibular joint is subdivided into two joints, separated by an articular disc – an upper joint between the disc and the temporal bone, and a lower joint between the disc and the mandible. The fibrocartilage disc is thicker posteriorly than anteriorly, which helps to prevent the disc from moving too far forward and clicking out of place (Figure 15.1).

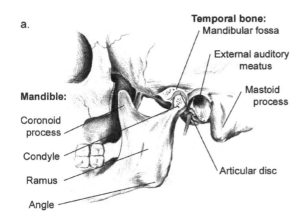

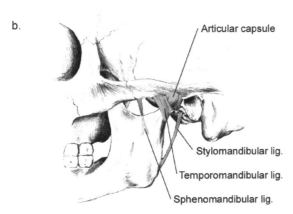

15.1 *(a) Each temporo-mandibular joint is formed between the condyle of the mandible fitting into the socket of the mandibular fossa of the temporal bone, separated by an articular disc*
(b) The joint is strengthened and stabilized by several ligaments

The disc receives attachment from the lateral pterygoid muscle (penetrating through the synovial capsule into the joint). When opening the mouth, the lateral pterygoid muscle draws the disc forward. On closing the mouth, elastic tissue attached to the posterior aspect of the disc draws it back into place. The correct balance of these tissue forces is essential in maintaining the appropriate position of the disc between the mandible and the temporal bone, and to the consequent freely moving fluent function of the joint.

The joint is strengthened and stabilized by several ligaments – the stylomandibular ligament (posteriorly), the temporo-mandibular ligament (anterolaterally), and the spheno-mandibular ligament (anteromedially) (Figure 15.1b).

There are also two smaller oto-mandibular ligaments – the disco-malleolar ligament which arises from the malleus within the middle ear and attaches into the retrodiscal tissue of the TMJ, and the anterior malleolar ligament which also arises from the malleus and connects to the mandible by blending with the spheno-mandibular ligament. These oto-mandibular ligaments may be involved in tinnitus and hearing disturbances associated with TMJ disorders.

Muscles of mastication

The temporo-mandibular joint is moved primarily by the muscles of mastication – the temporalis, masseter, lateral pterygoid and medial pterygoid muscles. All of these muscles can be highly significant in TMJ disturbances, as we have seen in Chapter 14:

> The medial and lateral pterygoid muscles are extremely important in TMJ and cranial dysfunction.[3]

> Relaxation of the lateral pterygoid muscle is essential to recovery.[4]

> Cranio-sacral system release and balancing of the lateral pterygoid muscles is essential for resolving TMJ syndrome.[5]

The movement of the articular disc is essential to the fluent opening and closing of the mouth; it is also essential that the capsule is drawn forward (by the lateral pterygoid muscle) to prevent it from becoming trapped as the mouth closes. Any excessive tension in the lateral pterygoid muscles may exert strain on the TMJ.

Various other muscles act on the mandible (sixteen altogether), and other muscles of the head, neck and back may also have a significant influence. Of particular relevance are the sterno-cleido-mastoid muscles, which are so often unbalanced and which readily draw the temporal bones out of alignment, with inevitable consequences on the temporo-mandibular joint. Involvement of the sterno-cleido-mastoid muscles in turn requires consideration of the spinal accessory nerves (Cr XI) which supply the muscles, and attention therefore also to the jugular foramina, the occipitomastoid sutures and the upper cervical spine, illustrating once again the need to take into account the infinite interactive ramifications through the body.

TMJ dislocation

The TMJ can be dislocated through injury, but dislocation occurs more commonly through opening the mouth too wide during activities such as yawning or dental treatment.

The TMJ is, broadly speaking, a ball and socket joint. When the mouth opens wide, the condyle moves out of its socket anteriorly, settling back into place when the mouth closes.

The TMJ becomes dislocated when the condyle moves too far forward and becomes stuck in front of the articular eminence (Figure 15.2). It is then unable to move back into place.

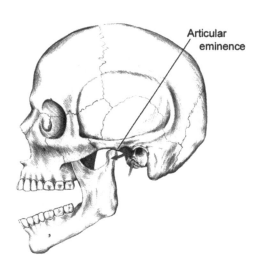

Articular eminence

15.2 The TMJ becomes dislocated when the condyle moves too far forward and becomes stuck in front of the articular eminence

This will often lead to spasm in the surrounding muscles, leaving the jaw locked open and unable to move, accompanied by considerable pain. The spasm may also render it difficult to return the condyle to its socket. In some cases, it may be possible to reposition the jaw without anaesthetics, particularly if action is taken immediately. However, in other cases, muscle relaxants and anaesthetics will be needed.

Following dislocation and subsequent relocation, the joint may be tender for a few days.

More significantly, the ligaments may remain loose, rendering the joint susceptible to repeated dislocation. Cranio-sacral treatment to restore the stability and integrity of the tissues can be helpful.

TMJ intra-articular disc displacement

(*Note:* TMJ disc displacement is also known as disc derangement, and also sometimes known as dislocation – which can be confusing since it may be unclear whether this refers to dislocation of the disc or the jaw.)

Disc displacement is common (affecting one third of the population), usually as an anterior displacement. It may lead to pain, especially on chewing, and may be accompanied by clicking, clunking or popping sounds (which sound loud to the individual, but are only slightly audible to others).

However, neither local pain nor clicking and popping sounds are diagnostic of a disc displacement. Some people have clicking TMJs which never cause any pain. Clicks and other joint sounds are common; they are not significant unless there are other symptoms:

> Studies using MRI and arthroscopy have shown displaced discs in those people who have symptoms of TMJ pain and dysfunction, as well as in those who had no symptoms. So in other words, many people without TMJ problems have displaced discs.[6]

According to Dr Louis Mercuri:[7]

> The accumulated scientific evidence in the 1990s appears to be showing that the disc, by itself, is not the sole culprit in TMJ and facial related pain, even when it is positioned off the condyle.

> A diagnosis of a displaced disc is not an indication for treatment. If the disc restricts movement and causes pain, treatment may be required. However, the two can be totally unrelated. If a displaced disc is present with no pain, then no treatment is needed. If the displaced disc is accompanied by pain, the pain may subside with or without treatment.

In the majority of cases, the disc will be self-reducing – in other words it will click back into place of its own accord.

In some cases, the disc may remain out of place ('without reduction') and may lead to an acute closed lock, with limited mouth opening (maximum 30mm), often accompanied by pain in the ear and around the TMJ, and capsulitis causing inflammation and pain in the soft tissues surrounding the joint. This most commonly occurs in a joint which has been clicking and self-reducing for some time.

In cranio-sacral practice, it is helpful to understand that clicking jaws are not necessarily an indication of a serious condition, particularly if they are painless. Many TMJ pains, clicking jaws, and disc displacements can resolve through the usual process of cranio-sacral integration, but as always we need to be alert to the possibility of a disc derangement which may need orthodontic attention.

TMJ syndrome

TMJ syndrome has many names, including temporo-mandibular joint dysfunction (TMD) and temporo-mandibular disorder.

The term TMJ syndrome is widely used in two different senses, to mean two very different scenarios:

1. A variety of *persistent symptoms involving the jaw and TMJ* – whatever their (unidentified) origin. ('My jaw hurts and I get headaches and earache, and I've had loads of dentistry and orthodontics but it doesn't seem to help.')
2. General *debilitation without local TMJ symptoms* – which turns out to be due to an unrecognized primary TMJ issue. ('I've been seriously ill for years and no one could find the cause – until a whole-person dentist identified that it was all coming from my TMJ.')

Distinguishing these different situations and addressing the root cause is the key.

Definition 1 is the more commonly used and most readily recognized definition. It is characterized by three principal symptoms: local pain in the jaw, face, ear, head and neck; limited mouth opening; and joint noises. It was formerly seen as a dental problem, but is now widely regarded as a 'multifactorial' condition, often described as 'poorly understood' – in other words a prime candidate for the more profound whole-person understanding of cranio-sacral integration:

> Most sources now agree that no irreversible treatment should be carried out for TMD.[8]

> It is better to consider all external factors before performing occlusal or other invasive work.[9]

Definition 2 is less widely recognized and is more the preserve of whole-person dentists. It is this version which requires more careful consideration and identification of the root cause, and the identification of potential dental primaries.

Symptoms

A more comprehensive account of symptoms which might more broadly be considered a part of TMJ syndrome, particularly in its second definition, or which might lead us to explore the TMJ more specifically, has been described previously (Chapter 6), and is summarized briefly here:

- jaw pain or TMJ pain, whether constant, intermittent, or on chewing
- noises of various kinds when opening or closing the jaw – clicking, popping, crepitus
- difficulty opening or closing the mouth fully
- asymmetrical movements of the jaw
- malocclusion and tooth pain
- earache, tinnitus, disturbances of hearing, pressure in the ear
- recurrent tonsillitis, difficulty swallowing
- headache, migraine, sinusitis, facial pain, head pain, neck pain
- general debilitation
- persistent or recurrent multiple symptoms of unidentified origin
- lack of lasting response to treatment.

All of these symptoms can have many other causes and are by no means diagnostic of TMJ dysfunction. Identifying whether a patient has a primary TMJ cause and needs whole-person dentistry can be enabled through the comprehensive assessment described in Chapter 6.

Primary TMJ dysfunction

Although most TMJ disturbances can be resolved through cranio-sacral integration, there will be circumstances when a primary dental disturbance is involved – particularly where the joint has degenerated, or there is persistent strain on the temporo-mandibular joint from local malformations.

The factors that might contribute to this have been covered comprehensively in Chapter 3 and, as we have seen, they may arise from developmental causes, growth patterns, genetic factors, birth trauma, long-term malocclusions, habit patterns, postural habits, injuries, dislocation, disc displacement or inappropriate dentistry. For convenience, these factors are once again summarized briefly here.

Growth and developmental causes

Many of the factors directly affecting the TMJ are secondary to maxillary and mandibular disturbance. This could be due to a developmental disturbance of the mandible, which may be too small, too large, displaced, protruded, retruded or underdeveloped.

Strain on the TMJ may also result from mandibular entrapment. This could in turn be due to developmental disturbances of the maxillae, which may be posteriorly compressed, laterally displaced, medially compressed, narrow-arched or too small, thereby restricting the mandible.

Crossbites and other developmental distortions of the teeth can also displace the mandible and put strain on the TMJ.

Inappropriate dentistry

Extractions of teeth, especially in childhood, can lead to overclosure of the bite, and also to retrusion of the mandible, with consequent strain on the TMJ.

Long-term malocclusions

If any malocclusion, imbalance, or disturbance to the jaw is left unresolved for long periods of time,

it can potentially put strain on the TMJ. If the bite is uneven and the teeth don't meet properly, the regular action of asymmetrical chewing can repeatedly exert unbalanced forces on the TMJs, leading to wear and tear and degeneration of the joint surfaces and tissues. Such malocclusion could be due to missing teeth, extractions, or a high filling. It could also be due to an anterior open bite, an overbite, or other occlusal disturbances.

Loss of vertical dimension

Loss of vertical dimension can also put strain on the TMJs. This could arise from persistent teeth grinding, or from missing teeth, again resulting in overforceful or asymmetrical chewing.

Habit patterns

An anterior open bite may arise as a growth pattern, but may also be due to excessive use of a dummy (pacifier) or excessive thumb-sucking, also putting strain on the TMJ.

Injury

Injury to the mandible may leave a persistent displacement of the jaw, or damage within the joint itself. Dislocation of the TMJ, whether through injury or through excessive opening – sometimes simply from yawning – can leave the joint weak, damaged or strained. Holding the mouth open during prolonged dental treatment may also strain the joint, particularly when combined with the tension induced by the stress of dental treatment.

If such injuries are resolved immediately through cranio-sacral integration, they may not lead to any long-term disturbance, but if they are left untreated and unbalanced then the persistent asymmetry may put strain on the TMJ.

Malformations, developmental disorders and long-term malocclusions which are continuously exerting strain on the TMJ need to be addressed through orthodontics, otherwise the disturbance will continue to exert strain and cause recurrent symptoms.

Persistent strain on the TMJ from any of the above causes may lead to joint degeneration, disc displacement and damage, and consequent persistent symptoms.

Intra-articular disc displacement, as we have seen above, may be symptomless, but may also be a significant cause of TMJ disturbance.

Where there is degeneration of the joint surfaces as a result of long-term wear and tear, the joint may sometimes need structural intervention – although it can often recover significantly through cranio-sacral balancing and appropriate care once any persistent structural strains and imbalances have been eliminated.

Non-dental factors affecting the TMJ

Non-dental factors that can lead to TMJ disturbance include stress, injury to the mandible, temporal bone imbalance, cranio-sacral imbalances throughout the system, muscular pulls and habit patterns.

Stress

Enough has been said already to emphasize that stress factors are the most common cause of TMJ disturbance (and health disturbances in general) and that the priority is always to address stress factors before embarking on extensive and often unnecessary orthodontics. In relation to the TMJ, this is particularly relevant where there is teeth clenching or teeth grinding.

Injury to the mandible

If TMJ discomfort is arising from direct trauma to the mandible, whether recent or past, the first priority is overall reintegration and resolution of the structural disturbances resulting from the trauma through cranio-sacral integration. In most cases this will be enough to resolve any resultant TMJ disturbances.

Temporal bone imbalance

The temporal bones are clearly fundamental to the function of the TMJs. Many TMJ disturbances will be associated with a temporal bone imbalance. But a temporal imbalance could be coming from anywhere in the body.

Cranio-sacral imbalances anywhere in the body

TMJ disturbances could be arising from imbalances anywhere in the body – the face, the cranium, the neck, the pelvis, the feet, the diaphragm, the organs, or anywhere else. Again, the priority is to bring the system as a whole into balance rather than carry out local orthodontic work within an unbalanced system.

Muscular pulls

Addressing muscular pulls is an integral part of addressing cranio-sacral system imbalances, and muscular imbalances anywhere in the body may affect the TMJ. It is of course particularly relevant to consider the pterygoid muscles, the other muscles of mastication, other muscles acting on the mandible, and other muscles acting on the head, neck and the rest of the body, such as the sterno-cleido-mastoid muscles, any of which may be creating asymmetry of the temporal bones and consequent unbalanced forces through the TMJs.

Habit patterns

Many different habit patterns may lead to strain on the TMJ. Once again it is essential to maintain a broad perspective, to look for, identify and address such habit patterns, rather than merely trying to address local symptoms. Such habit patterns include postural imbalances, leaning the head on the hands, emotional posturing, stress habits, and other behavioural patterns as described in Chapter 3.

The common tendency is to react to discomfort by simply thinking locally and wanting symptomatic relief from a medical practitioner (even at great expense and invasive treatment) rather than taking responsibility for one's own health. It can of course be far more productive to reflect on potential underlying causes of the discomfort, recognizing and addressing obvious lifestyle factors which can not only relieve symptoms and save substantial expense and unnecessary treatment, but also bring far more beneficial results.

IV

15

Splints

Splints, also known as bite plates, may be prescribed by dentists, whether for TMJ disturbances or for worn teeth. The purposes of a splint are:

- to reduce strain on the TMJ (particularly the impaction of the condyle into the joint) when there is loss of vertical dimension in the molars

- to prevent further wearing and damage to the teeth

- to retrain the muscles to operate within a correctly balanced bite. If the muscles are not retrained, they will persistently draw back into the distorted pattern to which they are accustomed.

Many patients find that splints are uncomfortable and disruptive to their system, causing headache, compression, and sometimes a sense of their whole system being closed down or clamped in a vice. They may be informed by their dentist that it is necessary to put up with the symptoms and keep using the splint in order to restore a balanced bite. However, if they persist with the splint, they may develop more severe symptoms which can lead to depression, persistent irritation and mental debilitation.

This is particularly true of splints to the upper jaw, which may lock up the system and prevent free mobility of the maxillae, with inevitable repercussions on the system as a whole. John Upledger suggests that if splints are restricting cranio-sacral motion, then they are not properly fitted. He also suggests that splints should only be used on the lower jaw, and not on the upper jaw.

The effects of a splint can be assessed by testing for cranio-sacral quality, motion and response with and without the splint in place.

Contacts

Since one of the principal priorities in addressing TMJ disturbance is integration of the system as a whole, a wide range of contacts may be appropriate according to the overall needs of the individual situation.

With regard to local contacts, the mandible contact (Figure 15.3) is clearly particularly relevant (Chapter 13), and contacts for the maxillae, palatines and vomer (Chapters 16, 17 and 18), the muscles of mastication (Chapter 14), and the temporal bones (see *Cranio-Sacral Integration – Foundation*) are also likely to be significant.

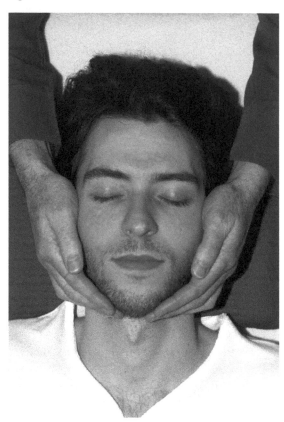

15.3   The mandibular contact is one of the most effective means of addressing TMJ disturbances

Contact can also be taken up on the TMJs themselves, with the hands resting gently on the sides of the head and the tips of the curled fingers resting on the surface of the skin over the TMJs (directly anterior to the ears). Through this contact, you can allow the inherent treatment process to take its course around the fulcrum of your contact. It may also be useful to include *energy drives* through the TMJ, visualizing the internal anatomy of the joint, identifying disturbances and directing the energy drive as appropriate (Figure 15.4).

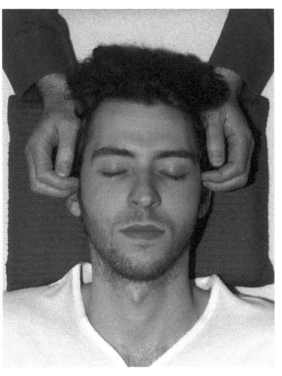

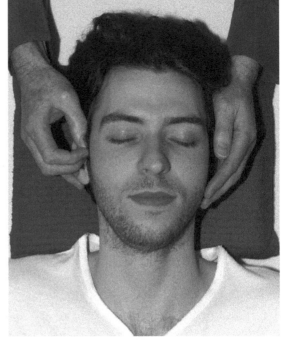

15.4 (a) External contact for the temporo-mandibular joints   *(b) Energy drive through the temporo-mandibular joint*

Even where there is damage and deterioration of the joint itself due to persistent wear and tear and prolonged unbalanced forces from a long-standing TMJ disturbance, the TMJ has potent potential for repair – given appropriate conditions. Once the body as a whole is restored to a state of balance and any sources of strain are removed, the joint has the ability to regenerate and recover, and energy drives can contribute to this process of repair.

Among the many contacts that may be relevant, the mandible contact is likely to be the most valuable in restoring balance and integration to the TMJ and its surrounding structures. This contact is also a very effective means of addressing and balancing the whole system.

Through overall cranio-sacral integration, a great many TMJ disturbances will be resolved, saving many patients from extensive dental and orthodontic treatment. It is preferable to choose the less invasive option of cranio-sacral integration first, in order to restore balance and integration to the system as a whole and probably resolve any TMJ issues in the process, moving on to dentistry and orthodontics only where this is

specifically indicated through accurate whole-person diagnosis and where there is a clearly identified primary dental cause.

Summary: Overall approach to TMJ disturbances

- When a patient has TMJ symptoms, evaluate the whole person as in previous chapters – evaluating from a cranio-sacral perspective, addressing any stress, identifying any dental primaries, and integrating the whole system through cranio-sacral integration. This is likely to resolve the situation in most circumstances.

- Always consider carefully and meticulously any dental or orthodontic assessment.

- Where there are clearly identified dental primaries, refer for whole-person dentistry accordingly.

- In all patients, remain alert to the possibility that symptoms elsewhere in the body, or debilitating disease, might be due to a primary TMJ disorder.

- Where the TMJ itself has been damaged, has become worn, or has deteriorated, firstly ensure that the TMJ itself is restored to a balanced state; secondly, ensure that the whole person is restored to a balanced state, thereby eliminating any further strain on the TMJ from elsewhere; thirdly, work cranio-sacrally on the TMJ itself in order to promote and enhance repair and regeneration.

Chronic conditions

- Bear in mind that, in some cases, the patterns are very deeply ingrained – whole-body imbalances, or stress habit patterns – and may take a significant length of time and many treatment sessions to change. In some cases, even when they do improve, they may need continuing maintenance and balancing.

- But also bear in mind that:
  - not only is cranio-sacral integration usually the most effective option
  - even long-term cranio-sacral treatment is generally significantly cheaper than orthodontics
  - it is also non-invasive
  - and it is usually addressing the cause rather than merely adapting and compensating.

- Understandably, when symptoms are persisting, recurring, or taking time to resolve (due to the chronic nature of the condition), patients tend to wonder if they should be getting something else done, or if orthodontics would sort it out, or whether they should follow the recommendations of their dentist or orthodontist. They are likely to be very tempted to follow that path – but once again what is needed is accurate diagnosis and explanation, not merely trying different approaches (especially invasive approaches) in the vain hope of a quick solution.

Chapter 16

The Maxillae

The maxillae (maxillary bones) are the pivotal bones of the face. They are located centrally, forming the main foundation around which the face is structured. They articulate with every other bone of the face, and with certain bones of the cranium as well.

They therefore have widespread significance for the overall balance of the face and a wide range of conditions affecting the face, including sinusitis, ear infections, nasal congestion, mucus congestion, allergic reactions, facial pain, dental and jaw disturbances, swallowing and breathing patterns, Bell's palsy, trigeminal neuralgia, disturbances to the eyes including lacrimal gland secretion, and many other local conditions. But their influence inevitably extends far beyond the face and may sometimes be the underlying source of headaches, migraine, hormonal imbalance and severe debilitation. They are of course very relevant to resolving many of the dental-related issues mentioned in previous chapters.

They are subject to restriction, compression and displacement from birth trauma, dentistry and facial injuries – to which they are particularly susceptible.

The maxillae, palatine bones and vomer have a close relationship and are often described collectively as 'the mouth parts' – because in some respects they operate as one unit and exert direct influence on each other. They move together in cranio-sacral motion, are often disturbed together and may release together. But they are also separate bones with separate identities and characteristics, and can therefore also be displaced or disturbed individually.

Working with the maxillae can have profound effects on the whole system, often giving a sense of lifting of pressure, weight, tightness, restriction or congestion, which may have affected the patient for decades, potentially influencing their whole nature and personality, particularly where restrictions have arisen from early injuries or childhood dentistry, leaving patterns to which the individual has become accustomed, experiencing them as 'normal'.

Anatomy

The maxillae (*maxilla* is Latin for the upper jaw) form the main central portion of the face (Figures 16.1 and 16.2), articulating with all the other bones of the face, including the nasal bones, the zygomata, the ethmoid, the lacrimal bones and the inferior nasal conchae, as well as the palatine bones and the vomer. They form the medial rim and part of the inferior rim of the orbits. They also meet the frontal bone through the frontal processes of the maxillae which pass up between the orbit and the nasal bones. They may sometimes form an articulation with the sphenoid (variable from one individual to another) and will at any rate always be intimately related to the sphenoid through the palatine bones and vomer (Figures 16.4 and 16.5).

The maxillae are hollow bones containing the *maxillary air sinuses* – the most common site of pain due to sinusitis (Figure 16.5).

The horizontal portions of the two maxillae together form the anterior two thirds of the hard palate, meeting centrally at the *inter-maxillary suture* (Figure 16.6). They articulate posteriorly with the two palatine bones (which together form the posterior one third of the palate) at the *maxillary-palatine suture*. The cross-shaped junction formed where the two maxillary bones and the two palatine bones meet is the *cruciate suture*, which can often be palpated in the roof of the mouth as a shallow concavity. Sometimes a ridge or lump may be palpated along this central suture of the hard palate. This is known as a *torus palatinus*. It may be a bony growth or may indicate that the vomer is pressing down through the roof of the mouth reflecting undue compressions in the facial structures (perhaps due to birth trauma).

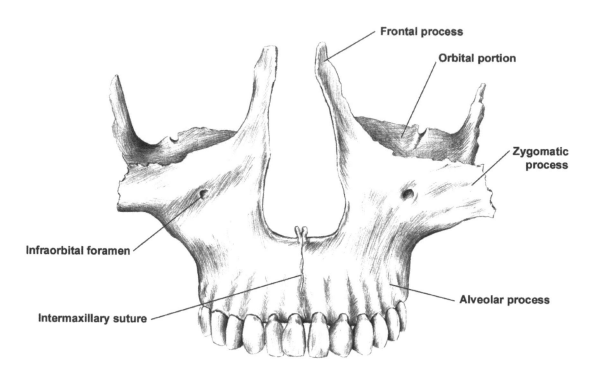

16.1   The maxillae form the central portion of the face

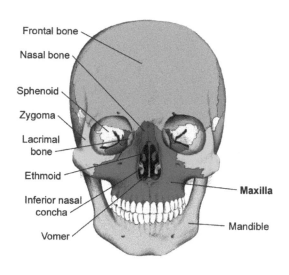

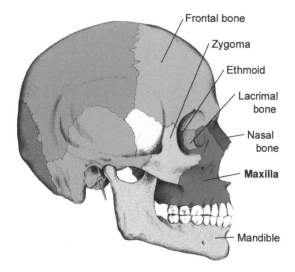

16.2   The maxillae articulate with all the other bones of the face

16.3   The maxillae – in situ – lateral view

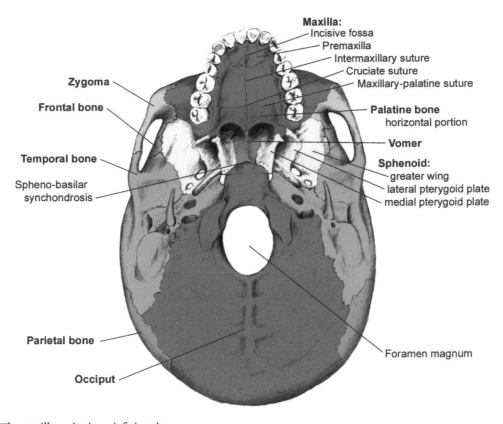

Maxilla:
Incisive fossa
Premaxilla
Intermaxillary suture
Cruciate suture
Maxillary-palatine suture

Zygoma

Frontal bone

Palatine bone
horizontal portion

Temporal bone

Vomer

Spheno-basilar synchondrosis

Sphenoid:
greater wing
lateral pterygoid plate
medial pterygoid plate

Parietal bone

Foramen magnum

Occiput

16.4   The maxillae – in situ – inferior view

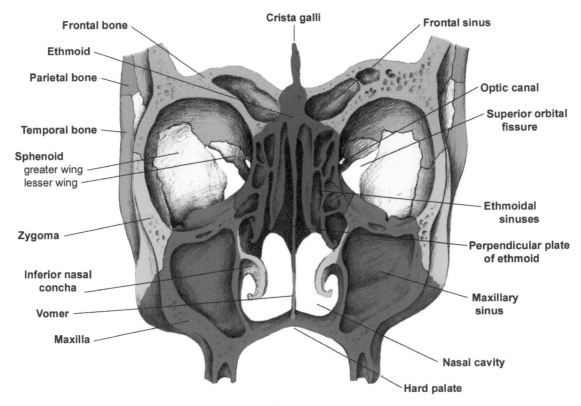

Crista galli

Frontal bone

Frontal sinus

Ethmoid

Parietal bone

Optic canal

Superior orbital fissure

Temporal bone

Sphenoid
greater wing
lesser wing

Ethmoidal sinuses

Perpendicular plate of ethmoid

Zygoma

Maxillary sinus

Inferior nasal concha

Vomer

Maxilla

Nasal cavity

Hard palate

16.5   The maxillae are hollow bones containing the maxillary air sinuses

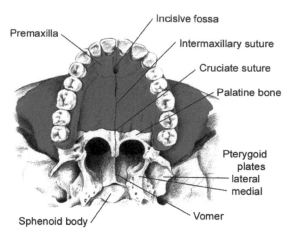

16.6   The maxillae form the anterior two thirds of the hard palate, each maxilla divided by a suture into a premaxilla and posterior maxilla

Premaxilla

The term maxilla is often used to include the whole upper jaw. However, the anterior portion of each maxilla is a separate bone known as the incisive bone or *premaxilla.* (The term premaxilla is used both for each individual incisive bone, and also for the premaxillary unit comprising both incisive bones.) There is a suture running medially from between the lateral incisor and the canine tooth on each side (the second and third upper teeth), separating the premaxilla from the posterior maxilla. These sutures persist into adult life and their mobility (along with the mobility of the intermaxillary suture) is essential to cranio-sacral motion and to healthy function. The incisive bones contain the two upper incisor teeth on each side, so the premaxilla is vulnerable to injuries and disturbances to the upper front teeth (a common occurrence arising from falls, blows or dentistry).

The *incisive canal* passes through the palate, with its superior opening close to the anterior end of the intermaxillary suture, at the junction between the premaxilla and posterior maxilla. On the inferior surface of the palate, it widens into the incisive fossa. It enables passage of the descending palatine artery and the nasopalatine nerve, a branch of the maxillary division of the trigeminal nerve, passing down along the nasal septum and through the incisive canal to provide sensory supply to the inferior surface of the palate.

On the external surface of each maxilla below the orbit is an *infraorbital foramen*, for the emergence of the maxillary division of the trigeminal nerve (Figure 16.1). The maxillary division exits the base of the cranium through the foramen rotundum, enters the orbit through the inferior orbital fissure, gives off alveolar branches to the upper teeth, and passes along a groove in the floor of the orbit (which is also the roof of the maxillary sinus). The groove deepens to become a tunnel, enabling the nerve to penetrate the floor of the orbit before emerging to the surface of the face at the infraorbital foramen. This nerve receives sensation from the maxillary portion of the face as well as the upper teeth, and may be involved in trigeminal neuralgia.

Various other neurological pathways, including autonomic nerve supply to the glands and mucous membranes of the nose and mouth and sinuses, may be compromised by disturbances to the maxillae, contributing to rhinitis, excessive mucus production and allergic reactions.

The *alveolar processes* of the maxillae are the bony ridges which contain the upper teeth, and consequently one of the main causes of disturbance to the maxillae and to the whole maxillary–palatine–vomer complex is dentistry, with resultant repercussions through these structures into the whole system. Disturbance to the maxillae as a result of dentistry is far more disruptive to the cranio-sacral system than dentistry to the mandible, since the maxillae are more intimately connected to the cranium, whereas the mandible is free to move and adapt to trauma, thereby reducing the degree to which trauma may be transmitted into the cranium and the system as a whole. All the teeth, both adult and deciduous, are present or forming at birth, with the upper teeth contained within the maxillae, waiting to descend at the appropriate time (Figure 16.7).

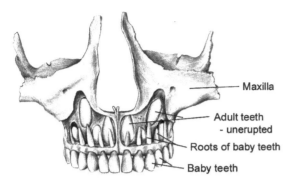

*16.7   All the teeth, both adult and deciduous, are present
or forming at birth, with the upper teeth contained
within the maxillae, waiting to descend at the
appropriate age*

Cranio-sacral motion

During the expansion phase (flexion phase) of cranio-sacral motion, the anterior portion of the maxillae (the upper incisor teeth) rises superiorly, coming up to meet the frontal bone as it arcs forward and down. At the same time, the two maxillae spread laterally, separating slightly at the posterior part of the intermaxillary suture (the back teeth moving apart slightly). The whole maxillary–palatine–vomer complex may also be pushed slightly anteriorly with each expansion phase as it arcs up to meet the frontal bone. During the contraction phase (extension phase) the opposite occurs.

In order to understand the interaction between the face and the cranium more fully, it is helpful to consider the cranio-sacral motion of the whole face in relation to the sphenoid and occiput. As the sphenoid arcs forward and down during the expansion phase of motion, it pushes the ethmoid forward. As the ethmoid, together with the rest of the facial structures, is pushed forward, the whole facial complex rotates in the opposite direction from the sphenoid, the anterior portion rising anteriorly, as if hingeing around the sphenoid–ethmoid articulation (Figure 16.8).

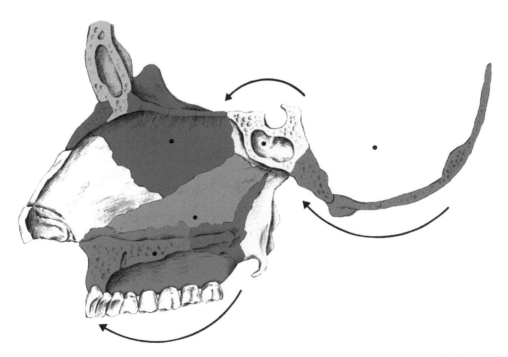

*16.8   Cranio-sacral motion of the face – the whole facial complex rotates in the opposite direction from the sphenoid, the
anterior portion rising anteriorly during the expansion phase of motion*

Maxilla

Adult teeth
- unerupted

Roots of baby teeth

Baby teeth

Contacts for the maxillae

Within the context of an overall integrated treatment, having established underlying vitality and overall balance of the system as a whole, identified relationships between the face and the rest of the body, and established a diagnosis and appropriate approach to overall treatment in accordance with the history of the patient and the findings within the cranio-sacral system as a whole, specific contacts for the maxillae may be appropriate.

This could be due to local symptoms, history of trauma to the area, impressions gained through engagement with the cranio-sacral system as a whole, or simply to explore the area.

General face contact

The general face contact, described in Chapter 12, engaging with the whole system through the face, provides a valuable overview and insight into the maxillae within the context of the rest of the face. As the face responds to this contact and to the inherent treatment process, the maxillae will naturally rebalance along with the rest of the face. Working with the general face contact can also prepare the way for more specific contacts.

This may be all that is needed for the integration of the maxillae. Alternatively, a particular fulcrum of resistance, or pattern of injury to the maxillae, may indicate that a more individual contact on the maxillae could be helpful.

External maxillary contact

This contact is similar to the general face contact, but more specific to the maxillae. Let your fingers come to rest lightly onto the cheeks bilaterally, taking care to place the fingers within the margins of the maxillae. With this contact you can engage more particularly with the maxillae and allow the continuing evolution of the inherent treatment process through points of stillness and release (Figures 16.9a and b).

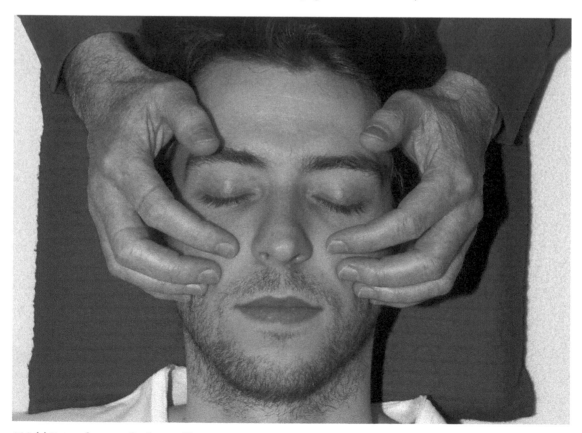

16.9 (a) External contact for the maxillae

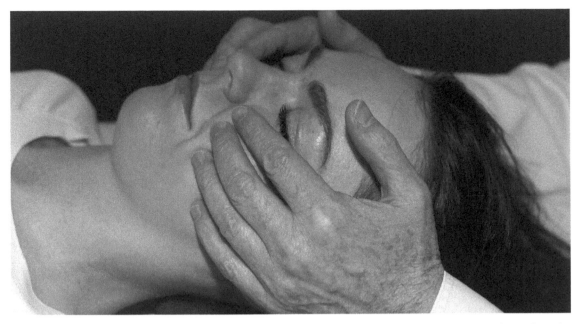

16.9 (b) Where there is a narrow maxillary arch, the forces held within the tissues may draw the maxillae (and your fingers) medially into compression

This contact is particularly valuable for patterns of medial compression, including a narrow maxillary arch with crowded teeth. In such cases, the forces held within the tissues may be drawing the maxillae medially into compression. Having followed the spontaneous responses within the maxillae, you can explore the possibility of medial compression, unilateral or bilateral, asking yourself whether there is any tendency for the maxillae to draw medially, and following the consequent responses to stillness and release. This release can often lead to a profound expansion of the maxillae – which can be allowed and encouraged – and a significant sense of relief and ease for the patient, possibly after years of medial compression arising from birth or childhood dentistry. It is also a valuable contact to explore with children whose maxillary arch is narrow and whose teeth are crowded, in order to release the compressive forces and restore balance and free mobility to the area, potentially saving them from extensive dental and orthodontic work. It can also be helpful in maxillary sinus congestion and nasal congestion.

Alveolar arches

This contact is similar to the previous contact, but with the fingers positioned a little lower on the maxillae, along the alveolar processes. It can again be useful where there is narrowing of the maxillary arch, with consequent crowding of the teeth and other repercussions (Figure 16.10).

Some systems will respond more readily to this finger position, others to the previous position. Engage with the system and feel which point of contact feels most responsive, again exploring specifically for the presence of medial compression.

It can be useful to follow these external contacts with a specific intraoral contact inviting a gentle lateral expansion of the narrow maxillary arch. This can be particularly helpful in children, since their young systems tend to be more malleable and responsive. Both the compressive and expansive contacts can be very beneficial in children who are wearing an expansion device (a dental appliance for widening the maxillary arch), greatly assisting the progress of the treatment process. Ideally, the compressive forces within the maxillae would be addressed cranio-sacrally before embarking on dental procedures, and the expansive aspects of the cranio-sacral treatment would be maintained regularly throughout the course of any dental treatment.

IV

16

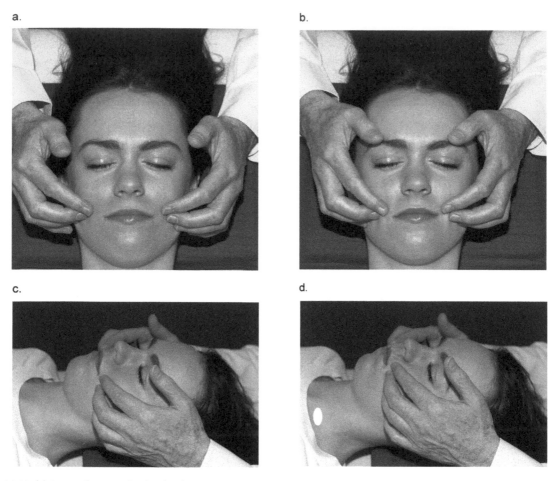

16.10 (a) External contact for the alveolar processes
   (b) A narrow maxillary arch may draw the alveolar processes medially into compression
   (c) External contact for the alveolar processes – lateral view
   (d) The alveolar processes drawing into medial compression – lateral view

Intraoral contacts

Even where there is no particular need for maxillary expansion, an intraoral contact is often the most effective contact for addressing specific restrictions of the maxillae, using the upper teeth as the point of contact (Figures 16.11–16.13). This is particularly relevant because much of the trauma and displacement of the maxillae arises as a result of forces exerted through the teeth – biting, chewing, teeth clenching and grinding, as well as dentistry. It also enables very precise and specific identification of patterns of resistance and their fulcrums. Also, by maintaining a dual contact between the cranium and the mouthparts, it enables a clear evaluation of the relationship and interaction between the maxillae and the rest of the cranium.

Standing upright and relaxed beside the patient's head, allow both your arms to hang loosely from the shoulders. When you are ready, let one hand come in softly through the energy field to rest gently over the spheno-frontal area, settling into engagement with the system as a whole before taking up the second contact. Once engaged, invite the patient to open their mouth and slide your index and middle fingers (one on each side of the mouth) along the biting surface of the upper teeth, until the pads of the fingers are resting approximately onto the seventh tooth (the second molar) on each side (Figures 16.11 and 16.12). Allow the palmar surface of your fingers to rest softly along the surface of the other upper teeth (Figure 16.13). The exact degree to which the fingers project into the mouth will depend on the relative size of fingers and mouth, and most of all on patient comfort. If necessary, one can engage with the fingers placed less deeply into the mouth, but where possible it is preferable to take the fingers as far back towards the seventh teeth as is comfortable for the patient, in order to enable as comprehensive a contact as possible on the maxillae.

Once in position, invite the patient to close their mouth gently, letting their lower jaw come to rest lightly onto your fingers, and to relax completely. (Some patients will be very concerned for your fingers and will hold their mouth open slightly to avoid squashing your fingers, thereby holding on to tension in their jaw. It is therefore helpful to check that the patient does relax their jaw completely, without undue concern for your fingers.)

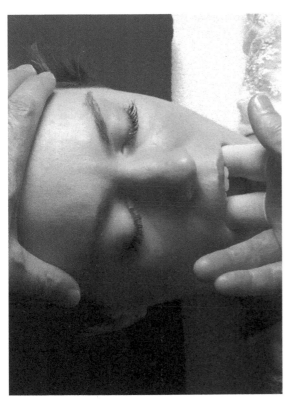

16.11 Intraoral contact for the maxillae

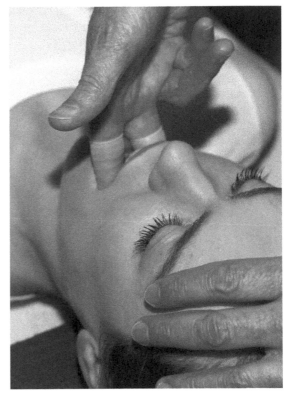

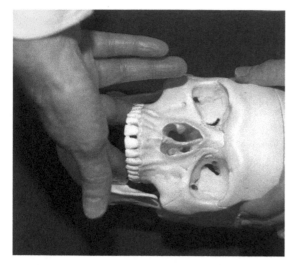

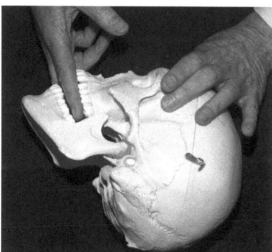

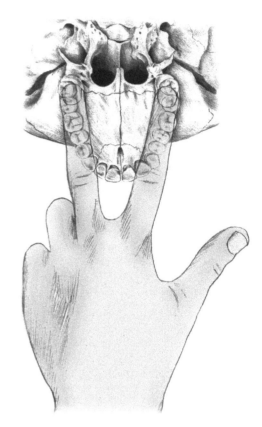

16.13 Slide your index and middle fingers along the biting surface of the upper teeth

Remind them to let you know if at any time they feel uncomfortable or if they need you to remove your fingers. (Since they are not likely to be able to speak with your fingers in their mouth, they could raise a hand, or grunt, or whatever other form of communication they prefer.)

Be sure to relax both your arms completely. Concern for the patient's comfort and the sensitivity of the face can sometimes lead practitioners to be tentative, holding their hand up in order not to weigh heavily onto the patient's face. It is of course essential not to weigh heavily onto the patient's face, but it is equally essential for the practitioner's arms and hands to be completely relaxed, the arm hanging loosely from the shoulder (if standing) or the hand hanging loosely from the wrist (if sitting). It is possible to work from a sitting position (described below).

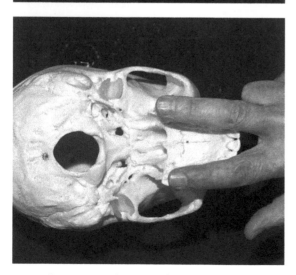

16.12 Finger position for intraoral contact on the maxillae

The inherent treatment process

Having established an appropriate and comfortable position, settle into engagement and allow the inherent treatment process to evolve. Evaluate quality, symmetry and motion, feel the expression of rhythmic motion both in the maxillae and in the cranium, as the maxillae rise to meet the frontal bone during the expansion phase (flexion phase) – the upper incisors rising, the upper molars widening. Observe and allow the responses in both your hands – the cranial contact and the mouth contact – feeling the interaction between them and following the response of the whole system as the therapeutic process evolves around the fulcrum of your contact and your attention.

As always there may be any number of different responses – systems that are freely mobile, systems that are rigidly stuck, systems that swirl around in a multitude of different directions, systems that draw very specifically in a particular direction. As always, all you need to do is allow the process to evolve round the fulcrum of your own stillness.

A common scenario is that initial movements will gradually settle and the system will gradually draw towards a particular fulcrum, reaching points of stillness and eventual release. This process may occur several times, whether returning to the same deeply ingrained fulcrum repeatedly, or following a more complex journey moving from one fulcrum to another as each one releases. The primary fulcrum may turn out to be, not within the maxillary complex, but somewhere else in the body, but can of course still be engaged with and addressed through this contact, and may indeed be specifically brought to light by this contact. However, if you have chosen to use this contact, it may be because you have already identified a fulcrum or restriction here, so the system is likely to draw towards this local fulcrum in order to enable release.

It may also be appropriate, particularly where there has been medial compression of the maxillae, as mentioned above, to invite a gentle lateral expansion of the narrow maxillary arch, as if your two fingers are gradually drawing apart (maxillary arch expansion). This can be most effective following an external maxillary contact which has enabled release of any compressive forces.

Ramifications throughout the system

As described previously in relation to the mandible, a blow or trauma to the face can have far-reaching consequences – mechanically, emotionally, and on many other levels throughout the system. The more you can identify and engage with these deeper far-reaching patterns, the more profound will be the response and the release. Maintain awareness of the repercussions, physical and emotional, of any forces exerted throughout the system, bearing in mind that the patterns manifesting at the maxillae may be arising from the pelvis, the solar plexus, the neck, the cranial base or anywhere else in the system.

As releases occur, the effects may be felt throughout the system, either because the maxillary pattern was causing repercussions through the body, or because the source of the maxillary pattern elsewhere in the body has responded. Emotional releases may also occur, with potentially profound changes to the whole system and the patient's sense of themselves.

Such emotional patterns may relate to suppressed fear or anger relating to an injury, or may relate to emotional tensions held in the mouth, or deeply embedded emotional patterns from birth or early childhood, perhaps relating to breastfeeding, dentistry or abuse.

Experienced practitioners

Experienced practitioners are likely to be able to engage with the system and follow the spontaneous responses as necessary without any particular format, following into flexion patterns, extension patterns, torsions, side-bendings and side-shifts and any combination of these according to the demands of the system, allowing the system to express its own needs and travel along its own journey. Allow the mouth to express itself. This may be all that is necessary.

Less experienced practitioners

Less experienced practitioners may find it helpful, in order to develop that skill, to explore the patterns of asymmetry (described below) within the system more methodically, to ask questions of themselves as to what patterns or combinations of patterns they are encountering. This may particularly be relevant if you are not feeling any response in the system. Specific exploration of these patterns may also be useful where the maxillae are severely locked from trauma, or where they remain persistently agitated and unsettled.

Exploring the different possibilities can enable the practitioner to identify subtle hidden patterns that were previously unnoticed, and can also elicit a response from the system, enabling the system to reveal and express underlying patterns that are not manifesting readily. It may also initiate a more comprehensive process of release.

Patterns of asymmetry

The patterns of asymmetry commonly described within the maxillary complex are similar to those found at the spheno-basilar synchondrosis (see *Cranio-Sacral Integration – Foundation*) and may be explored and addressed in a similar way:

- maintaining contact with the cranium as a point of reference
- monitoring the movement of the maxillary complex relative to the sphenoid and the rest of the cranium
- asking yourself if there is any indication of each of the various standard patterns
- exploring each pattern in turn
- observing and allowing the response in each case
- allowing the process to evolve into a more comprehensive integrated treatment process.

It is possible to proceed methodically through each pattern, assessing and taking note, and then treating the patterns or combinations accordingly (the traditional method as devised by Sutherland and described in Magoun).[1] However, it is probably more appropriate to work in a more spontaneous, less mechanical, manner more suited to the specific needs of the patient and the responses within the system. If necessary, you can start by exploring individual patterns, but as soon as you encounter a response, allow that response to lead into whatever journey may be appropriate. As always, the more familiar you are with the various patterns within the system, the more readily you will engage with them spontaneously.

Standard patterns of asymmetry

With one hand over the spheno-frontal area, the movements of the maxillae can be monitored in relation to the sphenoid and cranium. The standard patterns of distortion for the maxillae are (Figure 16.14):

Hyperflexion

- The anterior portion of the maxillary complex rises superiorly towards the frontal area, as the frontal area arcs forward and down.
- At the same time, the maxillary complex flares, particularly in its posterior portion.
- In other words, the upper incisors rising, the upper molars widening.

Hyperextension

- The anterior maxillary complex drops inferiorly away from the frontal area, as the frontal area arcs back and up.
- At the same time, the maxillary complex narrows, particularly in its posterior portion.
- In other words, the upper incisors falling, the upper molars narrowing.

Side-bending left

- The anterior maxillary complex turns in a horizontal plane towards the left (the front of the mouth turning to the left) relative to the sphenoid (as in a blow from the right, to the right side of the mouth).

Side-bending right

- The anterior maxillary complex turns in a horizontal plane towards the right, relative to the sphenoid.

Torsion left

- The left side of the maxillary complex rises superiorly towards the frontal bone, while the right side drops inferiorly (as in a blow from below to the left side of the jaw).
- The whole maxillary complex rotates around the horizontal antero-posterior axis of the intermaxillary suture while the cranium rotates in the opposite direction around the same axis.

a. Hyperflexion:

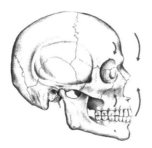

b. Hyperextension:

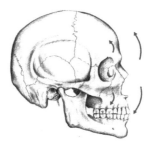

c. Sidebending Left:

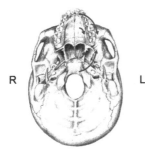

R   L

d. Sidebending Right:

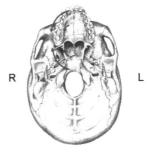

R   L

e. Torsion Left:

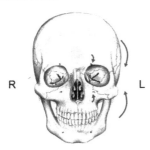

R   L

f. Torsion Right:

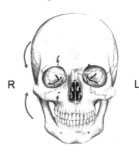

R   L

g. Impaction (Compression):

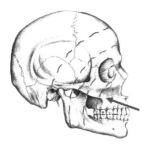

h. Disimpaction (Decompression):

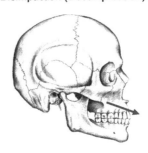

16.14 Standard patterns of asymmetry for the maxillae

Torsion right

- The right side of the maxillary complex rises superiorly towards the frontal bone, while the left side drops inferiorly.

Side-shift left

- The whole maxillary complex shifts to the left, relative to the sphenoid (as in a blow to the right side of the face – further back than the mouth).

Side-shift right

- The whole maxillary complex shifts to the right, relative to the sphenoid.

Impaction (compression)

- The maxillary complex is compressed posteriorly towards the sphenoid (as in a blow to the front of the mouth from the front; as if the practitioner's two hands – on the maxillae and sphenoid respectively – are being compressed towards each other).

Disimpaction (decompression)

This is not a pattern of injury or distortion, but a direction which might be invited (particularly following a compression) in order to enhance the release of deeply ingrained impaction forces.

- The maxillary complex draws out anteriorly away from the sphenoid (off the front of the face).

As with the spheno-basilar patterns, it is often therapeutic to follow any exploration of impaction (compression) with disimpaction (decompression) in order to enable maximum opening out into free movement following the release of a chronic compressive pattern.

Although directions of asymmetry have, as a means of clarification, been described here in relation to blows to the face, these patterns are not necessarily caused by direct injury. They may be caused by many other forces from different sources within or outside the body – whole-body imbalances arising from the pelvis, injuries elsewhere in the body, birth patterns, and so on.

The contact over the spheno-frontal area acts as a point of reference, in relation to which movements of the maxillae can be identified. This does not mean that it is held rigid – all contacts need to remain fluidic – but the movements of the maxillae are observed relative to the movements within the spheno-frontal contact. The cranium can usually be felt moving in the opposite or corresponding direction. For example, in a torsion pattern the mouthparts will twist one way and the sphenoid will twist in the opposite direction around the same axis. In flexion, the anterior maxilla will rise while the sphenoid arcs forward and down. In a side-bending pattern, the maxillae and sphenoid will side-bend towards the same side.

Each of these patterns is likely to have a corresponding pattern reflected at the spheno-basilar synchondrosis.

Whether working spontaneously or methodically, engage with the system in whatever way is appropriate, allowing the inherent treatment process to take its course, reaching fulcrums of restriction and in due course releasing, eventually settling to a balanced neutral state. This might be a brief release of a specific fulcrum, or it might be a long and profound treatment of the whole system, or it might lead into any number of other possibilities. When the process feels complete and the system feels settled, you can move on as appropriate.

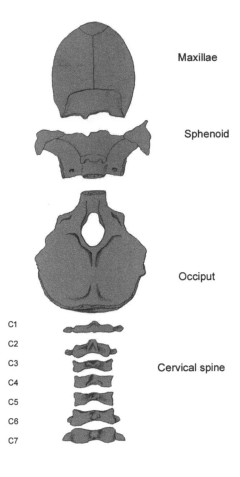

Maxillae

Sphenoid

Occiput

C1
C2
C3
C4   Cervical spine
C5
C6
C7

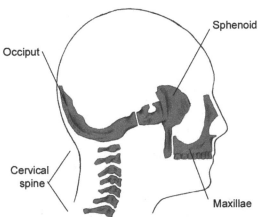

Sphenoid

Occiput

Cervical
spine

Maxillae

*16.15 Terminology for torsion and side-bending for the
maxillae can be more clearly understood when
the maxillae, sphenoid and occiput are viewed as
extensions of the spine*

Contacts for the premaxilla

Each maxilla includes a premaxilla anteriorly –
with a suture running between the lateral incisor
and the canine tooth on each side. Mobility at this
suture (as well as at the suture between the two
maxillae) is essential to cranio-sacral mobility and
healthy function. Restriction may be caused by
dental appliances crossing the suture (as described
in previous chapters) as well as due to injuries
to the upper front teeth, perhaps unrecognized
trauma going back to childhood. Intraosseous
restriction may also occur as a result of birth
compression or facial injury.

In order to engage with the premaxillae and
assess their mobility in relation to the cranium and
cranio-sacral system as a whole, take up contact
with one hand over the spheno-frontal area, and
take up contact on the premaxillae with the pads
of the index and middle fingers on the biting
surface of the upper incisors. Engage with the
system and assess mobility, allowing the process
to evolve appropriately (Figure 16.16).

You can also evaluate and address the mobility
of the premaxillae in relation to the posterior
maxillae by taking up contact with one hand over
the maxillae externally – the fingers on one side,
the thumb on the other side – and again take up
contact on the premaxillae with the pads of the
index and middle fingers on the biting surface
of the upper incisors. Engage with the system
and allow the process to evolve appropriately
(Figure 16.17).

IV

16

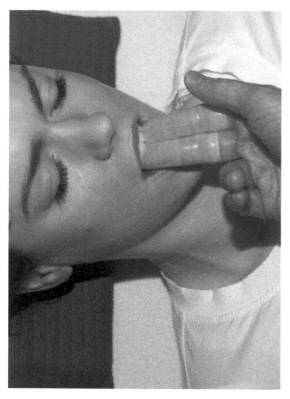

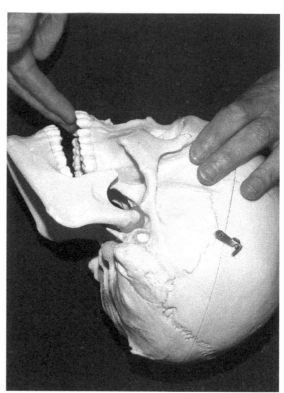

16.16 Contact for the premaxilla

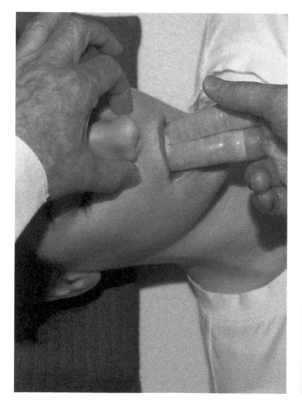

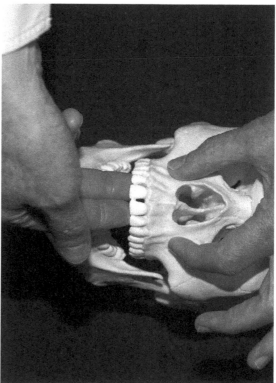

16.17 Contact for addressing the mobility of the premaxilla in relation to the posterior maxilla

Maxillary-frontal contacts (external)

Where the maxillae have been compressed superiorly towards the frontal area, whether bilaterally or unilaterally, more specific contacts between the frontal area and the maxillae may be beneficial:

With one hand over the frontal area, take up contact with the other hand over the maxillae (externally) – the fingers on one side, the thumb on the other side. Engage and assess the relationship between the frontal area and the maxillae. Explore compression between the two areas, feeling whether your two hands are being drawn together, bilaterally or unilaterally. This can be followed by inviting decompression (Figure 16.18).

If there is specific compression between the maxilla and frontal area on one side, contact can be taken up specifically on the affected side both on the frontal area and the affected maxilla, again exploring the response and exploring compression and decompression as appropriate (Figure 16.19).

The whole mouth

In working with the maxillae, we are not of course merely working with the bones. All the structures of the mouth – soft tissues, nerve pathways, glandular secretions (both salivary and mucous), teeth, tongue – will be involved and resolved through these contacts. As we explore these other structures in subsequent chapters, the overall significance of working with the maxillary area will become more apparent.

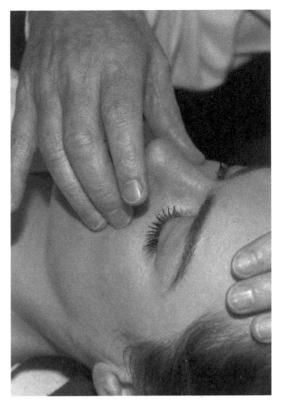

16.18 Maxillary-frontal contact – bilateral

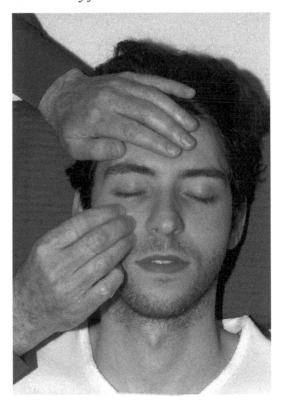

16.19 Maxillary-frontal contact – unilateral

IV

16

The tongue

Issues involving the tongue often relate to its nerve supply and the pathway of these nerves through the cranial base, and this will be dealt with in Chapter 31 on the hypoglossal nerve (Cr XII). It can also be beneficial to engage with the tongue directly through fascial unwinding. This may be relevant in some speech and language difficulties in which the tongue is implicated, in breastfeeding issues in babies or unresolved breastfeeding trauma in adults, or following trauma to the tongue. It may also be beneficial for a stutter, or any issues involving the tongue and self-expression. The responses to tongue unwinding, both physical and psycho-emotional, can be profound and sometimes challenging.

In order to unwind the tongue, engage with the system through the cranium with one hand under the occiput. When ready, take hold of the tongue between the fingers and thumb of the other hand, with the fingers on the superior surface and the thumb on the inferior surface. It is necessary to hold the tongue fairly firmly and relatively far back, in order to prevent it from slipping out from your fingers. Ensure that the patient knows to communicate with you if they feel a need to stop for any reason (since they will obviously be unable to speak). Allow the inherent treatment process to take its course, letting the tongue express its needs through whatever movements arise. A slight thought of traction can help to contain and maintain focus (Figure 16.20).

Patient responses to intraoral contacts

Patients may have various perspectives on the idea of having the practitioner's fingers inside their mouth. For some it will be perfectly comfortable. Others may be wary at first but soon find that any concerns were unwarranted. Some patients may find it difficult, particularly if they have a history of oral trauma or traumatic dentistry which may lead to a consequent fear or unexplained emotional reaction to anything associated with intraoral contact. Most patients, once they have become accustomed to the contact and have felt the therapeutic benefits, will be perfectly comfortable with it and may find it a particularly soothing and profoundly therapeutic contact. As long as the process is handled appropriately, with gentle fingers, soft contacts and taking care not to be invasive in any way, then there is no reason why there should be any difficulties. It is of course essential that the therapist approaches the situation without any apprehension, anxiety or tentativeness, as this will inevitably be transmitted into the process and increase the possibility of discomfort.

Some patients may find that they swallow repeatedly, possibly through dryness in the mouth, but more probably from tension. Encouraging the patient to relax the throat and neck and breathe freely may ease this tendency. If necessary, placing a higher cushion under the head, thereby taking the neck and throat into slight forward bending, can be helpful.

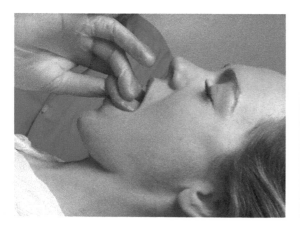
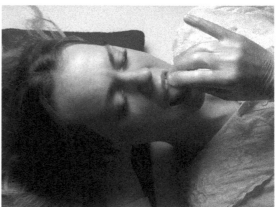

16.20 Unwinding the tongue can be beneficial for speech and language difficulties, or any issues involving trauma to the tongue

It is customary for the practitioner to wear protective gloves or finger cots for any procedure inside the mouth.

Sitting or standing?

For these intraoral contacts, the practitioner can be either sitting or standing beside the patient's head. In a sitting position, the arm contacting the mouthparts will need to be held high, and this can become strenuous, leading to tension in the arm, which may reduce sensitivity and be projected into the treatment process. The advantage of standing is that both arms can hang loosely from the shoulders and may therefore be more comfortable and relaxed.

Although the contact is generally comfortable for the patient, it is nevertheless preferable to keep the process relatively brief, so that the patient does not spend too long with fingers in their mouth. However, there are times when the process settles into a deeply engaged profound and prolonged whole-person treatment process and it may be appropriate to stay there at great length. Be prepared to hold into patterns for a long time, particularly with chronic deeply ingrained patterns. A gentle contact maintained over a longer period of time is much more profound and effective than a stronger force exerted for a short time, particularly as a gentle contact will not induce defensive resistance and reaction, and will therefore engage more deeply. Some patients may fall asleep during this process (with potential ramifications that we will look at shortly).

Oral trauma

If a patient does have significant concerns about having fingers in the mouth, this may reflect some specific issue associated with the mouth, whether from dental trauma, trauma associated with breastfeeding, abuse, or other oral trauma. Memories of the trauma, together with associated emotions, can be triggered by the oral contact – or even the thought of it.

In such cases, there are various considerations. On the one hand, it is of course essential to be sensitive to the patient's situation, not introducing contacts which will cause significant disturbance

to their emotional wellbeing. On the other hand, these contacts can be particularly relevant, providing an opportunity for the patient to engage with the past trauma more fully, discussing it, expressing it, dealing with the suppressed emotions, releasing the trauma and freeing themselves from the restrictive effects which the suppressed trauma may be exerting on their life. This does of course need to be handled with great sensitivity and care and with a comprehensive understanding of the whole process of addressing trauma.

Jaw clenching and finger preservation

In some cases you may notice the patient's lower jaw clenching firmly on to your fingers, sometimes to the point of significant discomfort. This is usually an indication of tension held in the jaw and indicates a need to address the underlying emotional tensions contributing to the jaw clenching, perhaps through the mandible, the muscles of mastication and through directly addressing the underlying emotional patterns. Clearly whilst carrying out the maxillary contact, you do not need to endure undue discomfort. It will be necessary, not only for the welfare of your own fingers, but also for the benefit of the patient, to keep reminding them to relax their jaw and let go of their jaw muscles. Perhaps a different contact may be more appropriate initially.

Ivo was in his fifties and had a long history of severe jaw pain and complex associated symptoms that had been troubling him for years. He had undergone extensive dentistry and orthodontics (which he claimed were responsible for his pain) in an attempt to resolve the issues, but without any success, and substantial cranial treatment also without any relief. He expressed strong resentment towards the dental profession and practitioners in general for causing his discomfort and failing to relieve it. He needed a lot of treatment. During his initial sessions, as I worked inside his mouth, he would very soon fall asleep. As he slept, his jaw would gradually but inexorably tighten, biting into my fingers with ever-increasing force. At regular intervals, I had to wake him and remind him to relax his jaw, before my fingers were completely severed. The underlying cause was of course stress factors – which had not been addressed by his dentists, orthodontists or other practitioners.

In young children, for whom this intraoral contact can often be very relevant, you need to be even more wary. Sometimes they may unintentionally bite your fingers, and occasionally some of them may quite deliberately decide to bite your fingers just for fun. This should not deter practitioners from using this contact with children, as it can be a very valuable means of addressing the many dental and jaw disturbances which contribute to the far-reaching consequences described in earlier chapters.

Cleft palate

Cleft lip and cleft palate are among the most common birth defects worldwide, with 1 in 600 children affected[2] (Figure 16.21). A baby may be born with a cleft lip, a cleft palate, or both cleft lip and cleft palate, either unilateral or bilateral. The birth defect develops during early pregnancy.

The cause is unknown, but is believed to be an interaction between genetic and environmental factors. The majority of cases are from the lower socio-economic classes.[3]

If untreated, cleft palate leads to difficulties with feeding, breathing, speaking, hearing and dentition, as well as the major psycho-social implications of appearance and disability.

In the developed world, cases are not widely seen these days as, in recent decades, cleft palate has become eminently treatable through plastic surgery. (My grandfather, Professor Thomas Kilner, was one of the pioneers in the development of plastic surgery in the 1920s and 1930s.)

Surgery is generally carried out in the first few months of life, and before 18 months if possible. Many children will need additional surgery as they grow older. Following surgery, children generally do well, and there may be no visible sign of the defect, but they may be prone to ear infections and hearing difficulties and sometimes speech and language issues. These persistent symptoms, particularly the recurrent ear

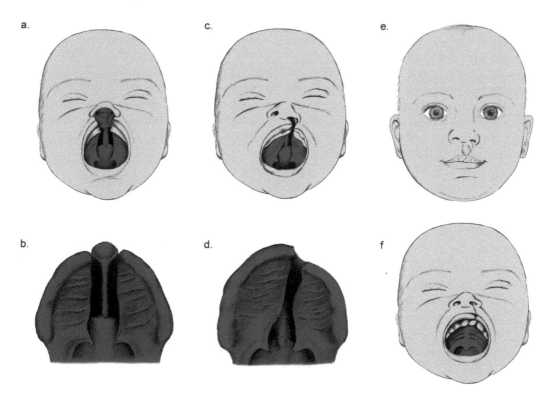

16.21 (a) Bilateral cleft lip and palate – anterior view
(b) Bilateral cleft lip and palate – inferior view
(c) Unilateral cleft lip and palate – anterior view
(d) Unilateral cleft lip and palate – inferior view
(e), (f) Following surgical repair

infections, are the usual reason why these children may be brought for cranio-sacral therapy.

Maya was four years old when I first saw her, and had been born with a cleft palate. Surgical repair had been successful, but she remained prone to frequent ear infections, glue ear and consequent significant hearing loss. She was a very willing and cooperative patient and within two sessions of cranio-sacral integration, her ears cleared, her hearing was fully restored, and her propensity to recurrent ear infections and glue ear disappeared permanently.

In India and other developing countries (with limited medical resources and a large proportion of the population living in poverty in remote areas) it is still common to see children and adults with untreated cleft palates. Every year 35,000 children in India are born with clefts.[4] Without surgery, these children would be condemned to a lifetime of isolation and suffering.

Fortunately, there is a marvellous arrangement in India known as Smile Train.[5] A fully equipped hospital train travels around India, stopping off for a week or two at various remote rural locations. Surgeons volunteer for one or two weeks at a time, performing around forty operations a day restoring cleft palates and changing the lives of people who would otherwise go through life with the severe limitations of a cleft palate.

Chapter 17

The Palatine Bones

The palatine bones are intimately related to the maxillae, and much of what has been said in relation to the maxillae will also apply to the palatines in terms of their significance within the face and in terms of related conditions and symptom pictures.

The palatine bones do, however, also have additional individual features of significance, positioned as they are between the maxillae and the sphenoid, forming a bridge between the cranium and the face. This crucial position can lead to various possible consequences:

- the *transmission of forces* of facial trauma from the maxillae into the sphenoid via the palatine bones

- or, alternatively, the palatine bones acting as *shock absorbers*, absorbing the impact of injuries to the face and preventing the transmission of forces into the sphenoid (a possibility which led Sutherland to describe the palatine bones as 'speed reducers')[1]

- or, the potential for the palatine bones to become *trapped* between the maxillae and the sphenoid, blocking cranio-sacral motion between the cranium and the face, and therefore throughout the system.

Restrictions of the palatines can affect local structures, leading to local symptoms, including disturbance of autonomic nerve pathways to the nose, mouth and face (particularly via the pterygopalatine ganglion), contributing to nasal allergies, rhinitis, dry eye, excessive lacrimation, and other disturbances of glandular secretions of the face.

Of greater significance is their potentially far-reaching restrictive effect on the system as a whole. In any patient whose system feels locked, blocked or stuck, or who is experiencing long-term, perhaps lifelong, symptoms of feeling tight, compressed, held in a vice, perhaps with severe headaches, migraine, or cluster headaches, it is advisable to check the mobility of the palatine area. The palatine bones can also be the source of other severely debilitating conditions including ADHD, hyperactivity and learning difficulties.

Symptoms of palatine restriction will not always be so severe, so it is also relevant to check the palatines in many other situations, and as a matter of course.

The palatines may be adversely affected as a result of all the usual causes – birth patterns, facial injury, and dental work on the upper jaw (particularly the extraction of upper wisdom teeth). If the maxillae are compressed as a result of any of the above causes, then the free mobility of the palatine bones may be compromised. The palatines may be trapped as a result of impaction forces (compression of the maxillae posteriorly towards the sphenoid) or by medial compression of the maxillae (a narrow maxillary arch) – since the palatines are contained between the posterior portions of the maxillary alveolar processes (between the wisdom teeth).

When we work with the palatine bones, we are as always concerned with the overall integration of the system rather than with adjustment of a specific bone, and with the overall effects that this bone or this region may have on the system as a whole rather than merely with local symptoms.

The whole maxillary–palatine–vomer complex operates to some extent as one unit and may become unbalanced or disturbed as one integrated unit. In such cases, treatment through the maxillae may sometimes resolve the overall patterns within the whole complex, including the palatines. Lateral expansion of the maxillae in particular may enable greater freedom of movement of the palatines. However, individual patterns of imbalance, restriction and resistance may occur separately in the palatines and may consequently need to be addressed individually.

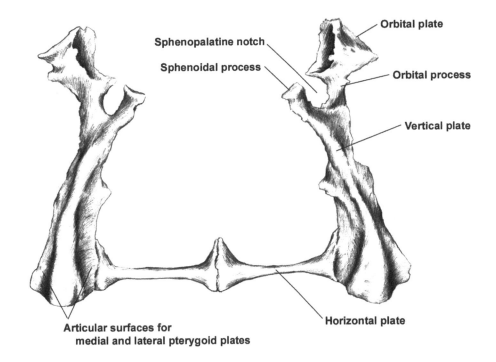

17.1 *The two palatine bones from the posterior part of the nasal cavity. Each palatine bone consists of a small horizontal plate and a larger vertical plate*

Anatomy

Each of the two palatine bones consists of a small *horizontal plate* and a larger *vertical plate*. Together they form the posterior part of the nasal cavity (Figure 17.1).

The horizontal plates form the posterior third of the hard palate, articulating with the maxillae anteriorly at the *maxillary–palatine suture*, and contained between the posterior extensions of the maxillary alveolar processes which house the wisdom teeth (the third molars) (Figure 17.2). The two horizontal plates meet centrally at the *interpalatine suture*, where they also articulate with the vomer which passes down from the sphenoid to rest on to the superior surface of the suture. The cross-shaped junction between the two palatine bones and the two maxillae is the *cruciate suture*.

The vertical components form the lateral walls of the posterior nasal cavity, passing up towards the back of the orbit. At the top of each vertical portion is a tiny *orbital plate* (Figure 17.1) which forms a very small portion of the floor of the orbit (just below the optic canal) (Figure 17.3). This orbital plate (orbital process) also forms a small articulation with the ethmoid via the ethmoidal crest onto the middle nasal concha.

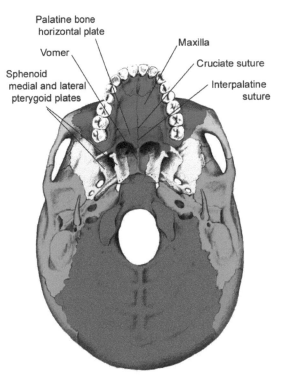

17.2 *The horizontal plates form the posterior third of the hard palate*

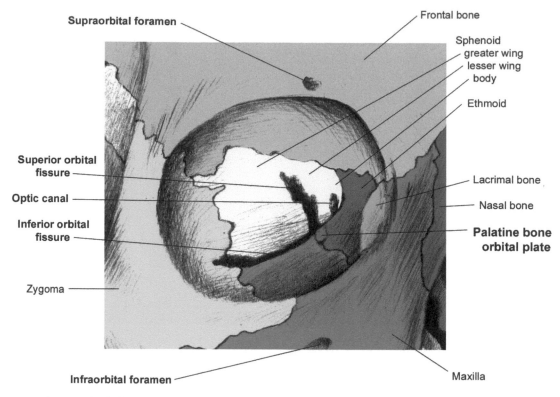

17.3 *The tiny orbital plate forms a very small portion of the floor of the orbit – just below the optic canal*

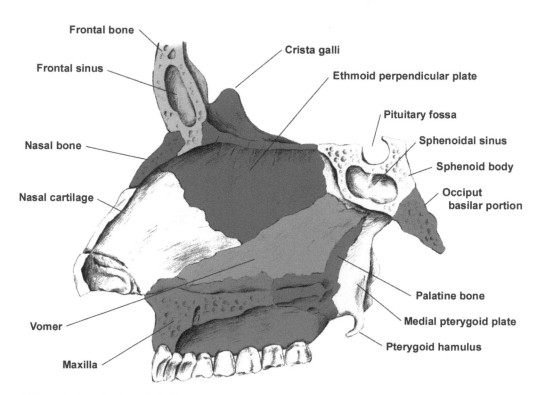

17.4 *Midline sagittal section through the face*

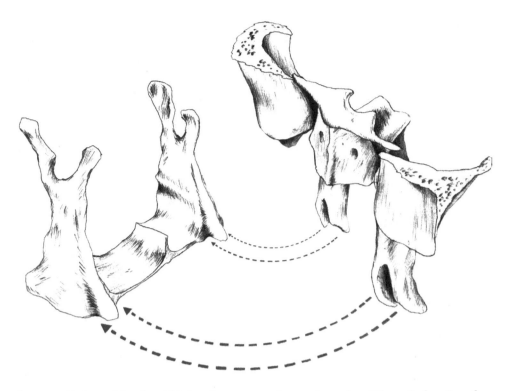

17.5 *The pterygoid plates of the sphenoid fit into the grooves on the posterior surface of the vertical portion of each palatine bone*

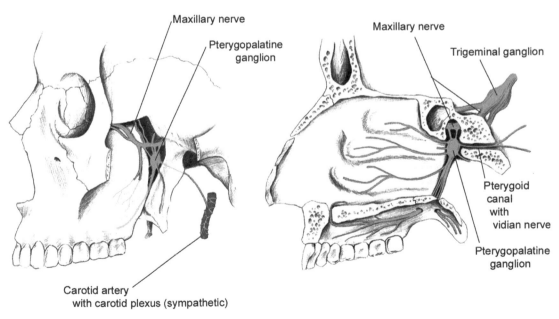

17.6 *The pterygopalatine ganglion is located within the pterygopalatine fossa and can have widespread effects on conditions affecting the face*

The vertical plates articulate posteriorly with the pterygoid processes of the sphenoid. This is a highly significant articulation (Figure 17.4).

On the posterior surface of the vertical portion of each palatine bone are two grooves, into which the medial and lateral pterygoid plates of the sphenoid sit. The surfaces of these grooves are smooth in order to allow the free gliding movement of the pterygoid plates within the grooves as the sphenoid and palatines move in relation to each other (Figure 17.5).

Since the sphenoid and the mouthparts rotate in opposite directions during rhythmic motion (as described earlier in Chapter 16), restriction of the palatine bones, particularly at the sphenopalatine articulation, can block this motion, locking up the whole cranio-sacral system with profound ramifications for the nature and personality of the individual.

Restriction of the palatine bones can also impinge upon the pterygopalatine ganglion (also known as the sphenopalatine ganglion) located in the pterygopalatine fossa. The pterygopalatine fossa is a space beneath the apex of each orbit, bounded by the sphenoid body superiorly, the lateral pterygoid process of the sphenoid posteriorly, the vertical component of the palatine bone medially, and the maxilla anteriorly (Figure 17.6). Through this ganglion pass various nerve fibres, including the sympathetic and parasympathetic nerve supply to the face, with widespread effects on glandular secretions, allergic reactions, hypersensitivities, and other disturbances throughout the face. Details of these repercussions will be explored more fully within the sections on the cranial nerves and autonomic nerve supply to the face.

Cranio-sacral motion

During rhythmic motion, the palatine bones move with the maxillae and the rest of the face, the anterior portion of the face rising with each expansion (flexion) phase and falling with each contraction (extension) phase – in other words rotating in the opposite direction to the sphenoid. The most evident aspect of this within the palatine bones is that they flare slightly away from each other (along with the posterior maxillae) so that the lateral edge of the horizontal portion of each palatine bone lifts slightly as they flare.

Contact

The palatine bones are not palpable externally. It is of course possible to engage with them through indirect contacts, such as the general face contact, taking your attention to the palatine area, visualizing and surveying the internal anatomy, and perhaps being drawn to fulcrums around the palatine area through the cranio-sacral system as a whole.

It can also be useful, particularly where there is specific trauma or restriction to the palatine bones themselves, to engage with the palatines more directly through an intraoral contact.

Since the palatine bones are so far back in the mouth, forming the posterior edge of the hard palate, it is not on the whole comfortable to contact both palatines simultaneously. It is therefore preferable to address each palatine separately.

In order to take up contact on each palatine bone, take up position standing beside the head (as for the maxillae). As with the maxillae, first take up contact with one hand over the spheno-frontal area, settling into engagement with the system as a whole before taking up the second contact.

Once engaged, invite the patient to open their mouth and slide the palmar surface of your index finger along the biting surface of the upper teeth as far as the position of the eighth tooth (the third molar or wisdom tooth) on the side of the mouth closest to you. Then move the pad of your finger medially, off the tooth, onto the surface of the hard palate on the near side (Figures 17.7 and 17.8). Exact positioning is crucial. The horizontal portion of the palatine bone is very small. The suture between the palatines and the maxillae is in line with the junction between the seventh and eighth teeth. If your finger is not far enough back, it will not be on the palatine bone, but on the maxilla. However, if you take your finger too far back, it will be on the soft palate, which is not only uncomfortable for the patient, but may potentially bring up unwanted reactions through the gag reflex.

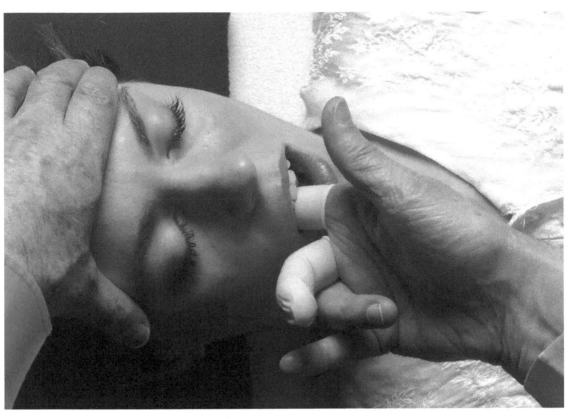

17.7   Intraoral contact for the nearside palatine bone

Having established a comfortable position, invite the patient to close their mouth, letting their lower jaw come to rest lightly onto your finger, and to relax completely.

Feel the increasing sense of engagement with the system through both hands, feeling the interaction between the cranial contact and the mouth contact. Maintain awareness of the response throughout the system. Follow the inherent treatment process on whatever journey it may lead you – through motion to stillness, release and resolution.

Because the palatine is so small, patterns of motion within the bone itself may not be easy to distinguish, but a sense of motion can be gained through overall engagement with the system, and within this wider sense of motion the relative mobility or restriction in the palatine region can become apparent.

The most notable impressions within the palatine bone itself may be its quality – restricted or mobile, agitated or calm – and its mobility, as the palatine flares out and lifts laterally, within the context of the surrounding structures.

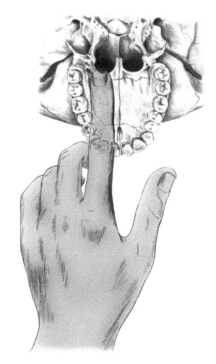

17.8   In order to contact the palatine bone, exact positioning needs to be very precise

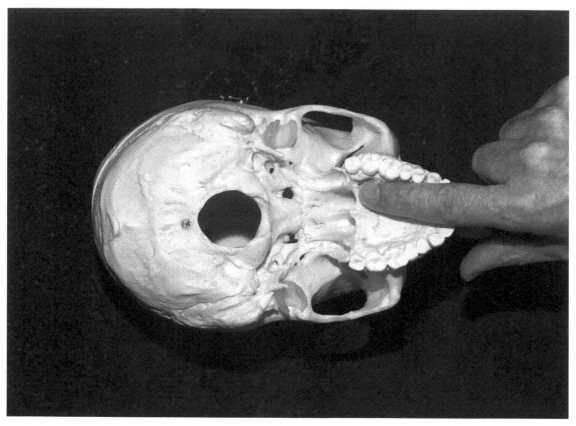

17.9   Contact for the palatine bones

Through this contact you can monitor the responses, both locally and throughout the system.

Feel the overall sense of mobility between the cranial contact and the mouth contact. If there is restriction, evaluate whether it is within the palatine area itself or drawing to a fulcrum elsewhere. If the restriction is within the palatine itself, explore with your attention the anatomical relations of the palatine bone relative to the maxilla anteriorly, or to the other palatine bone medially. In particular, survey the relationship between the palatine bone and the pterygoid plates of the sphenoid, feeling whether there is free gliding motion as the sphenoid arcs forward and down and the palatine (with the rest of the face) rotates in the opposite direction.

Whether the fulcrum is local or elsewhere, you can engage with the whole system through this contact and allow the inherent treatment process to take its course, monitoring responses throughout the system as a whole and following to resolution.

When the process is complete, ask the patient to open their mouth slightly, so that you can slide your finger across the back of the hard palate to the other palatine bone on the far side of the mouth. You can then continue the process as previously, comparing the responses within the two palatine bones and following the inherent treatment process wherever it may take you.

Once the process is complete, you can ask the patient to open their mouth and remove your finger, or move on to assess and address the vomer.

Chapter 18

The Vomer

The vomer is a delightfully delicate bone, with significance well beyond that which its apparent weightlessness might suggest.

It shares many features with the palatines:

- It is another component of the maxillary–palatine–vomer complex, and may therefore be disturbed – or released – in conjunction with the maxillae and palatines.

- It has its own individual characteristics and significance, and may therefore be disturbed separately and need to be addressed individually.

- It also forms a bridge between the maxillae and the sphenoid and therefore exhibits the same possible influences on the system – transmitting forces, acting as a shock absorber, or potentially locking the whole system.

Anatomy

The term *vomer* is Latin for ploughshare, and the vomer is similar in shape to the blade of a plough, angled down as if to plough a furrow in the roof of the palate along the intermaxillary suture (and it sometimes does exactly that).

The vomer is a thin slice of bone, formed by two layers of even thinner bone side by side, flaring at the top to form two small *alae* (wings) with a groove between them (Figure 18.1).

It passes down from the inferior surface of the sphenoid body to the superior surface of the hard palate, forming the lower portion of the nasal septum which divides the two halves of the nasal cavity along the midline (Figure 18.2).

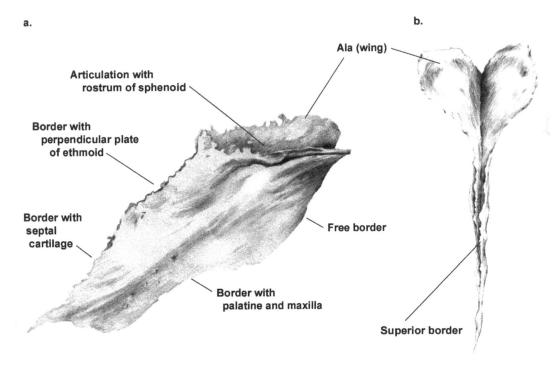

a.

Articulation with rostrum of sphenoid

Border with perpendicular plate of ethmoid

Border with septal cartilage

Free border

Border with palatine and maxilla

b.

Ala (wing)

Superior border

18.1   The vomer
(a) Lateral view
(b) Superior view

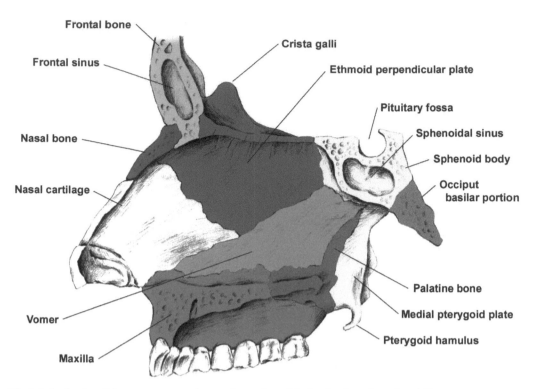

18.2   The inferior border of the vomer rests on the superior surface of the hard palate, along the midline

Along the top of its upper border, the rostrum on the inferior surface of the sphenoid body fits into the groove formed by the two alae, allowing a free gliding motion of the rostrum within the groove of the vomer (Figure 18.3).

At its lower border, the vomer rests on the superior surface of the hard palate, running along the superior surface of the intermaxillary and interpalatine sutures (Figures 18.2 and 18.4).

At the nasal septum, it articulates anteriorly and superiorly with the perpendicular plate of the ethmoid, which forms the superior portion of the septum (Figures 18.2 and 18.4).

Deviation

The vomer is often deviated. This reflects its function as a shock absorber, absorbing forces between the maxillae and the sphenoid, and also indicates the prevalence of such forces. These intraosseous distortions are particularly liable to be imposed during birth or childhood injuries. Ossification of the vomer is not complete until teenage years, leaving the bone soft and malleable and more readily distorted during these early years. This again emphasizes its function as a shock absorber, the delayed ossification specifically allowing for adaptation rather than fracture. Early treatment, releasing the surrounding forces, can

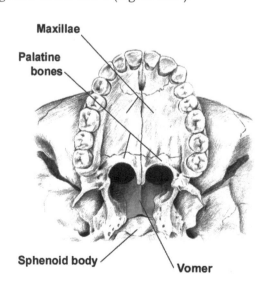

18.3   Superiorly, the vomer articulates with the sphenoid

enable resolution of the deviation. Once ossified, the deviated septum is less likely to rebalance, but the underlying compressions can still be addressed.

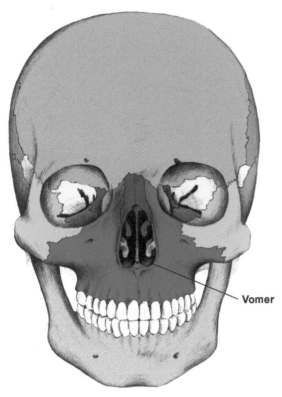

18.4 *The vomer forms the lower portion of the nasal septum, dividing the two halves of the nasal cavity along the midline*

Torus palatinus

Torus palatinus is an abnormal bony protrusion on the roof of the mouth, of variable size and shape.

It is a bony growth, probably brought on by unusual forces exerted on the palate by the surrounding structures. These forces include the pressure of the vomer pushing down on the intermaxillary suture, sometimes 'ploughing' through the suture. The initial forces may arise from birth, and may be aggravated by subsequent forces from injury or teeth grinding. It can often be responsive to cranio-sacral treatment, particularly through release of the underlying forces imposed on the area.

Locking up

Forces through the maxillae may be imposed into the sphenoid via the vomer. This can lead to restriction of the smooth gliding motion between the vomer and the sphenoid where the rostrum fits into the groove between the alae, preventing free expression of cranio-sacral motion between the cranium and the face. As with the palatines, this can also potentially lock up the whole system, with similar consequences and symptoms as described for the palatine bones (Chapter 17). Release of a restricted vomer can sometimes bring substantial relief from severe debilitation.

Cranio-sacral motion

During rhythmic motion, the vomer moves together with the maxillae and the rest of the face, the anterior portion rising up to meet the frontal bone (as it arcs forward and down) during the expansion (flexion) phase of motion, and the axis of rotation passing transversely through the centre of the bone. Since this is opposite to the movement of the sphenoid, the vomer needs to glide freely at the vomer–sphenoid articulation in order to avoid blocking the motion of the whole cranio-sacral system (Figure 18.5).

Contact

The vomer is not directly palpable externally, so contact with the vomer is most effectively enabled intraorally through the hard palate at the midline.

In order to contact the vomer, take up position standing beside the head (as for the maxillae). Take up contact with one hand over the spheno-frontal area, settling into engagement with the system as a whole before taking up the second contact (Figures 18.6 and 18.7).

IV

18

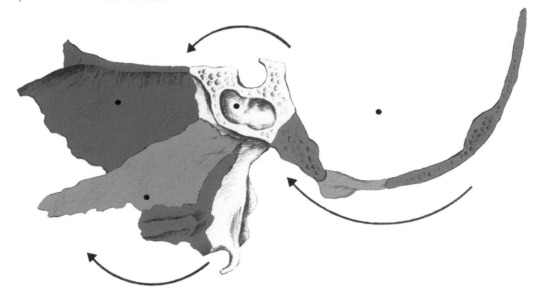

18.5 During rhythmic motion, the vomer moves together with the rest of the face, the anterior portion rising up to meet the frontal bone during the expansion phase

Once engaged, invite the patient to open their mouth and slide the palmar surface of your index finger along the midline of the palate until the pad comes to rest at the cruciate suture – the cross-shaped suture where the maxillae and palatine bones meet (Figure 18.8). There is often a slight concavity or indentation in the palate at this point – although as we have seen, there can also be a ridge or lump in cases of torus palatinus, which may enable more direct contact with the vomer and the compressive forces which have pushed it down through the palate.

Having established a comfortable position, with the patient's upper incisors resting lightly onto your index finger, invite the patient to close their mouth, letting their lower jaw come to rest lightly onto your finger, and to relax completely.

Allow the inherent treatment process to evolve, as with the maxillae and palatines, through motion to stillness, release and resolution.

Engage with the system through both hands, feeling the interaction between the cranial contact and the mouth contact, and maintaining a spacious awareness of responses throughout the system. Rhythmic motion is often particularly clearly palpable through the vomer, as the whole face rises and falls in relation to the frontal region.

Explore the surrounding area with your attention, visualizing the detailed anatomy, giving particular attention to the relationship between the vomer and the sphenoid at the vomer–sphenoid articulation, feeling the free gliding motion of the bones in relation to each other, visualizing the joint and the movement at the joint.

Patterns of asymmetry

The patterns of asymmetry described for the maxillae (Chapter 16) – hyperflexion, hyperextension, torsion, side-bending, side-shift, impaction – are often also apparent through this vomer contact and can be identified and addressed in the same way. They may arise spontaneously or can be surveyed methodically.

Impaction

Impaction is of particular significance in relation to compression of the vomer up into the rostrum of the sphenoid, and it is often relevant to explore this particular pattern, especially where there has been trauma to the face (from birth, injury, or dentistry) or where there is a deviated septum or a torus palatinus (Figure 18.9).

Where indications of compression are present, such as a deviated nasal septum or a torus palatinus, it is of course essential to be addressing the compressions throughout the system, in order to create greater spaciousness and enhanced mobility through the whole area, rather than merely attempting to correct the local distortion.

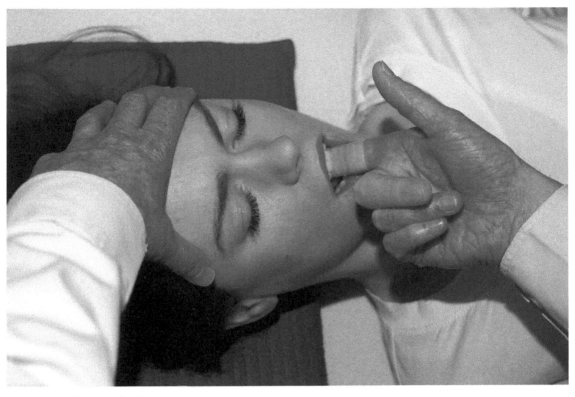

18.6   Intraoral contact for the vomer

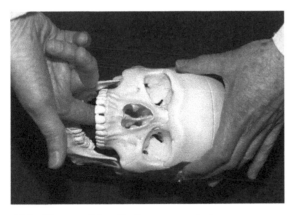

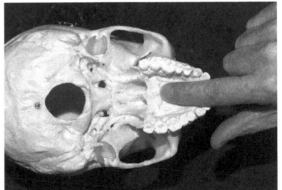

18.7   Finger positions for the vomer contact

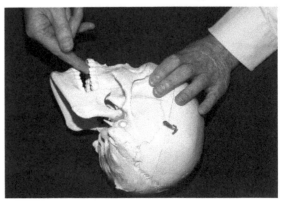

IV

18

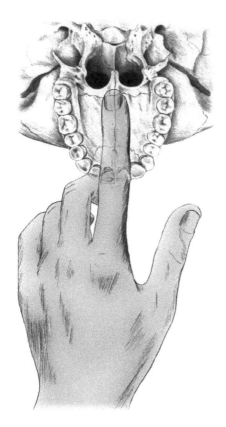

18.8 The pad of the index finger rests lightly on the cruciate suture

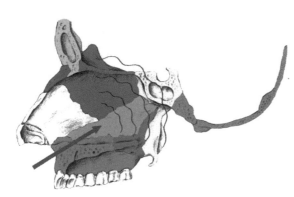

18.9 Impaction of the vomer may lead to compressive forces and shock effects in the face, the sphenoid, and the cranium

Pituitary hypophysis

In this position, with the finger at the cruciate suture, the point of contact is also as close as you can be to the pituitary gland and it provides a useful point of contact from which to take your attention to the pituitary hypophysis, or to introduce an energy drive into the pituitary where appropriate.

Rocking the vomer

Rhythmic motion is often clearly palpable through the vomer contact, providing a clear insight into the quality and nature of the system. Simply engaging with the rhythmic motion with our attention is likely to enhance its expression. The amplitude and strength of the motion can be further emphasized by rocking the vomer – engaging with the rhythmic motion through the vomer and the sphenoid and gently enhancing the motion with each phase. This can be likened to observing a child on a swing, swinging back and forth, and expanding the amplitude of swing by stretching out her legs on the forward movement and curling the legs under on the backward movement.

This can also be helpful where the vomer is severely restricted, or in a system where the rhythmic motion is weak, depleted and lacking vitality, for example in debilitating conditions such as chronic fatigue or post-viral syndrome, or in a newborn baby whose system lacks vitality, or simply as a means of energizing the cranio-sacral system as a whole.

Completion

As always, the emphasis is on overall integration. Once the therapeutic process at the vomer has come to resolution, ensure that the system comes into balance, ease, and neutrality, and ensure that the system as a whole has integrated any local changes, bringing the overall treatment process to a well-integrated and settled conclusion.

Chapter 19

Individual Teeth

Engaging with an individual tooth can be relevant where there is persistent pain, or in engaging with past trauma to the tooth, and can also be useful for diagnosing the source of a disturbance.

A common site of injury might be an upper incisor, or both upper incisors, following a fall. This could be a recent injury, or could be addressing the long-standing repercussions of trauma to the tooth and face from a childhood fall many years ago – potentially imposing force vectors deeply embedded into the tissues together with consequent facial symptoms. Contacting the affected tooth may also engage with the emotional patterns and effects on personality that have been ingrained in the system as a result of that childhood injury.

It can also be useful where there is persistent sensitivity or inflammation in an individual tooth which is not responding to dentistry, or for a tooth which remains painful following dental treatment – helping to integrate the surrounding tissues and dissipate the trauma of the dentistry, or to resolve the effects of trauma held in a particular tooth as a result of traumatic dentistry in the past. It is equally effective to take up contact on a crown, and this might be particularly relevant where there is an implant, helping the body to adapt to the new situation. Ideally, it is preferable to treat every tooth, crown or implant cranio-sacrally following dental treatment, in order to dissipate any shock in the system.

Hannah had been to the dentist three weeks earlier for some relatively straightforward dental treatment. But ever since, her tooth had been intensely painful, the pain increasingly spreading through her jaw and face.

She had been back to the dentist, but he said that there was nothing wrong. She was finding life unbearable, unable to think straight or concentrate due to the intense pain. As she was unable to get an appointment for a full cranio-sacral session, we were only able to have a brief emergency treatment. Within twenty minutes of cranio-sacral engagement with the affected tooth, jaw and cranium, her pain had gone, and she didn't need any further treatment.

This is not of course a magic solution to every tooth pain. Appropriate diagnosis is necessary, and where there are cavities, exposed nerves, abscesses, or NICOs (cavitations), dentistry is likely to be needed.

Tooth abscesses sometimes respond to cranial treatment and, as mentioned previously, can also respond well to homeopathy. Homeopathy is most effectively carried out within the context of an overall constitutional assessment, but tooth abscesses often respond well to the remedy Hepar Sulphuris 30. However, abscesses need to be monitored carefully and referred for dentistry where necessary.

In any persistent tooth pain, once the need for dentistry has been eliminated, the first priority is to integrate the whole jaw, face and cranio-sacral system, rather than merely treating the individual tooth locally, and to address any underlying causes anywhere in the body which might be causing disturbance. It is always essential to bear in mind that even something as specific as an individual tooth pain could be coming from the hip, the foot, or anywhere else in the body (as demonstrated so graphically in Chapter 8 by Dr Wojciech Tarnowski).

Contacts

Upper teeth

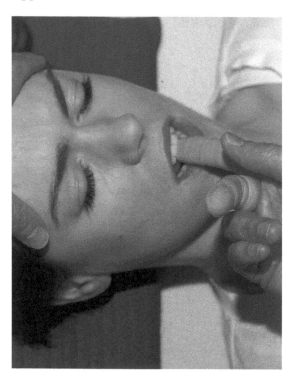

19.1 *Contact for an individual tooth in the upper jaw*

In order to contact an individual tooth, take up position as for the maxillae, palatines and vomer, with one hand over the spheno-frontal area to monitor the system as a whole. Take up contact on the individual tooth as appropriate, with the pad of your index finger resting lightly on the biting surface of the tooth (Figures 19.1–19.3). In cases of acute pain, the contact may need to be extremely light or even off the body. Sometimes it can be more appropriate to contact the gum at the base of the tooth.

Engage with the tooth, observe any responses, allow the evolution of the inherent treatment process. Survey with your attention through the tooth itself, the periodontal membrane, the nerve root, the surrounding gum and the jaw bone. Allow any unwinding that arises. Identify the effects of any forces exerted through the tooth, compressing into the tooth socket or in any other direction, monitoring the responses throughout the system through your spheno-frontal contact and your wide perspective.

It can be useful to engage with several different teeth in turn, to see whether the affected tooth feels different from the other teeth.

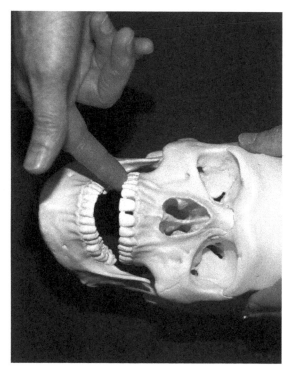

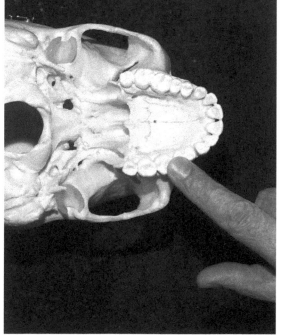

19.2 *Finger positions for individual teeth in the upper jaw*

It may also be helpful to introduce an energy drive into the tooth, perhaps targeted specifically towards a focal point of restriction or inflammation that has been identified.

Lower teeth

For a lower tooth, it may be preferable to cradle the mandible with one hand and take up contact on the individual tooth with the index finger of the other hand, in order to integrate the tooth and any associated trauma within the mandible (Figure 19.4). Pain in a lower tooth is less likely to be related to whole-body patterns since the mandible is less firmly attached to the cranium.

John Upledger reports the following experiences:[1]

> My clinical observations suggest that energy drives through a tooth, performed regularly, may vitalize the pulp of the tooth and obviate the need for extraction or root canal work.

> Gentle mobilization of the teeth in their sockets will enhance their ability to adapt to occlusal changes.

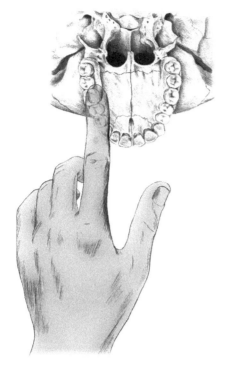

19.3 The pad of the index finger can contact the affected tooth

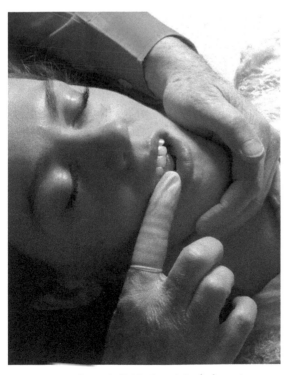

19.4 Contact for an individual tooth in the lower jaw

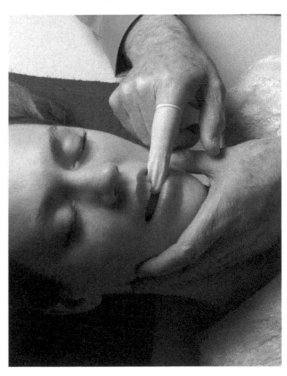

Diagnosis

Local quality

Engaging with an individual tooth can also be useful from a diagnostic perspective, feeling each tooth in turn, identifying any differences between them and any indications of trauma or disease. This may help to identify compressions and injuries, perhaps discovering the hidden source of some other health issue through an asymptomatic tooth, and may also identify abscesses and cavitations – recognizing the nature of the disease through the qualities expressed through the contact.

Be alert to the possibility of abscesses and NICOs (cavitations)

Particularly in patients with persistent and recurrent long-term symptoms of headache, neck pain and debilitation which are not responding consistently to treatment, it is essential to remain alert to the possibility of abscesses and NICOs (cavitations) as the possible source, and to ensure that these possibilities are fully investigated, even in patients who have already undergone thorough dental assessments, since such things can often be missed.

Laura suffered from frequent persistent headaches, neck pain, upper back pain and exhaustion, and spent much of her time feeling very unwell. She had seen many different therapists without success. She experienced slight discomfort in her jaw, but this was not a significant symptom compared with her other discomforts. She had been receiving regular dental treatment as a matter of course and had mentioned her symptoms to the dentist, but he had not discovered any explanation for her situation.

There were various possible factors contributing to Laura's symptoms. She was under a great deal of stress and was not managing it well. There was a great deal of tension in her head, neck and upper back.

She always felt much better after her cranio-sacral sessions, but her symptoms returned each time within a few days. There was clearly some underlying factor that was not being identified. In view of the recurrent symptoms and lack of lasting relief, a more thorough exploration was required. Individual assessment of each tooth revealed a specific disturbance in her first upper molar on the left – something that had not been immediately apparent under the many layers of tension throughout her system. I suggested that she ask her dentist for a more thorough investigation of the tooth, or if necessary visit a different dentist. This very quickly revealed an abscess, and once the abscess had been addressed, her many symptoms disappeared immediately and she did not need any further treatment.

Bear in mind that tooth pain may also be due to something much simpler, such as a high filling that needs to be adjusted by a dentist.

Distant sources

You can also engage with an individual tooth and ask the system where the disturbance is originating from – whether in the tooth itself, or anywhere else in the body, thereby identifying the primary source of an ascending pattern.

Part V

The Cranial Nerves

Chapter 20

Cranial Nerves – Introduction

Without our cranial nerves, we would not be able to see, hear, smell, chew, swallow, smile or frown. Our faces would be impassive and immobile. Our digestive system would be severely compromised, and our heart and lungs would not function. Cranial nerves are vital to day-to-day survival and play a major part in our overall health.

They are also involved in many specific conditions and disturbances affecting the face – including visual disturbances, squints, dry eye and photosensitivity, ear conditions such as tinnitus, deafness and vertigo, toothache, difficulties in swallowing, loss of smell, mucus congestion, sinusitis, ear infections, glandular imbalances, skin conditions, facial paralysis, torticollis – and they may be intricately involved in speech, language and learning difficulties. They can also be the bearers of severe pain.

Cranial nerves may be disturbed by physical injury to the face and head, compression or trauma during the birth process, infection, inflammation, bony restrictions, membranous tension and sclerosis, the after-effects of meningitis, tumours, damage during surgery, high blood pressure and other abnormal fluid pressures – arterial, venous, cerebrospinal, lymphatic – and many other sources of imbalance and restriction throughout the body.

Understanding the cranial nerves is essential for an overall understanding of the way the body functions as an integrated unit. It also enables identification and appropriate treatment of the many conditions involving these nerves. A significant element in the cranio-sacral treatment of cranial nerve dysfunction involves tracing their pathways in detail with our therapeutic attention. Detailed knowledge of the nerve pathways provides the informed awareness which enables the practitioner to do this, identifying areas of disturbance or restriction that may be contributing to dysfunction. For example in trigeminal neuralgia, tracing the pathway of the nerve with one's attention may identify the site of impingement of the nerve and enable the release of any restriction and the consequent relief of pain. In order to enable this, we need to have a clear visual impression of those pathways.

The twelve cranial nerves

There are twelve cranial nerves. Although generally referred to in the singular, each cranial nerve is a paired bilateral structure. They are numbered I–XII, with Roman numerals to distinguish them from spinal nerves. Each of them also has a name which partially describes its principal function or its nature. Many of the cranial nerves serve many different functions, but their principal functions can be summarized as follows:

Cr I	Olfactory	Smell
Cr II	Optic	Vision
Cr III	Oculo-motor	Eye movement
Cr IV	Trochlear	Eye movement
Cr V	Trigeminal	Sensation from the face
Cr VI	Abducent	Eye movement – abducts the eye
Cr VII	Facial	Motor to the muscles of the face
Cr VIII	Vestibulo-cochlear (formerly known as Auditory)	Hearing and balance
Cr IX	Glosso-pharyngeal	Sensory from the throat and tongue
Cr X	Vagus	Parasympathetic and sensory to most of the viscera
Cr XI	Accessory (Spinal Accessory)	Motor to sterno-cleido-mastoid and trapezius muscles
Cr XII	Hypoglossal	Tongue movement

Details of the many other functions of these nerves will be included in the more detailed description of each individual nerve that follows.

Numbering

Cranial nerves are numbered according to the location of their emergence from the brain and brainstem (Figure 20.1):

Cranial nerves I and II	emerge from the forebrain
Cranial nerves III and IV	emerge from the midbrain
Cranial nerves V, VI, VII, and VIII	emerge from the pons
Cranial nerves IX, X, XI, and XII	emerge from the medulla

Sensory, motor, sympathetic, parasympathetic

Cranial nerves (like nerves throughout the body) may carry sensory fibres, motor fibres, autonomic fibres (sympathetic or parasympathetic) or combinations of any or all of these.

Sensory fibres receive sensations:

- pain, temperature, touch, proprioception
- or the special senses of smell, vision, hearing, and taste.

Motor fibres induce movement:

- of the muscles of facial expression, the eyes, the tongue, the throat for swallowing and speaking, the neck.

Parasympathetic fibres induce autonomic responses:

- glandular secretions – tears, mucus, saliva, digestive juices
- pupil constriction, lens accommodation

Cranial nerves:

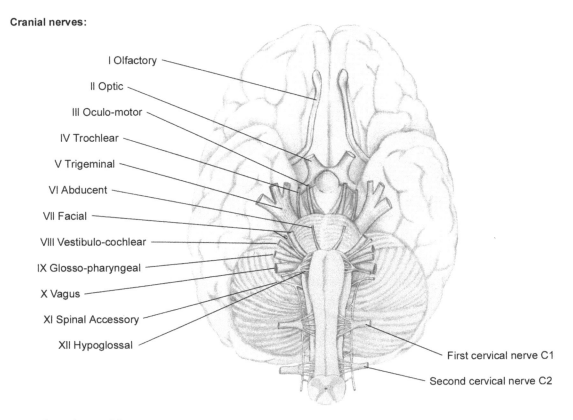

I Olfactory
II Optic
III Oculo-motor
IV Trochlear
V Trigeminal
VI Abducent
VII Facial
VIII Vestibulo-cochlear
IX Glosso-pharyngeal
X Vagus
XI Spinal Accessory
XII Hypoglossal

First cervical nerve C1
Second cervical nerve C2

20.1 The twelve cranial nerves

- various other autonomic responses maintaining the function of the heart, lungs and digestive system.

Sympathetic fibres carry out a wide range of functions, including:

- pupil dilation
- vasoconstriction
- sphincter constriction
- and also influence glandular secretions.

Cranial nerves may be:

sensory	carrying sensory fibres only
motor	carrying motor fibres only
sensory and motor	carrying a mixture of sensory and motor fibres
sensory, motor and parasympathetic	carrying a mixture of sensory, motor and parasympathetic fibres

In addition, most cranial nerves will be joined by sympathetic fibres, which originate in the upper thoracic spine (T1 and T2), pass up the neck, synapse at the superior cervical sympathetic ganglion, enter the cranium through the carotid canal, and join with the cranial nerves and their many branches, travelling along the same pathways as the cranial nerves to their various destinations. Sympathetic nerve supply is necessary in all parts of the body.

- Cranial nerves I, II and VIII are purely sensory.
- Cranial nerves IV, VI, XI and XII are purely motor.
- The other cranial nerves carry combinations of fibres.
- Four of the cranial nerves carry parasympathetic fibres – cranial nerves III, VII, IX, X.

Ganglia

There are two types of ganglia in the head:

- sensory ganglia
- parasympathetic ganglia.

Sensory ganglia

- These are the sites of synapse for sensory fibres bringing sensation towards the central nervous system.
- They are usually located just outside the central nervous system.
- They are equivalent to the dorsal root ganglia in the spine.
- They do not involve motor fibres (which synapse inside the central nervous system in their respective nuclei) so there are no sensory ganglia for the cranial nerves which are purely motor (IV, VI, XI, XII).
- All the true sensory nerves have ganglia.

(Illustrations for these ganglia are included with the detailed description of each nerve.)

Location of sensory ganglia

- The superior and inferior ganglia of the vagus nerve are located within and immediately below the jugular foramen.
- The superior and inferior ganglia of the glosso-pharyngeal nerve are also located within the jugular foramen.
- The large trigeminal ganglion is located in the cavum trigeminale, on the apex of the petrous portion of the temporal bone.
- The vestibular ganglion is located just inside the internal auditory meatus.
- The cochlear ganglion is located within the cochlea.
- The geniculate ganglion, receiving sensory branches of the facial nerve, is located at the geniculum of the facial canal within the temporal bone.

Variations

- Some of these sensory ganglia may have other fibres (motor and parasympathetic) passing through them without synapse, merely for convenience of distribution.
- The olfactory and optic nerves, although sensory, do not have ganglia or synapses outside the central nervous system, which is why they are generally considered not to be true cranial nerves.

Parasympathetic ganglia

- These are sites of synapse for parasympathetic fibres on their way to the glands of the face and the smooth muscle of the eyes.
- They are located outside the central nervous system, usually some distance away (as terminal ganglia) close to their destination.
- There are four pairs of parasympathetic ganglia relating to the face:
  - ciliary ganglia
  - otic ganglia
  - pterygopalatine ganglia
  - submandibular ganglia (also known as submaxillary ganglia).
- These ganglia also contain other fibres which are passing through merely for convenience of distribution. These other fibres do not synapse within the ganglia. They include sympathetic fibres, and sensory fibres from various cranial nerves.

(The parasympathetic ganglia will be described in greater detail in Chapter 32 on the autonomic nerve supply to the face.)

Nuclei

A nucleus is the location for cell bodies of motor nerve fibres. Nuclei are always located within the central nervous system. The nuclei of cranial nerves are located within the brain and brainstem (midbrain, pons or medulla). Motor nerve fibres emerge from the nucleus as nerve roots and travel to their destination along their individual pathway. There are somatic motor nuclei and also parasympathetic motor nuclei.

Nerves and tracts

- A nerve is a nerve pathway outside the central nervous system.
- A tract is a nerve pathway within the central nervous system.

However, there are occasional misnomers, such as the optic nerve which is inside the central nervous system.

Nomenclature

Many small branches from the main nerves have their own names. These named nerves may contain combinations of fibres from several different cranial nerves, may contain sympathetic and/or parasympathetic fibres, may change their name in different sections of their pathways, may give off branches with different names, and may have different names in different texts.

For example:

- The short ciliary nerves are primarily carrying parasympathetic fibres to the eyeball, but also contain sympathetic fibres, and some sensory branches of the trigeminal nerve.
- The parasympathetic division of the facial nerve is initially named the nervus intermedius; it then becomes the chorda tympani (travelling with sensory fibres of the facial nerve) and finally travels as part of the lingual nerve (a sensory branch of the trigeminal nerve).

Interconnectedness

The cranial nerves are generally presented as twelve distinct items, each with their respective pathway and functions. As an initial introduction, this basic framework provides a useful foundation through which to gain an understanding of each nerve. In reality, however, the picture is much more complex.

Fibres from different nerves join together, cross over and intermingle for convenience of distribution. Consequently, many named nerves are combinations of branches from several nerves. For example, the trigeminal nerve (Cr V) at various points along its pathway combines with fibres from Cr III, IV, VI, VII, IX, X and XI, as well as with parasympathetic and sympathetic fibres.

Many of the cranial nerves also make extensive interconnections, both with each other and with associated areas of the brain, including the thalamus, the cerebellum, the limbic system, and the central nervous system as a whole, in order to coordinate function and enable appropriate reflexes and responses to circumstances.

Our eyes, ears and other senses are intricately connected to our muscular and coordinating systems through reflex associations which enable us to respond rapidly and appropriately to stimuli, dodging flying missiles and flying fists, or reacting to loud noises.

Complex interactions between eyes, ears, balance, equilibrium and muscle function enable us to carry out activities from the simplest action of picking up a cup of tea to complex coordinated tasks. This also includes emotional responses to sensations through connections with the limbic system, and through memory associations, and to the reticular alarm system, activating appropriate (or sometimes inappropriate) reactions and responses to circumstances. Many of these interconnections relate to basic survival strategies such as are found in more phylogenetically primitive animals. Others are more highly developed sophisticated interactions relating to the cerebral cortex and complex emotional and psychological functions.

For example:

- The olfactory nerve (Cr I) receives sensations of smell, transmits these messages to the vagus nerve (Cr X), stimulating responses in the digestive system, and also stimulates responses in the limbic system, stimulating emotional responses to fragrances and odours.

- The glosso-pharyngeal, vagus and accessory nerves (Cr IX, X and XI), although usually presented as three separate nerves, are in fact so closely interrelated as to be potentially considered as one nerve complex, with fibres intermingling, crossing over, travelling to the same destinations and serving similar functions.

- The vagus nerve (Cr X) is a large and far-reaching nerve with many functions. Recent developments on polyvagal theory have postulated different levels of function within the vagus nerve, with significant implications for health and personality.

Nerve fibres unrelated in their function may travel together and be described as one nerve; for example, the parasympathetic fibres which contract the pupil and adjust the lens travel almost their whole journey with the third cranial nerve and are generally described in association with Cr III, although they have a separate nucleus, separate fibres and separate functions.

The whole picture could be compared to an intricate railway system, in which trains predominantly travel along main lines, but may diverge along branch lines, connect with other main lines, where they may encounter local trains from other branch lines, cross from one line to another, or rejoin other main lines. The trains may also reach railway stations or junctions (like the ganglia of the face) where they can either pass straight through without stopping, or transfer their cargo of goods or passengers onto a different train.

In order to understand this complexity, it is helpful to start with the usual standard framework of the twelve cranial nerves in order to establish an understanding of the main pathways and functions.

Appreciating the complexity of the cranial nerves can help us to understand the intricacies of such things as speech and language difficulties which may involve many different cranial nerves and complex interactions between them.

It also emphasizes the need for total integration of the system and the value of cranio-sacral integration, allowing the inherent treatment process to do whatever is necessary to resolve the multitude of complex disturbances – bony restrictions, compression of foramina, membranous tensions, impingement of nerves, and many other sources – evolving around the fulcrum of our therapeutic presence and our informed awareness.

Chapter 21

Foramina of the Face and Cranium

Foramen (singular) is Latin for a hole; *foramina* (plural) are holes.

Most of the structures of the face receive their nerve supply via cranial nerves.

Cranial nerves have their nuclei in the brain and brainstem. They pass in and out of the cranium through various foramina in the skull – which may be potential sites of compression or constriction.

In order to understand the cranial nerves, it is helpful to be familiar with the foramina through which they pass. In this chapter, the emphasis is on the foramina themselves, with a brief mention of the structures passing through them. Further detail of the cranial nerves themselves will be provided in the subsequent sections covering each cranial nerve.

Some of the foramina also carry arteries and veins along with cranial nerves.

Foramina at the base of the skull (starting at the anterior cranium) (Figures 21.1, 21.2, and 21.3)

(All these foramina are *bilateral* paired structures, apart from the cribriform plate and the foramen magnum.)

Foramina of the anterior cranium

The **cribriform plate** is the roof of the ethmoid bone, permeated with a pepper-pot array of tiny holes, through which the fibres of the *olfactory nerve* (Cr I) pass up from the nasal cavity. (*Cribriform* is Latin for 'in the form of a sieve'; *ethmoid* is Greek for 'sieve-shaped'.)

The **optic canal** is located between the body of the sphenoid and the lesser wing of the sphenoid on each side, and carries the *optic nerve* (Cr II) travelling from the retina of the eye to the brain, together with the *ophthalmic artery* carrying arterial blood supply to the orbit.

Fissures in the back of the orbit

There are two fissures (narrow elongated slits) in the back of the orbit: the *superior orbital fissure* and the *inferior orbital fissure* (Figure 21.2).

The **superior orbital fissure** is a fissure in the back of the upper orbit, between the sphenoid lesser wing (above) and sphenoid greater wing (below), providing passageway into the orbit for four cranial nerves and the ophthalmic vein. The cranial nerves are:

- the *oculo-motor nerve* (Cr III)
- the *trochlear nerve* (Cr IV)
- the *abducent nerve* (Cr VI),

enabling movement of the eyeball, and

- the *ophthalmic branch of the trigeminal nerve* (Cr V),

receiving sensation from various parts of the orbit and the forehead. The *ophthalmic vein* carries venous drainage from the orbit, draining into the cavernous sinus.

The sphenoid is in three separate portions at birth. The superior orbital fissure and optic canal may therefore be susceptible to distortion due to compressive forces imposed during birth trauma.

The **inferior orbital fissure** is a similar fissure in the lower part of the back of the orbit, between the sphenoid greater wing (above) and the maxilla (below), enabling the entry of the *maxillary branch of the trigeminal nerve* (Cr V) into the floor of the orbit.

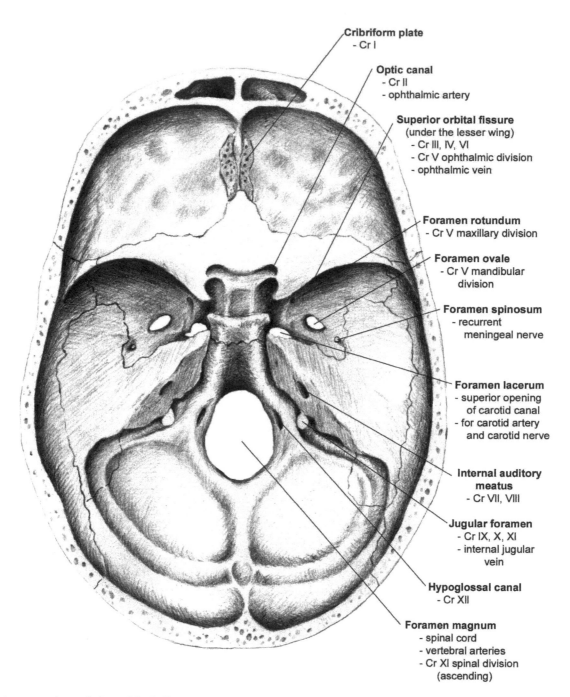

Cribriform plate
- Cr I

Optic canal
- Cr II
- ophthalmic artery

Superior orbital fissure
(under the lesser wing)
- Cr III, IV, VI
- Cr V ophthalmic division
- ophthalmic vein

Foramen rotundum
- Cr V maxillary division

Foramen ovale
- Cr V mandibular
  division

Foramen spinosum
- recurrent
  meningeal nerve

Foramen lacerum
- superior opening
  of carotid canal
- for carotid artery
  and carotid nerve

**Internal auditory
meatus**
- Cr VII, VIII

Jugular foramen
- Cr IX, X, XI
- internal jugular
  vein

Hypoglossal canal
- Cr XII

Foramen magnum
- spinal cord
- vertebral arteries
- Cr XI spinal division
  (ascending)

21.1   Foramina at the base of the skull – superior view

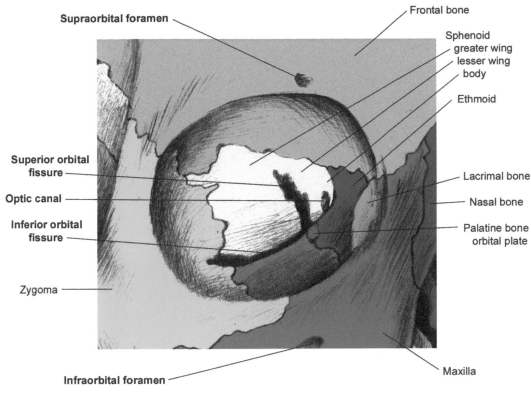

Supraorbital foramen

Frontal bone

Sphenoid
greater wing
lesser wing
body

Ethmoid

Superior orbital fissure

Optic canal

Inferior orbital fissure

Lacrimal bone

Nasal bone

Palatine bone
orbital plate

Zygoma

Infraorbital foramen

Maxilla

21.2   Foramina of the orbit

Foramina within the greater wing of the sphenoid

There are three foramina within the greater wing of the sphenoid: the *foramen rotundum*, the *foramen ovale* and the *foramen spinosum* (Figure 21.1).

The **foramen rotundum** is a small round hole within the greater wing of the sphenoid, through which the *maxillary branch of the trigeminal nerve* (Cr V) exits from the cranium (before entering the orbit through the inferior orbital fissure as described above).

The **foramen ovale** is a larger oval-shaped hole in the greater wing of the sphenoid (posterior to the foramen rotundum) through which the *mandibular branch of the trigeminal nerve* (Cr V) exits from the cranium, together with the *motor branch of the trigeminal nerve* (Cr V).

The **foramen spinosum** is a small hole in the greater wing of the sphenoid (posterior to the foramen ovale) through which the *middle meningeal artery* passes up into the cranium to provide arterial supply to the meninges, together with the *recurrent meningeal branch of the trigeminal nerve* – a small branch of the mandibular branch of the trigeminal nerve, which branches off from the

main mandibular branch shortly after it exits from the cranium (as described above) and immediately returns into the cranium to receive sensory input from the meninges.

Foramina within the temporal bone

There are two foramina within the temporal bone: the *internal auditory meatus* (Figure 21.1) and the *stylomastoid foramen* (Figure 21.3).

The **internal auditory meatus** is located within the medial wall of the petrous portion of the temporal bone, providing entry into and exit from the structures contained within the interior of the temporal bone.

The *vestibulo-cochlear nerve* (Cr VIII) passes from the inner ear (within the temporal bone) to the brainstem through this foramen.

The *facial nerve* (Cr VII), on its way to the face, passes from the brainstem into the temporal bone through the internal auditory meatus and travels along its own facial canal within the temporal bone (eventually exiting from the temporal bone at the stylomastoid foramen, before turning forward towards the face).

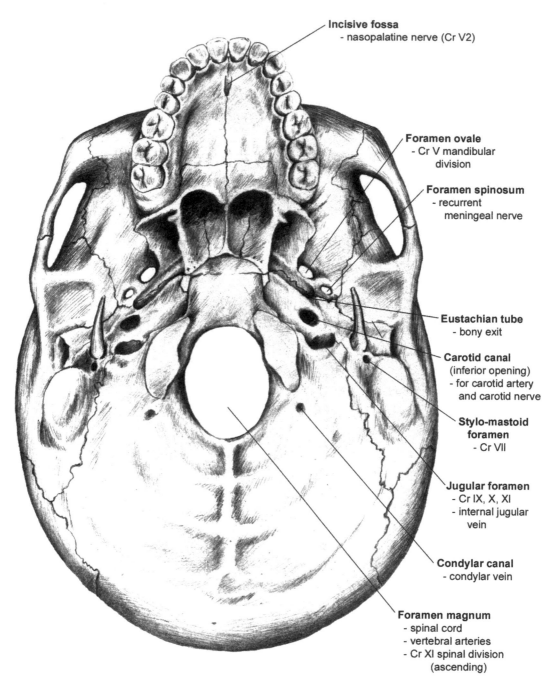

Incisive fossa
- nasopalatine nerve (Cr V2)

Foramen ovale
- Cr V mandibular
  division

Foramen spinosum
- recurrent
  meningeal nerve

Eustachian tube
- bony exit

Carotid canal
(inferior opening)
- for carotid artery
  and carotid nerve

**Stylo-mastoid
foramen**
- Cr VII

Jugular foramen
- Cr IX, X, XI
- internal jugular
  vein

Condylar canal
- condylar vein

Foramen magnum
- spinal cord
- vertebral arteries
- Cr XI spinal division
  (ascending)

21.3   Foramina at the base of the skull – inferior view

The **stylomastoid foramen** is a tiny foramen which, as its name suggests, is located between the styloid process (anteriorly) and the mastoid process (posteriorly) on the inferior surface of the temporal bone. The *main motor branch of the facial nerve* (Cr VII), having passed through the temporal bone, exits here before turning anteriorly to travel to the face (Figure 21.3).

Foramina between two bones

The **jugular foramen** on each side is located *between* two bones rather than within a bone (Figures 21.1 and 21.3). It is therefore particularly vulnerable and is commonly compressed and distorted, particularly through birth trauma, but also potentially through head injuries in early childhood and by muscular tensions at all ages. This is particularly relevant because it carries several highly significant structures.

It is located between the occiput and the mastoid portion of the temporal bone, in the floor of the posterior cranial fossa, where the occipitomastoid suture opens out to form the jugular foramen (like a river opening out into a lake). Through this foramen are passing:

- the *internal jugular vein*
- the *glosso-pharyngeal nerve* (Cr IX)
- the *vagus nerve* (Cr X)
- the *spinal accessory nerve* (Cr XI).

The *vagus nerve* is providing parasympathetic supply to most of the viscera of the body – heart, lungs and digestive system – so compression of the vagus nerve within this foramen is often implicated in visceral conditions – including asthma, colic and many other cardiac, digestive and respiratory conditions.

The *internal jugular vein* carries almost all of the venous drainage from within the cranium. The potential for restriction of venous drainage through compression of the internal jugular vein at this foramen is also significant, contributing to back pressure and stagnation of venous blood within the venous sinuses of the cranium which provide the majority of the venous drainage from the brain, with consequent impairment of fresh oxygenated arterial blood supply to the brain. This may result in a plethora of symptoms including poor memory, poor concentration, vagueness, congestion, headaches, migraine,

mental confusion and other mental dysfunctions, most notably in the elderly. If such compression is present from birth or early childhood (whether due to birth trauma or to an early injury to the head) then the venous congestion in the cranium may affect brain development.

The other significant foramen located between two bones is the **foramen lacerum,** which is covered below.

Foramina within the occiput

The **hypoglossal canal** is located within the condylar portion of the occipital bone and is not readily visible from above, as it is within the medial wall of the foramen magnum (Figure 21.1). It passes out anterior to the occipital condyle on each side, enabling passage of the *hypoglossal nerve* (Cr XII) from the brainstem to the tongue.

The **foramen magnum** (Latin for large hole) is the large hole at the base of the skull, formed within the occipital bone, through which the spinal cord passes up to be continuous with the brainstem and brain. This foramen carries:

- the *spinal cord*
- the spinal roots of the *spinal accessory nerve* (Cr XI)
- the *vertebral arteries.*

The occiput is in four separate portions at birth, surrounding the foramen magnum (fully fusing at around the age of six years). The foramen magnum is therefore particularly susceptible to distortion during severe birth trauma (and due to head injuries during the first six years of life), potentially impinging on the medulla and spinal cord.

Vertebral arteries

The two vertebral arteries not only provide the major arterial supply to the brain (together with the two carotid arteries), but also follow a tortuous and vulnerable S-shaped pathway (Figure 21.4). Passing up through the vertebral foramina within the cervical vertebrae, they turn medially at a right angle between the atlas (first cervical vertebra) and the occiput. They then turn through another right angle to pass up through the foramen magnum, before coming together to form the basilar artery. The basilar artery joins the

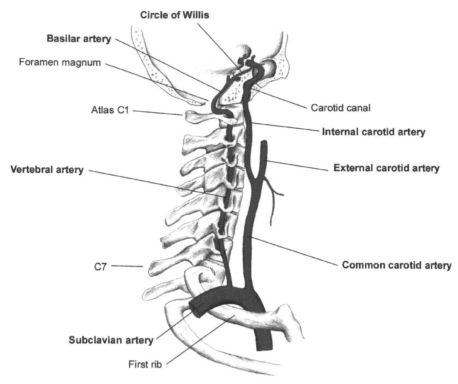

21.4   The carotid and vertebral arteries

Circle of Willis at the base of the brain, giving off branches to various regions of the cerebrum and cerebellum. The vertebral arteries are therefore particularly susceptible to compression between the occiput and atlas (leading to vertebro-basilar insufficiency), particularly in old age when postural collapse may contribute to compression, but also as a result of compressive head injuries (including birth trauma), neck injuries, and tension in the cervical and suboccipital regions.

Further foramina

There are various other foramina distributed through the cranium, which do not carry cranial nerves, but which are worthy of note for other reasons.

The **external auditory meatus** is the ear hole and will be covered in the chapter on the ear.

The exit for the Eustachian tube

The **Eustachian tube** (also known as the auditory tube or salpingo-tympanic tube) provides drainage from the middle ear into the nasopharynx. It is of vital significance in recurrent middle ear infections, glue ear and other ear conditions (as we will see in Chapter 35 on the ears). It passes as a bony canal within the temporal bone, continuing anteromedially as a cartilage-covered tube along the spheno-temporal suture, before emptying into the back of the nasal cavity. Its tiny opening (where the bony canal opens into the cartilaginous tube) can be seen on the inferior surface of the cranial base, along the spheno-temporal suture, medial to the temporo-mandibular joint, opening medially towards the nasal cavity. This opening is located between the carotid canal (posteriorly) and foramen ovale (anteriorly), emerging almost horizontally towards the nasopharynx (Figure 21.1).

Foramen lacerum and carotid canal

The **foramen lacerum** is another foramen which is located *between* two bones, rather than within a bone, leaving it potentially more vulnerable. It is located between the body of the sphenoid and the petrous portion of the temporal bone (Figure 21.1). It is the superior opening of the carotid canal, through which the *internal carotid artery* enters the cranium to provide a major part of the arterial blood supply to the brain. Also passing through this canal is the *carotid nerve*, which is the continuation of the sympathetic pathway from the upper thoracic spine via the neck through the carotid canal to the head.

The foramen lacerum and the carotid canal are significant and are more complex than they first appear. In a dry cranium, the foramen lacerum appears to pass straight down through the temporal bone (Figure 21.1). In a living skull, however, the foramen lacerum is not a true foramen, since its lower portion is filled with cartilage, so that nothing can pass through (Figure 21.6).

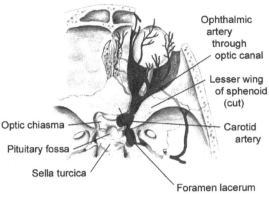

21.7 The internal carotid artery emerges from the carotid canal superiorly above the foramen lacerum, passing through the cavernous sinus on each side of the sella turcica

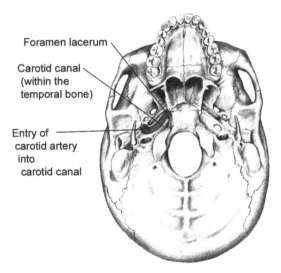

21.5 The internal carotid artery enters the temporal bone from below, passing through the carotid canal within the temporal bone, and emerges superiorly above the foramen lacerum

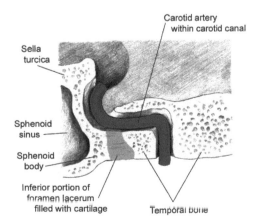

21.6 Carotid canal – lateral view. The lower end of the foramen lacerum is filled with cartilage

The **carotid canal** therefore follows a tortuous S-shaped pathway through the temporal bone. The entrance to the canal is on the inferior surface of the bone, passing into the interior of the temporal bone (Figure 21.5). This bony canal then passes medially within the temporal bone, emerging into the base of the cranium superiorly through the upper portion of the foramen lacerum, above the cartilage plug (where the medial projection of the petrous portion of the temporal bone meets the greater wing of the sphenoid) (Figure 21.7).

The *carotid artery* therefore travels up the side of the neck (in close association with the jugular vein and vagus nerve within the carotid sheath), dividing into an external carotid artery and an internal carotid artery on each side. The internal carotid artery passes up through the S-shaped carotid canal, emerging superiorly at the foramen lacerum, to feed into the Circle of Willis – an arterial ring at the base of the brain, from which branches emerge to supply the brain. The two carotid arteries (together with the two vertebral arteries) form the main arterial supply to the brain (Figures 21.4, 21.8 and 21.9).

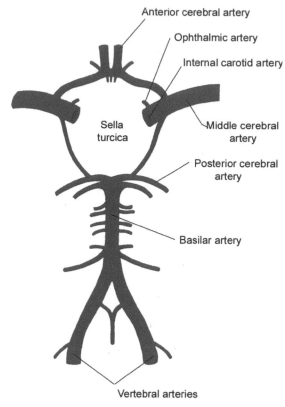

Anterior cerebral artery

Ophthalmic artery

Internal carotid artery

Sella turcica

Middle cerebral artery

Posterior cerebral artery

Basilar artery

Vertebral arteries

21.8 The Circle of Willis

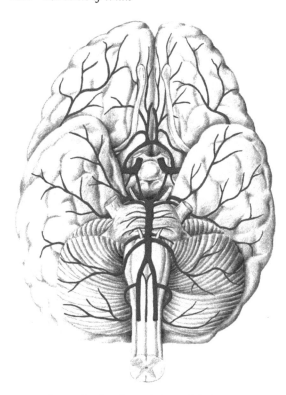

21.9 The Circle of Willis at the base of the brain

Carotid nerve

The sympathetic nerve pathway to the head and eyes travels up from the upper thoracic spine (T1 and T2) via the sympathetic chain in the neck, synapsing at the superior cervical sympathetic ganglion, continuing up through the carotid canal to provide the sympathetic supply within the cranium.

The *carotid nerve* is the portion of that sympathetic pathway which passes upward from the superior cervical sympathetic ganglion through the carotid canal on the surface of the carotid artery, where it also forms the carotid plexus (a network of sympathetic fibres) before being distributed through its various branches to different structures within the cranium, including the eyes.

Other minor foramina

Certain other minor foramina are visible in the base of the skull. These are variable foramina, mostly carrying small emissary veins. (Emissary veins enable drainage from the veins on the outside of the cranium into the venous sinuses inside the cranium.)

- The **mastoid foramen** is a small foramen in the mastoid process of the temporal bone, carrying the mastoid vein.

- The **condylar canal** is a small foramen within the occiput, posterior and lateral to the occipital condyle, lateral to the foramen magnum, carrying the occipital emissary vein.

- The **foramen caecum** is located at the junction of the frontal bone with the anterior ethmoid. It carries an emissary vein from the nose to the superior sagittal sinus. It is significant because it can be a passageway for infection from the nasal cavity into the cranium and the meninges.

- The **incisive fossa**, located close to the anterior end of the intermaxillary suture, is the inferior opening of the incisive canal which passes through the hard palate, allowing passage of the nasopalatine nerve (a branch of the maxillary division of cranial nerve V, receiving sensation from the roof of the mouth).

Foramina of the face

Most foramina are in the base of the skull. There are also three significant foramina on the anterior face (and a fourth on the medial aspect of the mandible), providing entry for the three main branches of the *trigeminal nerve* (Cr V), carrying sensation from the three corresponding regions of the face (Figure 21.10).

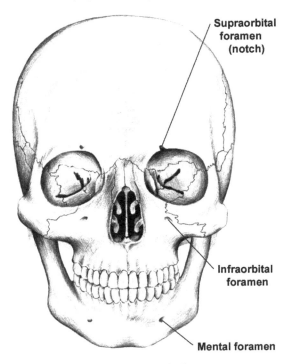

21.10 Foramina on the surface of the face

The **supraorbital foramen (supraorbital notch)** is a variable structure which may be formed as a foramen or as a notch in the superior rim of the orbit, sometimes as a foramen on one side and a notch in the other orbital rim. It carries the *frontal nerve – a terminal branch of the ophthalmic division of the trigeminal nerve.*

It can usually be palpated along the upper rim of the orbit. Pressing on this spot may induce a slight tenderness, but conversely pressing on this spot when it is painful (in headache or migraine, for example) may bring relief.

The **infraorbital foramen** is within the maxilla, just below the inferior rim of the orbit. The *maxillary division of the trigeminal nerve* passes down through the base of the cranium via the foramen rotundum, immediately turns forward to enter the orbit through the inferior orbital fissure, giving off alveolar branches to the upper teeth, travels along the floor of the orbit along a groove, which then becomes a tunnel passing beneath the inferior rim of the orbit, before finally emerging to the surface at the infraorbital foramen.

The **mental foramen** is within the mandible, on the anterior surface, on each side of the symphysis menti (chin). The *mandibular nerve* (the terminal branch of the mandibular division of the trigeminal nerve) passes down through the base of the cranium via the foramen ovale, enters the mandible through the mandibular foramen, in the medial wall of the ramus of the mandible, travels inside the mandible, giving off alveolar branches to the lower teeth, before finally emerging to the surface at the mental foramen.

The **mandibular foramen**, mentioned in the description of the mental foramen above, is on the medial surface of the ramus of the mandible and is the point through which the *mandibular nerve* enters the jaw.

V

21

Foramina of the face and cranium – an abbreviated summary for quick reference

Foramen	Principal structures passing through	Bone within which the foramen is located
Cribriform plate	Cr I Olfactory nerve	Ethmoid
Optic canal	Cr II Optic nerve Ophthalmic artery	Sphenoid
There are two fissures in the back of the orbit:		
Superior orbital fissure	Cr III Oculo-motor nerve Cr IV Trochlear nerve Cr VI Abducent nerve Ophthalmic branch of Cr V Trigeminal nerve Ophthalmic vein	Sphenoid
Inferior orbital fissure	Maxillary branch of Cr V Trigeminal nerve	Between sphenoid and maxilla
There are three foramina in the greater wing of the sphenoid:		
Foramen rotundum	Maxillary branch of Cr V Trigeminal nerve	Sphenoid
Foramen ovale	Mandibular branch of Cr V Trigeminal nerve Motor branch of Cr V Trigeminal nerve	Sphenoid
Foramen spinosum	Middle meningeal artery Recurrent meningeal branch of Cr V Trigeminal nerve	Sphenoid
Foramina within the temporal bone:		
Internal auditory meatus	Cr VII Facial nerve Cr VIII Vestibulo-cochlear nerve	Temporal
Stylomastoid foramen	Exit for Cr VII Facial nerve	Temporal
Foramen between the temporal bone and the occipital bone:		
Jugular foramen	Internal jugular vein Cr IX Glosso-pharyngeal nerve Cr X Vagus nerve Cr XI Spinal accessory nerve	Between temporal and occiput
Foramina within the occiput:		
Hypoglossal canal	Cr XII Hypoglossal nerve	Occiput
Foramen magnum	Spinal cord Spinal roots of Cr XI Spinal accessory nerve Vertebral arteries	Occiput

Summary of foramina – continued

Further foramina

There are various other foramina distributed through the cranium, which do not carry cranial nerves, but which are worthy of note for other reasons.

Foramen	Principal structures passing through	Bone within which the foramen is located
External auditory meatus	Entry to the external ear canal	Temporal
Eustachian tube (Auditory tube)	Exit of the Eustachian tube from the middle ear	Temporal
Foramen lacerum and carotid canal	Carotid artery Carotid nerve (sympathetic)	Between the temporal and sphenoid

Other foramina

Foramen	Principal structures passing through	Bone within which the foramen is located
Mastoid foramen	Mastoid emissary vein	Temporal
Condylar canal	Condylar emissary vein	Occiput
Foramen caecum	Emissary vein	Frontal/ethmoid
Incisive fossa	Nasopalatine nerve	Maxillae

Foramina of the face

Foramen	Principal structures passing through	Bone within which the foramen is located
Supraorbital foramen	Frontal nerve – a terminal branch of the ophthalmic division of the trigeminal nerve	Frontal
Infraorbital foramen	Maxillary nerve – the terminal branch of the maxillary division of the trigeminal nerve	Maxilla
Mental foramen	Mandibular nerve – the terminal branch of the mandibular division of the trigeminal nerve	Mandible
Mandibular foramen	Mandibular nerve – as described above	Mandible

V

21

Chapter 22

Cranial Nerve I – The Olfactory Nerve

Function

Sensory	Receiving olfactory sensations (smell)

Overview

Our olfactory nerves (Cr I) enable us to receive sensations of smell. They carry olfactory sensations from the nasal cavity to the brain (Figure 22.1). They are purely sensory.

Interconnections

Olfactory sensations also stimulate responses in various other parts of the brain, stimulating digestive function through connections with the vagus nerve, and emotional responses and memories through connections with the limbic system and associated areas of the brain. Loss of smell can therefore have significant effects on function and on quality of life. It may also diminish the sense of taste, since much of our perception of taste arises from our sense of smell. The nose can distinguish hundreds of substances, even in minute quantities, whereas the tongue can distinguish only five distinct qualities of taste.[1]

Olfactory sensitivity

The sense of smell in humans is much weaker than in many other mammals, but is nevertheless capable of sensing subtle olfactory sensations. In

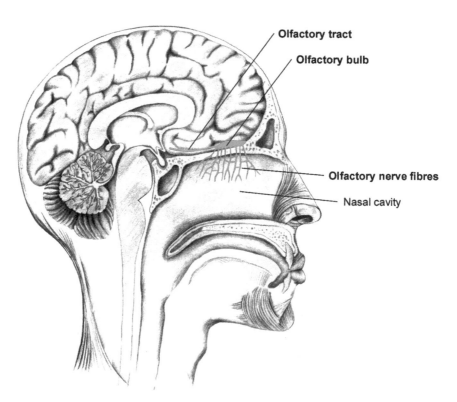

22.1   The olfactory nerve (Cr I) carries olfactory sensations from the nasal cavity to the forebrain

female humans, the sense of olfaction is strongest around the time of ovulation, significantly stronger than during other phases of the menstrual cycle and stronger than the sense in males.[2] Female humans are able to smell some aspect of the HLA genes of potential sex partners[3] and prefer partners with HLA genes different from their own – an evolutionary device to counteract incest and thereby strengthen the immune system and other functions in offspring.[4] Humans can detect individuals that are blood-related through olfaction. Mothers can identify their biological children but not their stepchildren. Pre-adolescent children can detect their full siblings but not half-siblings or step-siblings through their sense of smell.[5]

Insects smell via their antennae. Dogs have an olfactory sense up to a million times more acute than humans, and bloodhounds up to a hundred million times more sensitive than humans. Some bears have a sense of smell seven times stronger than that of the bloodhound and can detect the scent of food up to eighteen miles away, as well as underground.[6]

Pathway (Figure 22.2)

- Receptors within the *olfactory mucosa* in the upper part of the nasal cavity receive sensations of smell entering the nose.

- Fibres from these receptors travel up through the tiny holes in the *cribriform plate* (the roof of the ethmoid bone) in the roof of the nasal cavity.

- Emerging onto the superior surface of the ethmoid bone, these fibres enter the *olfactory bulbs* (two worm-like extensions of the forebrain lying on the superior surface of the cribriform plate) where they synapse.

- The neurological impulses are then transmitted posteriorly from the olfactory bulbs along the *olfactory tracts* into the forebrain.

Olfactory receptor neurons are unusual in that they can regenerate and are constantly reproduced throughout life.

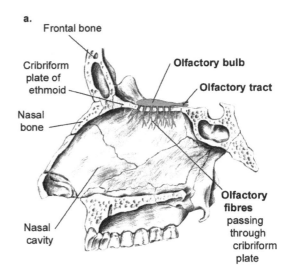

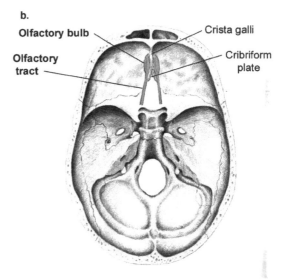

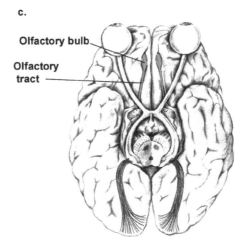

22.2   The olfactory nerve – lateral view, superior view, inferior view

Anosmia

Loss of smell (anosmia) may arise from various different causes:

- Fracture of the cribriform plate due to physical injury such as a blow to the face or a car accident, damaging the olfactory nerve fibres as they pass through the cribriform plate of the ethmoid bone.

- Lesser displacements or restrictions to the mobility of the ethmoid and its adjoining bones, including the frontal, sphenoid and vomer.

- Membranous tensions impinging on the olfactory nerve fibres as they pass through the dura on the superior surface of the cribriform plate.

- Congestion in the nasal cavity blocking the receptors; and congestion within the foramina of the cribriform plate impinging on the olfactory fibres.

Loss of smell can also arise with no identifiable physiological cause, and may be brought on by shock or an emotional event.

More transient loss of smell may be due to:

- excessive dryness of the nose, since the conversion of olfactory sensations to neurological stimuli is dependent on the dissolving of fragrant (or obnoxious) substances in the moist mucous membrane of the nasal cavity

- or more obviously may be due to blockage of the nasal passages as a result of a cold or nasal allergy.

Cerebrospinal fluid drainage

The olfactory nerve pathway is also significant for another crucial function. It provides the most significant pathway for drainage of cerebrospinal fluid from the brain. Cerebrospinal fluid drains from the subarachnoid space through several different outlets – through the arachnoid villi, through spinal nerve exits, and through cranial nerve exits – but the most significant and substantial of these drainage pathways is through the olfactory nerve outlets passing through the holes in the cribriform plate, ultimately draining into the lymphatic system. The health and mobility of this region and of the cribriform plate in particular is essential to cerebrospinal fluid flow throughout the cranium, and therefore to fluid pressures within the brain – arterial, venous and cerebrospinal fluid – and consequently to the overall function of the brain, brainstem, and all the cranial nerves.

Chapter 23

Cranial Nerve II – The Optic Nerve

Function

Sensory	Vision
	Visual reflexes

Overview

Our optic nerves enable us to see. They are concerned solely with vision and visual reflexes. They are purely sensory. Disturbances to the optic nerves may lead to loss of vision. There are many different potential sources of disturbance.

Light entering the pupil of the eye passes through the lens, the aqueous humour and the vitreous humour of the eyeball, and is focused by the lens onto the receptors (125 million rods and 7 million cones, approximately) within the retina of the eye. (Rods are for light and dark vision, cones for colour vision.) Fibres from these receptors come together as the optic nerve at the back of the eyeball – a relatively thick nerve (among the cranial nerves, it is second only to the trigeminal nerve in thickness). Each optic nerve carries approximately one million fibres, with the central artery of the retina and central vein of the retina travelling through the centre of the nerve.

Visual images are received at the retina of the eye and are processed in the *occipital lobe* of the brain. The optic pathway therefore travels from the front of the face to the back of the head, passing via the optic nerve, optic chiasma, optic

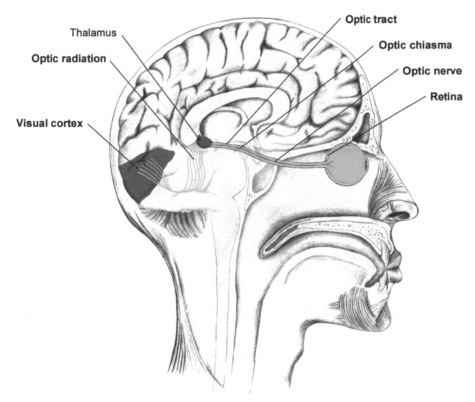

23.1 *The optic pathway passes from the retina of the eye via the optic nerve, optic chiasma, optic tract and optic radiation to the visual cortex within the occipital lobe*

tract and optic radiation to the visual cortex in the occipital lobe (Figures 23.1 and 23.2).

Pathway (Figures 23.1–23.7)

Each optic nerve:

- travels posteriorly from the back of the eyeball
- passes through the *optic canal* (between the body of the sphenoid and the lesser wing of the sphenoid)
- emerges medial to the anterior clinoid process, anterior to the pituitary gland
- here, the two optic nerves come together at the *optic chiasma*, where they partially decussate
- medial fibres from each optic nerve *decussate* (cross over to the opposite side), lateral fibres continuing on the same side
- the combined fibres (lateral fibres from the same side and medial fibres from the opposite side) continue posteriorly on each side as the *optic tract*

- giving off branches to the lateral geniculate body of the thalamus (enabling visual reflexes) and then continuing as the *optic radiation* to the visual cortex, located within the calcarine fissure of the *occipital lobe.*

Not a true nerve

The optic nerve is not generally considered to be a true cranial nerve. It is an extension of the brain; in fact, the whole eyeball is an extension of the brain and is completely enveloped within the meninges, the sclera (white) of the eye being a continuation of the meningeal membrane. Consequently, there is no synapse along the main pathway.

Decussation

Decussation of the optic nerves provides additional protection for the vital function of vision, so that damage – at least in certain areas – will still leave us with some vision in both eyes, rather than losing the sight of that eye completely.

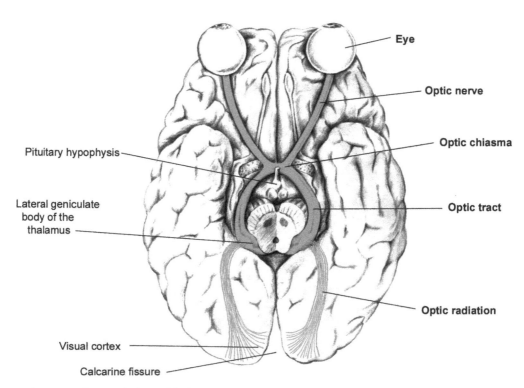

23.2 The optic pathway at the base of the brain

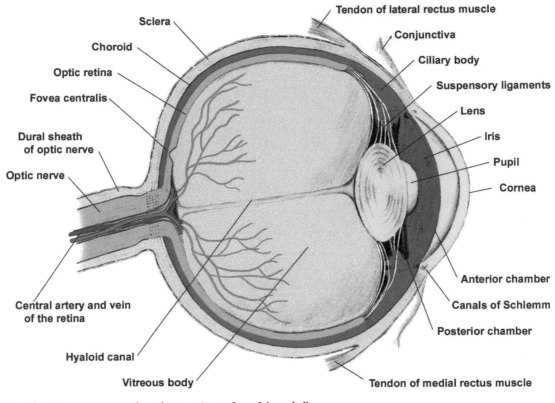

23.3 *The optic nerve emerges from the posterior surface of the eyeball*

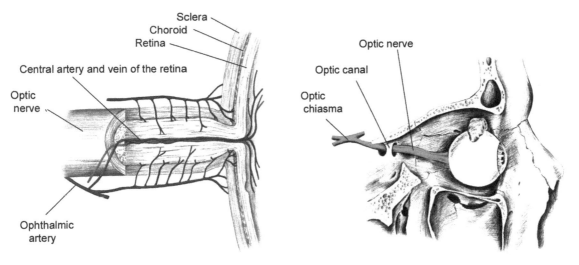

23.4 *The central artery and vein of the retina travel through the central core of the optic nerve*

23.5 *The optic nerve exits the orbit through the optic canal*

V

23

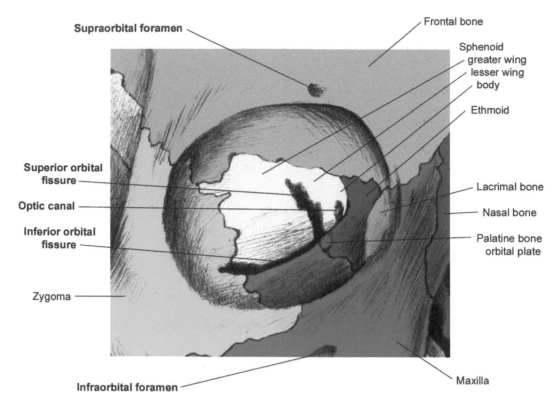

Supraorbital foramen

Frontal bone

Sphenoid
greater wing
lesser wing
body

Ethmoid

Superior orbital
fissure

Optic canal

Inferior orbital
fissure

Lacrimal bone

Nasal bone

Palatine bone
orbital plate

Zygoma

Infraorbital foramen

Maxilla

23.6   Foramina of the orbit – anterior view

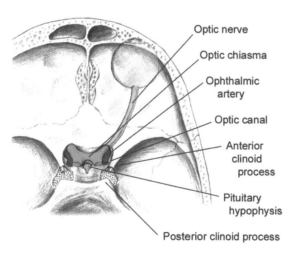

Optic nerve

Optic chiasma

Ophthalmic
artery

Optic canal

Anterior
clinoid
process

Pituitary
hypophysis

Posterior clinoid process

*23.7   The two optic nerves come together at the optic
chiasma, where they partially decussate*

Clinical considerations

Disturbances of optic nerve function can arise from many different sources. The nerve may be affected by:

- cranial bone displacement – particularly involving the sphenoid, but inevitably affected by the overall balance of the cranium as a whole and of the orbit in particular

- nerve compression – particularly within the optic canal and at the sella turcica

- membranous tension – due to meningitis, meningisms, meningeal inflammation, or meningeal contraction

- neuritis.

The optic nerve can also be affected by various pathologies, including diabetes, multiple sclerosis, a pituitary tumour, tumours elsewhere along the pathway, stroke and neurological damage.

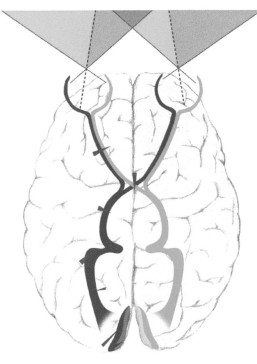

23.8 Neurological damage can occur at different sites within the optic pathway, with varying effects according to the site

Neurological damage can occur at different sites within the optic pathway, with varying effects according to the site (Figure 23.8):

- Damage to the *optic nerve* itself (between the eyeball and the chiasma) would cause loss of sight in the affected eye.

- The *optic chiasma* is located immediately in front of the pituitary gland. A pituitary tumour, potentially causing damage at the centre of the optic chiasma, may therefore lead to dysfunction in the medial fibres of both sides, leading to tunnel vision. (The medial fibres provide lateral vision, that is, perceiving the lateral part of the visual field, so lateral vision would be lost on both sides.) It is also possible for damage at the chiasma to be more widespread, affecting all the fibres, or to be unilateral, affecting all the fibres to one eye.

- Damage at the *optic tract* would lead to loss of vision in the medial fibres of one eye and the lateral fibres of the other eye, reducing the visual field on the opposite side. (Damage to the left optic tract reduces the visual field on the right.)

- Damage can also affect the *optic radiation* and the *visual cortex* with a variety of consequences according to the site of damage.

The optic nerve can be one of the first nerves to be affected in multiple sclerosis, so visual disturbances could potentially be an early sign of the disease. However, this is one of the rarer causes of visual disturbance, and not a factor that should arouse undue alarm whenever visual disturbances occur.

The eyes will be covered in greater detail in Chapter 34.

V

23

Chapter 24

Cranial Nerves III, IV, VI – The Oculo-Motor, Trochlear and Abducent Nerves

Principal functions

Nerve	Type	Function
Cr III Oculo-motor	Motor Parasympathetic	Eye movement Pupil constriction, lens accommodation
Cr IV Trochlear	Motor	Eye movement
Cr VI Abducent	Motor	Eye movement

Overview

These three nerves enable us to move our eyes, and are the nerves involved in squints. We will address them together, because they serve similar functions, and because they also follow very similar pathways from the brainstem to the orbit (Figure 24.1). They operate in conjunction with each other, in order to move the eyeball, and thereby direct the gaze in different directions.

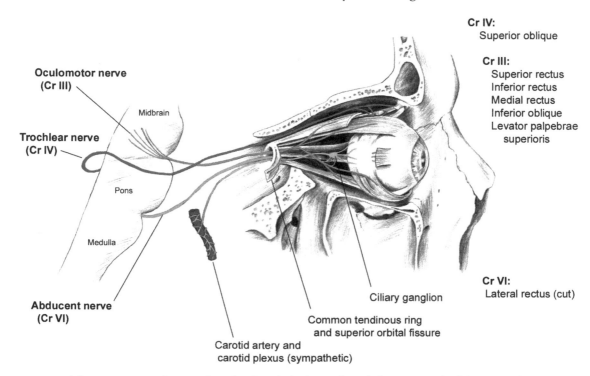

Cr IV:
Superior oblique

Cr III:
Superior rectus
Inferior rectus
Medial rectus
Inferior oblique
Levator palpebrae
superioris

Cr VI:
Lateral rectus (cut)

Oculomotor nerve
(Cr III)

Midbrain

Trochlear nerve
(Cr IV)

Pons

Medulla

Abducent nerve
(Cr VI)

Carotid artery and
carotid plexus (sympathetic)

Common tendinous ring
and superior orbital fissure

Ciliary ganglion

24.1   Cranial nerves III, IV and VI travel together from the brainstem through the superior orbital fissure into the orbit

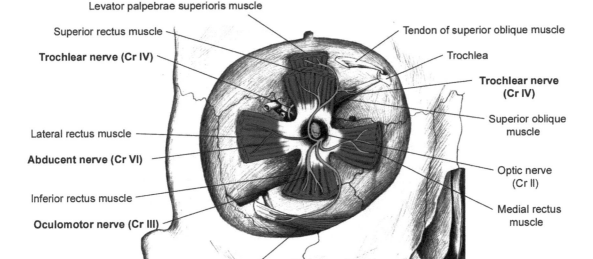

24.2   All three nerves provide motor supply to the extrinsic muscles of the eye

Functions

All three nerves are motor to the *extrinsic muscles* of the eyes – the muscles on the outside of the eyeball which move the eye (Figure 24.2).

All three nerves have their nuclei in the brainstem.

Cranial nerve III is distinctive in that it also carries *parasympathetic fibres* to the *intrinsic muscles* of the eyes – the muscles within the eyeball which constrict the pupil and adjust the lens for near or far vision.

The parasympathetic fibres arise from their own nucleus in the brainstem and join with the oculo-motor nerve in order to travel to the orbit.

There are six extrinsic muscles of the eye:

- superior rectus
- inferior rectus
- medial rectus
- lateral rectus
- superior oblique
- inferior oblique.

- *Cranial nerve VI* (the abducent nerve) supplies the *lateral rectus muscle*, enabling abduction of the eye.
- *Cranial nerve IV* (the trochlear nerve) supplies the *superior oblique muscle*, directing the gaze downward and outward.
- *Cranial nerve III* (the oculo-motor nerve) supplies the other four extrinsic muscles. It also supplies the levator palpebrae superioris muscle, which raises the upper eyelid. (The eyelid is also raised by the superior tarsal muscles which receive their innervation through sympathetic supply.)

Pathway

All three nerves travel from the brainstem to the orbit, running along the floor of the middle cranial fossa, passing through the *cavernous sinus*, and entering the orbit through the *superior orbital fissure* (Figure 24.1, 24.3 and 24.4):

- Cranial nerve III emerges from the anterolateral midbrain.
- Cranial nerve IV emerges from the posterolateral midbrain, and decussates. This is the only cranial nerve to emerge from the posterior brainstem, and the only cranial nerve apart from the optic nerve to decussate.
- Cranial nerve VI emerges from the anterior pons.

The three nerves travel together along the floor of the middle cranial fossa, on each side of the sphenoid body (Figure 24.4). They enter the posterior wall of the cavernous sinus (Cr III and Cr IV running close to the lateral wall of the cavernous sinus, Cr VI a bit further medially). They emerge together from the anterior wall of the cavernous sinus and pass into the orbit together through the superior orbital fissure (Figures 24.1, 24.2 and 24.4):

- Cr VI (abducent) enters through the medial part of the fissure, passes through the common tendinous ring, and travels directly to the lateral rectus muscle.
- Cr IV (trochlear) enters through the lateral part of the fissure and passes behind the superior rectus muscle directly to the superior oblique muscle (*not* through the common tendinous ring).
- Cr III (oculo-motor) enters through the middle of the fissure and passes through the common tendinous ring before giving off branches to the superior rectus, inferior rectus, medial rectus and inferior oblique muscles, and also to the levator palpebrae superioris muscle.

    It also carries parasympathetic fibres to the intrinsic muscles of the eye for pupil constriction and lens accommodation. The parasympathetic fibres branch away from the main nerve within the posterior orbit in order to synapse in the ciliary ganglion, just behind the eyeball, continuing into the eyeball independently as the short ciliary nerves (Figures 24.1 and 24.4).

a. Oculomotor nerve (Cr III):

Midbrain (anterior)

Muscles supplied:
Superior rectus
Inferior rectus
Medial rectus
Inferior oblique
Levator palpebrae superioris

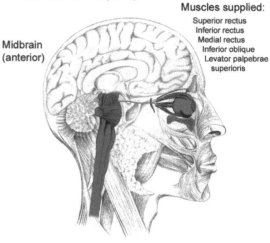

b. Trochlear nerve (Cr IV):

Midbrain (posterior)

Superior oblique

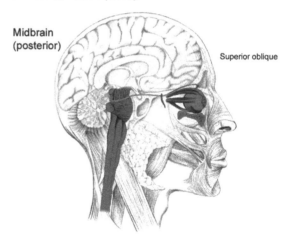

c. Abducent nerve (Cr VI):

Pons

Lateral rectus

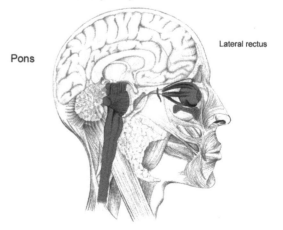

24.3   Cranial nerves III, IV and VI

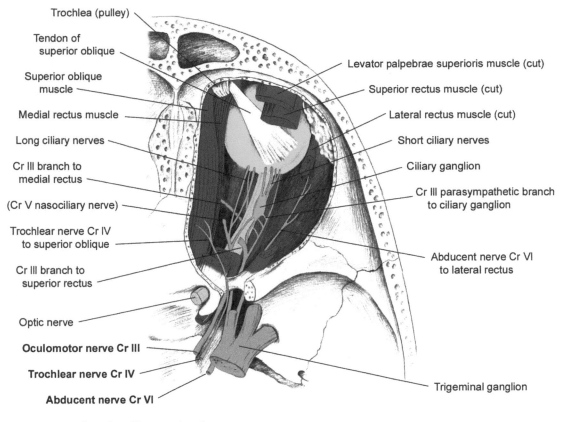

Trochlea (pulley)

Tendon of superior oblique

Superior oblique muscle

Medial rectus muscle

Long ciliary nerves

Cr III branch to medial rectus

(Cr V nasociliary nerve)

Trochlear nerve Cr IV to superior oblique

Cr III branch to superior rectus

Optic nerve

Oculomotor nerve Cr III

Trochlear nerve Cr IV

Abducent nerve Cr VI

Levator palpebrae superioris muscle (cut)

Superior rectus muscle (cut)

Lateral rectus muscle (cut)

Short ciliary nerves

Ciliary ganglion

Cr III parasympathetic branch to ciliary ganglion

Abducent nerve Cr VI to lateral rectus

Trigeminal ganglion

24.4 Nerve supply to the orbit – superior view

Function and dysfunction

The *oculo-motor nerve* (Cr III) serves three functions:

a) eye movement via the superior rectus, inferior rectus, medial rectus, and inferior oblique muscles

b) raises the upper eyelid via the levator palpebrae superioris muscle

c) pupil constriction and lens accommodation via parasympathetic fibres to the intrinsic muscles of the eye.

Injury may lead to strabismus (squint) and diplopia (double vision) on looking in any direction which involves the use of these muscles. The affected eye can only move outward and downward and will tend to be directed laterally, since the lateral rectus muscle (supplied by Cr VI) will now act unopposed.

Injury affecting the levator palpebrae superioris muscle may lead to a ptosis (drooping) of the eyelid, but because the eyelid is also supplied by sympathetic fibres to the tarsal muscles, the effect will be only partial.

Injury affecting the parasympathetic component of the nerve will leave the pupil unable to constrict, therefore leading to a persistently dilated pupil on the affected side, potentially causing photophobia.

It may also affect accommodation of the affected eye to near and far vision.

The *trochlear nerve* (Cr IV) is purely motor, enabling the eye to look downward and outward, via the superior oblique muscle. Injury may lead to strabismus and diplopia on trying to look down and out to the affected side.

The *abducent nerve* (Cr VI) is purely motor, abducting the eye in order to look laterally via the lateral rectus muscle. Injury may lead to strabismus and diplopia on trying to look laterally to the affected side. The eye will tend to be directed medially (convergent strabismus, cross-eyed) since the medial pull of the medial rectus muscles (supplied by Cr III) will now be unopposed by the paralysed lateral rectus muscle. Convergent strabismus is the most common type of squint, or cranial nerve disturbance of the eye.

Strabismus and diplopia

- *Strabismus (squint)* may indicate a fixed squint, where the eye is constantly directed out of alignment. Alternatively, it can indicate a transient squint, where one eye fails to follow the direction of gaze in certain directions.

- *Diplopia (double vision)* occurs as a result of a strabismus because the two eyes are not directed towards the same spot.

For example, damage to the abducent nerve (Cr VI) will result in loss of abduction of the eye on the affected side. If, for instance, the abducent nerve is damaged in the right eye, the patient's right eye will not turn to the right, so when the patient tries to look to the right, the left eye will look in the desired direction and the right eye will remain directed straight ahead, leading to a transient squint (strabismus). The patient will also experience double vision (diplopia) while trying to look in that direction, because their two eyes are not directed to the same spot. In practice, the patient soon learns to adapt by turning their head instead of turning their eyes.

Treatment

Squints are very common and have various causes, not all of which involve their cranial nerve supply.

Some cases will be very responsive to cranio-sacral integration, particularly where there are clearly evident cranial or membranous distortions, and where there is a history of birth trauma.

Squints are often addressed through an operation at an early age without any cranio-sacral assessment, so it is impossible to evaluate how many of those cases would have responded to cranio-sacral treatment. Operations may resolve the squint successfully, but will not address any other imbalances that may be contributing to the squint.

Cranio-sacral treatment involves:

- clear identification of the nerves, muscles or other structures involved through a clear understanding of their function

- accurate diagnosis of the location and source of the disturbance through cranio-sacral palpation and particularly by tracing the nerve pathways with your informed awareness

- cranio-sacral balancing of the orbit, the cranium, the membranes and any other structures involved

- identifying and addressing patterns throughout the body that may be contributing to the disturbance in the eye

- addressing birth trauma (and other injuries) as necessary

- and of course overall integration of the cranio-sacral system as a whole.

Cranial Nerve V – The Trigeminal Nerve

Principal functions

Sensory	to the face
Motor	to the muscles of mastication
	and other small muscles of the ear, palate and throat

Overview

The trigeminal nerve is perhaps best known for the extreme pain of *trigeminal neuralgia*, often described as one of the most excruciatingly painful conditions, and a condition which is not generally well understood or effectively treated but which can often be highly responsive to cranio-sacral integration.

The various branches of the trigeminal nerve also supply the teeth, and it is therefore the nerve through which we experience the agonies of toothache, and the nerve which is anaesthetized during dental treatment.

As well as transmitting pain, it is also of course serving many very useful purposes in carrying valuable and informative sensations from the face – from the forehead, nose, orbits, cheeks and throat (externally).

Function

The trigeminal nerve, as its name indicates, has three main divisions. In fact, it has three main *sensory* divisions. It also has a significant *motor* division (Figure 25.1).

It is primarily associated with receiving sensation from the face. The structures from which it receives sensation include the skin of the face from the top of the head down to the lower jaw and throat, the eyeball, conjunctiva, lacrimal gland, ear, external ear canal, nasal cavity, oral cavity, the sinuses, the teeth, the temporo-mandibular joint, the anterior tongue, the nasopharynx, and the meningeal membranes of the anterior and middle cranial fossae, including parts of the tentorium. It also receives proprioceptive input from the muscles of mastication, the muscles of facial expression, the extrinsic muscles of the eye, and the eyeball.

The motor branch supplies the muscles of mastication, enabling chewing and other movements of the lower jaw, along with several other smaller muscles – mylohyoid, the anterior belly of digastric, tensor tympani, and tensor veli palatini.

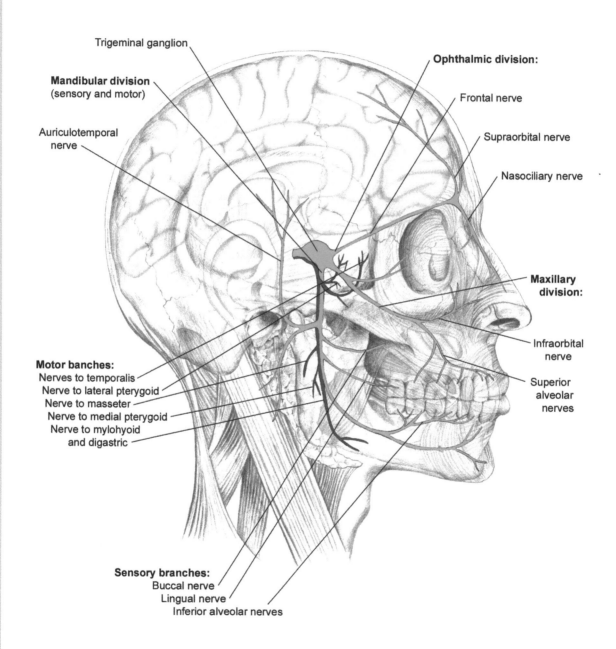

Trigeminal ganglion

Mandibular division
(sensory and motor)

Auriculotemporal
nerve

Ophthalmic division:

Frontal nerve

Supraorbital nerve

Nasociliary nerve

**Maxillary
division:**

Infraorbital
nerve

Superior
alveolar
nerves

Motor banches:
Nerves to temporalis
Nerve to lateral pterygoid
Nerve to masseter
Nerve to medial pterygoid
Nerve to mylohyoid
and digastric

Sensory branches:
Buccal nerve
Lingual nerve
Inferior alveolar nerves

25.1 *The trigeminal nerve (Cr V) has three sensory divisions and a motor division*

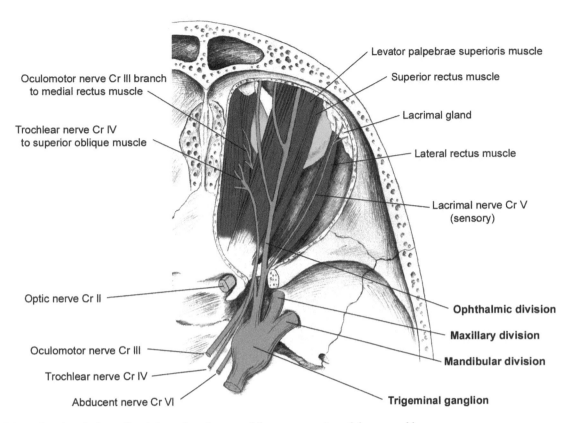

Levator palpebrae superioris muscle

Superior rectus muscle

Lacrimal gland

Lateral rectus muscle

Lacrimal nerve Cr V (sensory)

Ophthalmic division

Maxillary division

Mandibular division

Trigeminal ganglion

Oculomotor nerve Cr III branch to medial rectus muscle

Trochlear nerve Cr IV to superior oblique muscle

Optic nerve Cr II

Oculomotor nerve Cr III

Trochlear nerve Cr IV

Abducent nerve Cr VI

25.2   The trigeminal ganglion is located on the apex of the petrous portion of the temporal bone

Trigeminal ganglion (Figure 25.2)

(Also known as the semilunar ganglion, or the gasserian ganglion.)

There is a large trigeminal ganglion bulging out on each side of the brainstem, contained within the cavum trigeminale (a membranous cave encapsulating the ganglion and its roots). It is located on the apex of the petrous portion of the temporal bone, where there is sometimes a slight indentation in the bone. This ganglion, like other sensory ganglia, is the site of synapse for sensory fibres travelling in from the periphery. Preganglionic fibres of the three sensory divisions of the trigeminal nerve pass into the ganglion, where they synapse before relaying their sensory input into the brainstem via postganglionic fibres.

The motor division does *not* of course synapse in this sensory ganglion, but passes under the ganglion on its way out from the brainstem.

Divisions

The three sensory divisions – the ophthalmic, the maxillary and the mandibular (sometimes abbreviated to Cr V-1, Cr V-2, Cr V-3) – travel to three distinct regions of the face, receiving sensation from those areas (Figure 25.3).

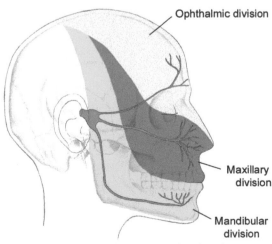

Ophthalmic division

Maxillary division

Mandibular division

25.3   The three sensory divisions travel to three distinct regions of the face

Each division passes through various foramina along its pathway, giving off many branches on the way, and intermingling with many other nerves, before emerging to the surface of the face at its own individual foramen (Figure 25.4):

- the *ophthalmic* division emerges at the *supraorbital foramen* (or supraorbital notch)
- the *maxillary* division emerges at the *infraorbital foramen*
- the *mandibular* division emerges at the *mental foramen*.

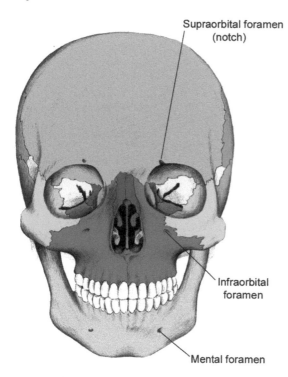

Supraorbital foramen (notch)

Infraorbital foramen

Mental foramen

25.4 Each division emerges to the surface of the face at its respective foramen

The motor division travels initially with the mandibular division, and is therefore usually described as part of the mandibular division. The motor and sensory components of the mandibular division travel together throughout much of their pathway, giving off branches which may also carry both motor and sensory fibres. Motor branches supply the muscles of mastication (chewing) and other smaller muscles of the ear, palate and throat.

Pathway

The three sensory divisions emerge together from the trigeminal ganglion (at the apex of the petrous portion of the temporal bone) before dividing along their individual pathways (Figure 25.5).

The ophthalmic division (Cr V-1)

After emerging from the trigeminal ganglion:

- the *opthalmic* division travels along the floor of the middle cranial fossa, together with cranial nerves III, IV and VI
- passes through the cavernous sinus, together with cranial nerves III, IV and VI
- enters the orbit through the *superior orbital fissure* (also with cranial nerves III, IV and VI).

Within the orbit, it gives off:

- a small *lacrimal branch* (sensory, *not* secretory) to the lacrimal area
- a *nasociliary branch*, which receives sensory input from the cornea, the iris, the ciliary muscles and the pupil dilator muscles and gives off branches which penetrate into the nasal cavity and pass to the frontal, ethmoidal and sphenoidal sinuses
- a main *frontal branch*, which emerges to the surface at the *supraorbital notch* to supply the frontal area, receiving sensation from the forehead, including the frontal sinus.

It receives sensation from the upper portion of the face, including the forehead, the eyes, upper eyelids and lacrimal glands, the nose, the nasal cavity and the frontal, ethmoidal and sphenoidal sinuses.

The maxillary division (Cr V-2)

After emerging from the trigeminal ganglion:

- the *maxillary* division travels anteriorly along the floor of the middle cranial fossa
- turns inferiorly through the floor of the cranium via the *foramen rotundum*
- on emerging to the inferior surface of the base of the cranium, it immediately turns anteriorly to enter the orbit through the *inferior orbital fissure*.

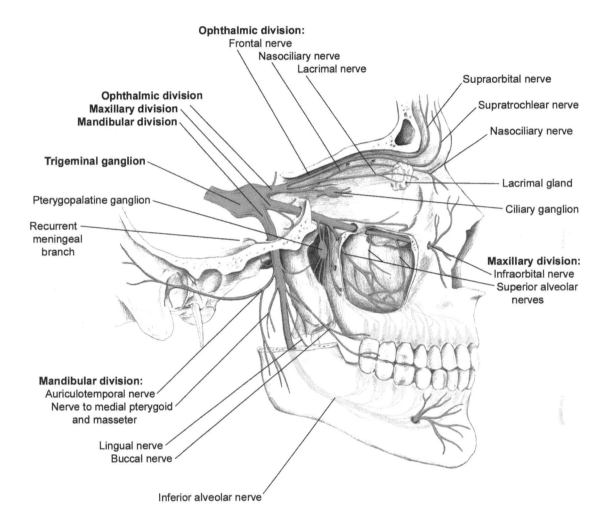

25.5   The trigeminal nerve (Cr V)

Within the orbit:

- it passes along a groove in the floor of the orbit (the groove then deepening to become a tunnel)
- giving off *alveolar branches* to the upper teeth
- and a branch to the maxillary sinus
- before emerging to the surface of the face at the *infraorbital foramen* below the inferior rim of the orbit.

It receives sensation from the middle portion of the face, from the lower eyelid to the upper lip, including the side of the nose, the mucous membranes of the nose and nasopharynx, the maxillary sinuses, the roof of the mouth and the upper teeth.

The mandibular division (Cr V-3)

After emerging from the trigeminal ganglion:

- the *mandibular* division turns immediately down through the *foramen ovale*
- gives off a *recurrent meningeal branch* (nervus spinosus) which passes back up into the cranium through the foramen spinosum (together with the middle meningeal artery) to supply the meninges of the anterior and middle cranial fossae and the mastoid air cells.

It then divides into four branches:

- an *auriculo-temporal branch* to the skin of the external ear, the ear canal, the tympanic membrane, and the temporal area
- a *buccal branch* – receiving sensation from buccinator muscle
- a *lingual branch* – receiving sensations of touch from the anterior tongue
- a main *inferior alveolar branch*
  - which enters the *mandibular foramen* on the medial surface of the ramus of the mandible
  - travels inside the mandible, giving off alveolar branches to the lower teeth
  - before emerging at the *mental foramen* on the anterior surface of the mandible.

The inferior alveolar branch is the nerve that is anaesthetized by a dentist before working on the lower teeth, the needle being inserted just above the point where the nerve enters the mandibular foramen.

The mandibular division receives sensation from the lower portion of the face including the mandible, the lower teeth, gums and lip, the anterior tongue, the TMJ, the mastoid air cells, and the skin of the ear, external ear canal and temporal area.

The motor division (Figure 25.1)

The motor division is generally described as part of the mandibular division, but in view of its distinct functions, it is helpful to look at it separately:

- it emerges from the pons, travelling beneath (*not* through) the trigeminal ganglion
- passes out through the *foramen ovale* (together with the sensory component of the mandibular division)
- joins with the sensory component of the mandibular division, the motor and sensory components travelling together throughout much of their pathway, giving off branches, each of which may also carry both motor and sensory fibres.

The motor branches primarily supply the muscles of mastication, and include:

- *two nerves (anterior and posterior) to the temporalis muscle*
- a *nerve to the lateral pterygoid muscle*
- a *nerve to the masseter muscle*
- a *nerve to the medial pterygoid muscle*
- a *nerve to the mylohyoid muscle and the anterior belly of digastric muscle of the throat.*

The nerve to the medial pterygoid muscle also gives off two smaller branches:

- a *branch to the tensor tympani muscle within the ear*
- and a *branch to the tensor veli palatini muscle of the palate.*

Clinical considerations

The *tensor veli palatini* muscle is involved in opening the Eustachian tube which drains the middle ear. Overstimulation of the mandibular division of the trigeminal nerve (including teeth grinding) may therefore be involved in recurrent middle ear infections and glue ear.

The *tensor tympani* muscle, as its name suggests, tenses the tympanic membrane, thereby dampening vibrations. This is useful in reducing auditory sensitivity when exposed to loud noise, and also comes into play in response to the sound of your own jaws when chewing, but disturbances of this mechanism could affect acuity of hearing and therefore potentially be involved in hearing disorders and learning difficulties due to disturbed auditory sensations.

The *tympanic reflex* helps in preventing damage to the inner ear by contracting the muscles within the middle ear – the tensor tympani and stapedius muscles – thereby dampening vibrations. Exposure to loud noise can lead to involuntary contraction of the tensor tympani muscle in order to reduce auditory input. This can sometimes be accompanied by earache, fluttering sensations, or a sense of fullness in the ear. In people with hyperacusis (auditory hypersensitivity) there may also be involuntary contraction of the tensor tympani muscle. In some cases, the tensor tympani muscle may contract just by thinking about a loud noise. Cranio-sacral engagement with the trigeminal nerve and other associated structures, including energy drives directed into the middle ear and specifically to the tensor tympani and stapedius muscles, may be helpful in such cases.

Trigeminal neuralgia

Trigeminal neuralgia is considered to be the most painful condition known to the medical world. It tends to occur as intermittent recurrent episodes of extremely severe facial pain which come and go unpredictably in sudden shock-like attacks, generally described as stabbing, shooting, excruciating, burning, or strong electric shocks. It affects one or more of the three areas of the face supplied by the trigeminal nerve, most commonly the maxillary or mandibular divisions.

Episodes are generally brief, lasting from a few seconds to about two minutes, but may involve many bursts of pain in quick succession. It may occur only occasionally, or it may occur frequently throughout the day and night. This can continue for weeks, months or years, and in severe cases can sometimes involve several hundred episodes a day.

Attacks can be triggered by the slightest stimulus – the lightest of touches, even a gentle breeze, eating, biting, brushing teeth, applying make-up, shaving, movement of the head – or can sometimes occur without any trigger at all. The condition can be so severe that the patient becomes fearful of eating, talking or even moving, and this can lead to weight loss, isolation and depression. There may be periods of remission for several months or even years, but periods of remission tend to become shorter as time goes on.

Trigeminal neuralgia affects approximately one person in every thousand, mostly over the age of 50, affecting women more than men.[1] It usually occurs on one side of the face only, most commonly the right-hand side. Occasionally it can involve both sides, but not usually at the same time.

The cause of trigeminal neuralgia is unknown. The most popular medical theory is that the pain is caused by pressure on the trigeminal nerve, probably in the region of the ganglion, usually from a blood vessel.[2] Compression causes the nerve to become irritated. Irritation can lead to damage to the myelin sheath.[3] The nerve then becomes more excitable and erratically fires pain impulses. However, this theory on its own is not entirely consistent, since other people with vascular pressure on the ganglion do not necessarily suffer neuralgia.

The nerve may also be compressed elsewhere along its pathway and may be damaged by injury, infection and in rare cases by a tumour or multiple sclerosis (although it tends to be a late symptom in multiple sclerosis).[4]

Another possible cause is the presence of a latent herpes virus.[5] The herpes simplex virus is mainly known as the cause of cold sores in and around the mouth. After infection, the virus becomes latent, usually lying dormant in the trigeminal ganglia or along the trigeminal nerve fibres, ready to emerge later in life as trigeminal neuralgia. This is similar to the way in which the herpes zoster virus, which causes chicken pox, subsequently lies dormant in the dorsal root ganglia of spinal nerves, emerging later in life as shingles. The herpes virus can also lie dormant in the ganglia of the facial and vestibular nerves, emerging later as Bell's palsy or vestibular neuritis.

The herpes simplex virus lives in the trigeminal nerves and usually remains dormant until activated at times of depleted health. Potential activating factors include ageing, stress (physical or emotional), illness, infections, fever and immunosuppressive medication.[6]

This theory is supported by the fact that the ophthalmic division is rarely involved, and herpes simplex infections mostly affect the mouth or the areas supplied by the maxillary and mandibular divisions.

Medical treatment for trigeminal neuralgia consists of medication or surgery. Medication is often found to have only limited benefits, and inevitably involves side effects which can be more troublesome than the neuralgia. Injections and minor surgical procedures may similarly have only limited benefits, and inevitable side effects such as loss of sensation in areas of the face. Major intracranial surgery to remove pressure due to a blood vessel carries severe risks – including deafness and even stroke. Trigeminal neuralgia has also been known to recur even after surgery to sever the nerve.

Cranio-sacral perspective

Cranio-sacral treatment can often prove beneficial. Cranio-sacral integration of the system as a whole and the local area in particular will inevitably eliminate restrictions, enable greater mobility and spaciousness, and restore fluent function, thereby potentially removing impingement on the nerve, whether due to bony restriction, membranous tension, vascular pressure, or any other cause, and will also enhance the body's ability to deal with any latent viral infection.

If there is pressure on the nerve at the ganglion, the increased mobility of the cranio-sacral system is likely to relieve the pressure. If there is impingement on the nerve anywhere along its pathway, the cranio-sacral process may identify and release the source of the restriction. If a dormant virus is involved, cranio-sacral integration can enhance immunity and address the various stress factors which may be contributing to the emergence of the virus. Whatever the causative factors, the cranio-sacral system will reveal any disturbances and potentially bring them to the surface for release and resolution. Also, all neurological activity, including neuralgia, can be increased by sympathetic overstimulation, so trigeminal neuralgia is likely to be aggravated at times of stress or other causes of sympathetic stimulation. Relief of stress and sympatheticotonia through cranio-sacral integration may therefore also contribute to relief of the neuralgia.

Since there is no single explanation, it seems likely that there are multiple contributory factors. So a possible scenario might be a combination of a dormant virus aggravated by pressure on the nerve (from many possible sources – bony, membranous or vascular) – emerging at a time of activation from various stress factors which are depleting the body's resources. The integrative approach of cranio-sacral integration can potentially address all of these factors.

Milosz was 67 and had been suffering from severe trigeminal neuralgia for over ten years. Initially, his condition had been diagnosed as a dental problem and he had undergone a great deal of dental treatment without any relief. Only some time afterwards did he discover by chance that his symptoms were classic indications of trigeminal neuralgia. This led him to try various other treatments, but all to no avail. When someone suggested cranio-sacral integration he was sceptical but prepared to try anything.

His trigeminal neuralgia was exclusively on the right side of his face, within the maxillary distribution, and exhibited all the typical symptoms of intermittent extreme sharp pain, triggered by the slightest movements or stimuli, or often by nothing at all.

The whole right side of his cranium was very restricted, with a quality of solidity which indicated that it had been like that for many years. Because the restriction was so deeply ingrained, progress was slow at first, but he enjoyed the relaxing effects of the treatment, and was reassured by the identification of a clearly evident potential cause for his condition, so he persisted with his sessions. Within a few sessions he began to feel distinct changes and a notable reduction in his symptoms. As the solidity in his cranium gradually released, his symptoms continued to decline, with a particularly significant shift after the seventh treatment.

Milosz's symptoms eventually cleared completely and he also reported a substantial change in his overall mood and feeling of wellbeing, not only due to the relief from his painful neuralgia, but also on a more profound and far-reaching level of being.

In many patients with trigeminal neuralgia there will be a similar quality of rigidity, solidity or compression in certain areas of the cranium or face and, even when the exact location of the impingement on the nerve may not be clearly evident, the process of cranio-sacral integration, opening up the cranium and the whole cranio-sacral system to a greater degree of mobility, spaciousness and fluency, will often bring relief along with many other associated benefits.

A cranio-sacral approach to trigeminal neuralgia

An appropriate cranio-sacral approach to trigeminal neuralgia could therefore involve the following:

- Engage and see what the system reveals – overall quality, shock and trauma, specific restrictions on various levels, allowing the expression and resolution of whatever issues may arise.
- Allow the inherent treatment process to address the system's needs, enabling greater mobility and fluent function of the system as a whole and the relevant local areas in particular.

- Explore specifically the most likely areas of impingement:
  - the area around the trigeminal ganglion at the apex of the petrous portion of the temporal bone, ensuring free mobility of the temporal bones and the sphenoid
  - the surrounding membranes, bearing in mind that the trigeminal ganglion is encased within the cavum trigeminale, a membranous sheath which is of course continuous with all the surrounding membranes, so membranous tensions are likely to be relevant, whether from contraction, inflammation, emotional tension, or perhaps a previous episode of meningitis.
- Trace the pathway of the affected division of the nerve with your therapeutic attention, through its respective foramina, or anywhere along the nerve pathway.
- Identify and address any trauma to the face and to the cranium as a whole. In contacting the face, it is useful to bear in mind that, although the neuralgia is triggered by the lightest of touches, it is not generally triggered by a firm touch, so a firmer touch on the face is likely to be perfectly tolerable and therapeutic.
- Enhance the immune system and the underlying vitality through the usual progression of the cranio-sacral process.
- Address any other factors that may be contributing to the emergence of a virus – stress, injury, medication, toxicity.

In other words, as always, allow the integrative process of cranio-sacral integration to take its course, in conjunction with your informed awareness.

V

25

Chapter 26

Cranial Nerve VII – The Facial Nerve

Principal functions

Motor	to the muscles of the face
Special sensory	to the anterior tongue (taste)
General sensory	to the external ear and mastoid region
Parasympathetic	to the glands of the face

Overview

Our facial expressions are enabled through our facial nerves – every smile, every frown, and a multitude of other reflections of our mood. The facial nerve is primarily concerned with *movement* of most of the muscles of the face – the muscles of facial expression.

It also has a *sensory* branch receiving sensations of taste from the anterior tongue, and some further lesser sensory branches.

It carries a significant *parasympathetic* component supplying most of the glands of the face (except for the parotid gland) and is therefore involved in the secretion of tears, mucus and saliva, and in disturbances affecting these secretions (Figure 26.1).

Its intricate pathways render it susceptible to disturbance from many different sources, including ear infections, mumps and palatine bone restrictions, as well as all the usual injuries, accidents, strains and cranio-sacral imbalances of the system as a whole, particularly involving the temporal and sphenoid bones, and of course facial injuries.

It is the nerve involved in the common condition of Bell's palsy.

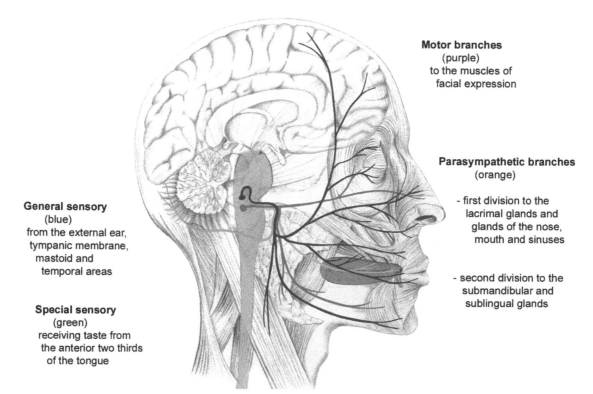

Motor branches
(purple)
to the muscles of
facial expression

Parasympathetic branches
(orange)

- first division to the
lacrimal glands and
glands of the nose,
mouth and sinuses

- second division to the
submandibular and
sublingual glands

General sensory
(blue)
from the external ear,
tympanic membrane,
mastoid and
temporal areas

Special sensory
(green)
receiving taste from
the anterior two thirds
of the tongue

26.1   The facial nerve (Cr VII) has motor, general sensory, special sensory, and parasympathetic components

Pathway

Overview

The facial nerve passes through the temporal bone, within its own facial canal, from the internal auditory meatus (Figure 26.2a) to the stylomastoid foramen (Figure 26.2b). Initially, the three components (motor, sensory and parasympathetic) travel together. The parasympathetic division and the sensory division to the tongue branch off within the canal. The main motor branch emerges at the stylomastoid foramen to be distributed to the muscles of the face. Part of its journey carries the nerve through the middle ear (the main trunk forming an indentation into the wall of the tympanic cavity, and the sensory branch to the tongue passing through the middle ear) (Figure 26.3).

Main trunk

The main trunk, comprising all three components (motor, sensory and parasympathetic):

- leaves the brainstem from the lower pons
- immediately enters the petrous portion of the temporal bone through the *internal auditory meatus* (together with Cr VIII)
- the combined nerve (all three components of the facial nerve) then travels through its own bony canal within the temporal bone – the *facial canal*
- the canal turns a 90 degree angle at the *geniculum* (*genu* is Latin for knee) within the petrous portion of the temporal bone
- several branches (parasympathetic, sensory, and one small motor branch) separate from the main trunk within the canal
- the main motor trunk emerges from the facial canal at the *stylomastoid foramen.*

a. Cranial base - superior view:

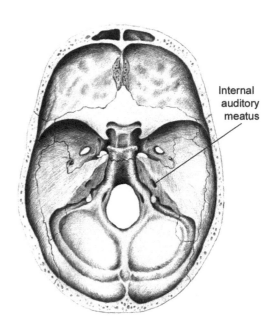

Internal auditory meatus

b. Cranial base - inferior view:

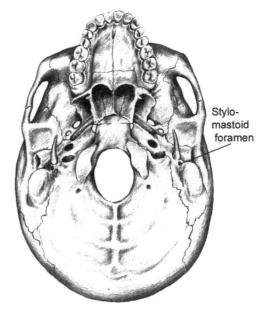

Stylo-mastoid foramen

26.2   The facial nerve enters the temporal bone via the internal auditory meatus and exits via the stylomastoid foramen

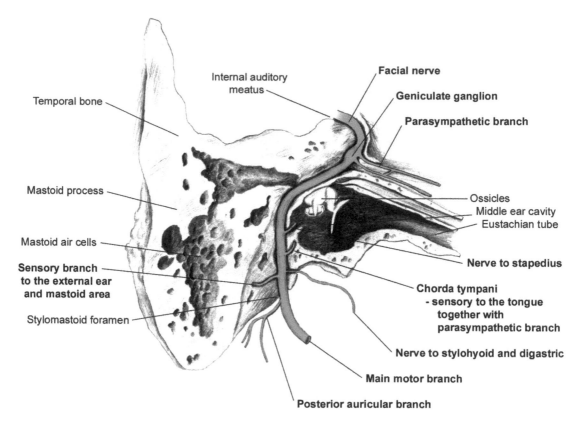

26.3 *The facial nerve travels through the facial canal within the temporal bone, giving off various branches*

Branches within the canal

Within the facial canal, the main trunk gives off various branches, each branch travelling through its own separate bony canal within the temporal bone:

- At the geniculum, the *first parasympathetic division* branches off to supply the glands of the upper face.

- Between the geniculum and the stylomastoid foramen, the facial nerve gives off:

  ○ a small *motor branch to the stapedius muscle* of the middle ear

  ○ a *sensory branch to the tongue*, together with the *second parasympathetic division* to the glands of the lower face.

Some further small sensory branches separate from the main trunk at the stylomastoid foramen.

Motor division

Overview

The motor division provides motor supply to most of the muscles of the face (excluding the muscles of mastication and levator palpebrae superioris) (Figure 26.4). It also provides a small motor branch to the stapedius muscle within the middle ear, a posterior auricular branch to the muscles behind the ear including occipitalis, and small motor branches to the digastric and stylohyoid muscles of the throat.

Pathway

The *nerve to stapedius* separates from the main nerve within the facial canal, passing through its own bony canal into the middle ear cavity to supply the stapedius muscle.

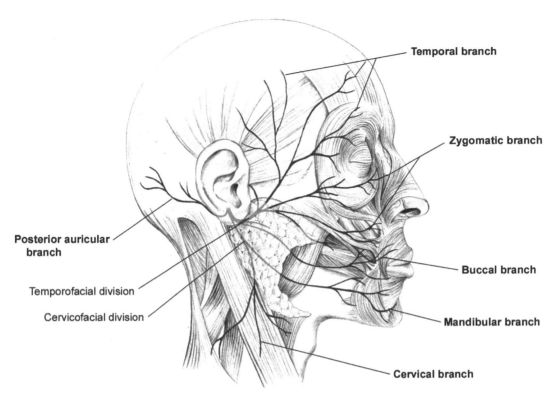

26.4 *The facial nerve has five main motor branches*

After emerging from the facial canal at the stylomastoid foramen, the nerve gives off:

- *motor branches to the digastric and stylohyoid* muscles of the throat
- the *posterior auricular nerve* to the muscles behind the ear.

The *main motor branch* then travels anteriorly across the angle of the jaw:

- It passes *through the substance of the parotid gland* (but does *not* supply it).
- Within the parotid gland, the nerve divides initially into two divisions (the temporo-facial and cervico-facial nerves) and then into five main branches to the various muscles of the face:
  - *temporal branch*
  - *zygomatic branch*
  - *buccal branch*
  - *mandibular branch*
  - *cervical branch.*

Clinical considerations

The pathway through the parotid gland can result in compression of the motor branch of the facial nerve during episodes of mumps (parotitis). This can lead to Bell's palsy – flaccid paralysis of the muscles of the face. This will usually be transient, recovering spontaneously once the infection, inflammation and swelling of the glands have passed, but can sometimes leave persistent symptoms. (Bell's palsy will be described in greater detail below.)

The *nerve to stapedius* is a small motor branch which separates from the main trunk between the geniculum and the stylomastoid foramen. Stapedius is the smallest muscle in the body. It is a tiny muscle, inside the middle ear, attaching onto the stapes (one of the three bony ossicles within the middle ear). Its role is to dampen vibrations of the stapes in response to loud noise, thereby protecting the inner ear from excessive levels of sound. Stapedius and its nerve supply may therefore be implicated in auditory disturbances, and in speech, language and learning difficulties.

Muscles of the facial area which are *not* supplied by the facial nerve include:

- the muscles of mastication (supplied by the trigeminal nerve – mandibular division, Cr V)
- the levator palpebrae superioris (supplied by the oculo-motor nerve, Cr III).

Parasympathetic division

Overview

The parasympathetic component arises from its own nucleus within the pons and travels with the main trunk as far as the geniculum. (The parasympathetic portion of the facial nerve between the brainstem and the geniculate ganglion is known as the nervus intermedius.) It then separates into two divisions:

- The *first division* passes through the pterygoid canal to synapse at the *pterygopalatine ganglion*, the postganglionic fibres supplying the lacrimal glands (tears) and the mucus glands of the nose, mouth and sinuses.
- The *second division* passes to the *submandibular ganglion* where it synapses with postganglionic fibres to the submandibular and sublingual glands (saliva and mucus).

Pathway

The first division separates from the main trunk at the geniculum, travelling anteriorly through its own bony canal within the temporal bone (at which point it is known as the greater petrosal nerve), emerging into the middle cranial fossa. Here it is joined by sympathetic fibres to form the vidian nerve (also known as the nerve of the pterygoid canal) which passes through the pterygoid canal to synapse at the pterygopalatine ganglion. The postganglionic parasympathetic fibres supply the lacrimal glands, nasal glands, and the mucosa of the nose and of the frontal, maxillary, ethmoid and sphenoid sinuses – for secretion of tears, nasal secretions and mucus from the various mucous membranes of the nose, mouth, sinuses and face.

The second division separates from the main trunk further down the facial canal between the geniculum and the stylomastoid foramen, along with the sensory branch to the tongue – together known as the chorda tympani nerve. The parasympathetic fibres branch off (travelling with the lingual nerve – a branch of the mandibular division of the trigeminal nerve) to synapse in the submandibular ganglion. Postganglionic fibres supply the submandibular and sublingual glands, enabling secretion of saliva and mucus from these glands and from the mucosa of the mouth.

(Note that the facial nerve does *not* supply the parotid glands, which are supplied by the parasympathetic branch of the glosso-pharyngeal nerve Cr IX.)

The pterygopalatine ganglion is located in the pterygopalatine fossa located between the lateral pterygoid plates of the sphenoid (posteriorly), the palatine bones (medially) and the maxilla (anteriorly), and is susceptible to compression, with potential repercussions on the glandular secretions of the face – lacrimal, nasal, salivary and mucosal. Free mobility of the palatine bones, along with the maxillae and vomer, as well as the sphenoid, can be crucial to a healthy balance of secretions from the facial glands, particularly as sympathetic fibres also pass through this ganglion. We will be exploring various contacts for addressing this area during subsequent chapters.

Sensory division

Overview

The *geniculate ganglion* (a sensory ganglion) is located within the facial canal at the geniculum. This is the site of synapse for the incoming sensory components of the facial nerve.

The main sensory branch carries *sensations of taste from the anterior two thirds of the tongue*. (Sensations of touch, temperature and pain from the anterior two thirds of the tongue are received via the trigeminal nerve Cr V-3.)

The other sensory branches leave the main trunk just below the stylomastoid foramen, branching off to receive sensation from the skin of the external ear canal, the tympanic membrane, and the mastoid and temporal areas behind the ear.

Pathway

The sensory branch to the tongue diverges from the facial canal between the geniculum and the stylomastoid foramen (half an inch above the stylomastoid foramen) together with the second division of parasympathetic fibres. It follows an intricate pathway, passing through the middle ear. Taste may therefore be affected by middle ear infections.

Having separated from the main trunk within the facial canal, it doubles back through its own separate bony canal, passes through the middle ear close to the malleus, and continues through another bony canal (the petrotympanic fissure), emerging into the infratemporal fossa between the mandible and the lateral pterygoid plate. It then joins the lingual nerve (a sensory branch of the mandibular division of the trigeminal nerve which carries general sensation from the anterior two thirds of the tongue) through which it reaches the tongue.

It is known as the chorda tympani during the portion of its pathway (together with parasympathetic fibres) from the geniculate ganglion until it joins the lingual nerve (just below the foramen ovale).

Clinical considerations

The principal consequences of facial nerve dysfunction include:

- Bell's palsy and other disturbances of muscle function in the face (motor branch)
- disturbed secretions of the lacrimal glands and the glands and mucous membranes of the eyes, nose, mouth, sinuses and face (parasympathetic division)
- disturbances of hearing and learning (nerve to stapedius)
- disturbances of taste (chorda tympani).

Factors which might affect overall facial nerve function include bony restrictions or imbalances, particularly involving the temporal and sphenoid bones, membranous tensions anywhere along the nerve pathway, and disturbance to the nerve root at the internal auditory meatus or at the pons. The nerve can also be affected by an acoustic neuroma in the region of the internal auditory meatus (where cranial nerves VII and VIII travel together) or by operations for acoustic neuromas potentially damaging the facial nerve. There may also be tumours or damage anywhere along its pathway.

If symptoms only involve the motor branches, this would suggest that the injury is outside the facial canal, either around the stylomastoid foramen, in the parotid gland (due to mumps), or along its pathway through the face.

If symptoms affecting the muscles of the face are accompanied by disturbances of taste and of the parasympathetic supply to the glands of the face (dry eye, facial secretions, etc.), this would indicate damage proximal to the emergence of the relevant branches – as with an acoustic neuroma or damage in the upper portion of the facial canal.

If only the parasympathetic supply to the glands of the face is affected without disturbance to motor function, this might suggest disturbance to the pterygopalatine ganglion, perhaps involving the palatine bones and the relationship between the palatines and the sphenoid, or imbalances of the autonomic nervous system.

Symptoms affecting taste only might involve middle ear infections.

Bell's palsy

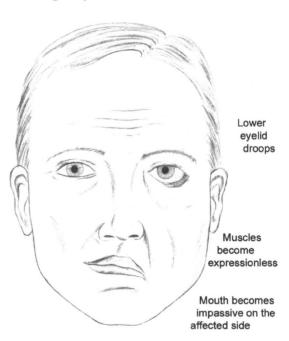

Lower eyelid droops

Muscles become expressionless

Mouth becomes impassive on the affected side

26.5 Bell's palsy involves flaccid paralysis on one side of the face

Bell's palsy (named after Scottish anatomist Sir Charles Bell, 1774–1842, who described the condition in 1829) involves flaccid paralysis of the face, usually unilateral, due to damage or impingement of the facial nerve (Figure 26.5).

Symptoms:

- The muscles on one side of the face droop and become expressionless.
- One side of the face remains immobile.
- The smile is crooked and one-sided.
- Tears tend to trickle from the affected eye, as the lower eyelid no longer contains them.
- Saliva may dribble from the affected side of the mouth.
- Food tends to collect in the cheek.

Bell's palsy can be transient, lasting weeks or months, or can be persistent, depending on the extent and nature of the damage. Strictly speaking, Bell's palsy is, by definition, of unknown origin, but with unilateral facial paralysis there will sometimes be a clearly identifiable cause, involving damage within or around the cranium. At other times it may arise spontaneously, perhaps following a viral infection. Causes of damage include stroke, tumours, surgery to remove tumours – particularly an acoustic neuroma – parotid gland surgery, head injury, nerve inflammation, middle ear infections, and latent herpes virus infection. Transient episodes may be brought on by cases of mumps (parotitis) since the nerve passes through the parotid gland.

Cranio-sacral approach

Cranio-sacral treatment for Bell's palsy will of course vary according to the nature and history of the condition, but would involve engaging with the system as usual and allowing it to reveal and resolve any restrictions or imbalances that may arise, whether in the cranium, the face or elsewhere. It would also involve identifying the site of damage both through the symptom picture and through palpation, tracing the nerve pathway with your therapeutic attention. It is also beneficial to engage with the muscles of the face, utilizing soft tissue stimulation and fascial unwinding to release and revitalize the muscles and helping to stimulate the nerve. It may be helpful to release restrictions within the parotid gland where appropriate. As always, it will be essential to ensure overall integration of the local area, the whole matrix, and the system generally in order to restore mobility and function insofar as possible.

Tracing the nerve pathway might lead you to the region of the internal auditory meatus in the case of an acoustic neuroma or nerve damage following an operation for acoustic neuroma, or might identify restrictions anywhere within the facial canal or along the nerve pathway.

Vera was 82 years old and she found her Bell's palsy very frustrating. It had started three years earlier following an operation for an acoustic neuroma and was showing no sign of abating. She found the cranio-sacral treatments very soothing and soon started to feel significant changes in her face from session to session. It was a slow process, but gradually her face became more active, more alive and more comfortable, and her eye in particular felt notably better. Unfortunately, the nerve damage was too great for a complete recovery, but she felt very pleased with the improvement that had been possible.

Associations with other cranial nerves

The facial nerve nucleus also makes connections with the second, third, fourth, fifth, sixth and eighth cranial nerves, coordinating movements of the eyelids and eyeballs, including the blink reflex in response to bright light or loud sounds.

Chapter 27

Cranial Nerve VIII – The Vestibulo-Cochlear Nerve

Principal functions

Sensory	Hearing
	Equilibrium

Overview

The vestibulo-cochlear nerve (Cr VIII) is the nerve which enables us to hear and also to maintain our balance. It may therefore be involved in hearing loss, tinnitus, vertigo and in Ménière's disease.

Formerly known as the auditory nerve, it is a purely sensory nerve receiving sensations of hearing and balance (through its cochlear division and its vestibular division respectively). The organs for both these functions are contained within the inner ear inside the petrous portion of the temporal bone.

The nerve has a short pathway, passing from the *inner ear*, within the temporal bone, through the *internal auditory meatus* (together with the facial nerve Cr VII) into the lower pons (Figure 27.1).

It consists of two separate nerves, travelling along very similar pathways, and therefore described as one single nerve.

Cochlear division

Sound waves entering the external auditory canal cause vibrations in the tympanic membrane (ear drum). These vibrations are transmitted through the malleus, incus and stapes (the ossicles) of the middle ear to the oval window, through which

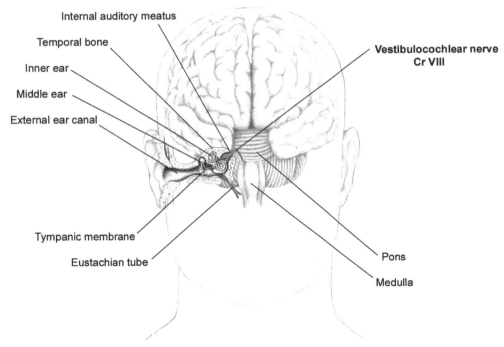

27.1   The vestibulo-cochlear nerve (Cr VIII) passes from the inner ear within the temporal bone to the lower pons

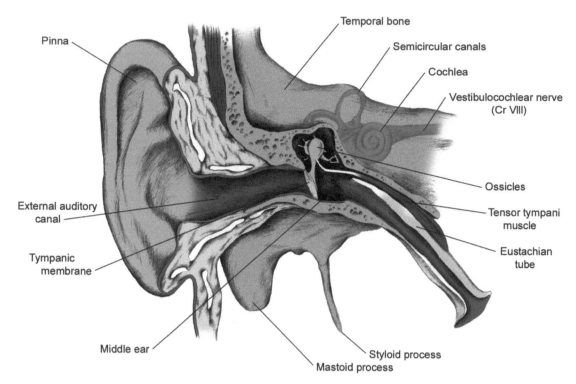

27.2   Sound waves entering the external auditory canal are transmitted via the tympanic membrane through the middle ear to the inner ear

they are transmitted to the cochlea of the inner ear (Figure 27.2). Hair cells of the organ of corti within the cochlea convert these vibrations into neurological stimuli, which are transmitted to the brain via the cochlear division of the vestibulo-cochlear nerve (Figure 27.3).

The sensory ganglion for the cochlear division is the *spiral ganglion*, located within the cochlea (Figure 27.3). The number of nerve fibres within the cochlear nerve averages around 30,000 in humans,[1] diminishing with age, leading to consequent hearing loss. Other species with more acute hearing have a greater number of fibres. For example, the domestic cat has around 50,000 fibres.[2]

Vestibular division

Vestibular sensations (balance and equilibrium) are picked up by tiny hair-like receptors within the vestibular system (from the ampullae of the semicircular canals and the maculae of the saccule and utricle) stimulated by the movement of fluid within the canals. These stimuli are converted into neurological impulses which are transmitted from the vestibular mechanism via the vestibular division of the vestibulo-cochlear nerve (Figure 27.3).

The sensory fibres of the vestibular nerve synapse at the *vestibular ganglion* (ganglion of Scarpa) located just inside the internal auditory meatus.

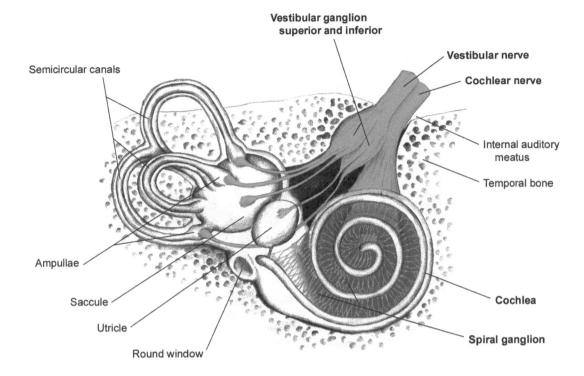

27.3   *The vestibulo-cochlear nerve carries sensations of hearing and balance from the cochlear and vestibular systems within the inner ear*

Pathway

The two divisions travel together from the *inner ear* as the vestibulo-cochlear nerve before emerging from the temporal bone into the cranial cavity through the *internal auditory meatus* (together with the facial nerve Cr VII) to enter the brainstem at the anterolateral pons (Figure 27.4).

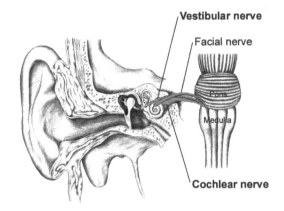

27.4   *The vestibulo-cochlear nerve passes from the inner ear through the internal auditory meatus to the pons, together with the facial nerve*

Clinical considerations

Disturbances to the cochlear division may lead to deafness and tinnitus. Disturbances to the vestibular division may lead to dizziness, vertigo and motion sickness.

Causes of damage to the vestibulo-cochlear nerve include infection of the inner ear, Ménière's disease, meningitis, encephalitis, head injuries, or prolonged exposure to loud noise. Other causes include acoustic neuromas (which may also affect the facial nerve as the nerves travel together through the internal auditory meatus) (Figure 27.5) and ototoxic antibiotics.

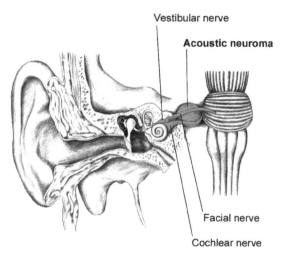

27.5 An acoustic neuroma may affect both the vestibulo-cochlear and facial nerves

Ototoxic antibiotics

One potential cause of damage to the vestibulo-cochlear nerve is exposure to ototoxic antibiotics, such as gentamicin and streptomycin.[3] These may be prescribed for various bacterial infections at any age. Gentamicin is used routinely in newborn babies as a prophylactic antibiotic, since it is effective against many bacteria. It is ototoxic and nephrotoxic. In other words it can damage the ears and the kidneys, and can lead to hearing loss. Its ototoxic effects are of course recognized. Levels are prescribed carefully to minimize risk, and babies are monitored carefully for any resulting neurological defects.

Cranio-sacral approach

The ears will be covered more fully in Chapter 35 exploring the structure and function of the ear in greater detail. The various disturbances involving the vestibulo-cochlear nerve and affecting the ears, including tinnitus, ear infections, glue ear, hearing loss, dizziness, vertigo, labyrinthitis, vestibular neuritis and Ménière's disease, along with an overall approach to working with the ears and conditions affecting the ears, will be addressed then, exploring how these conditions can be addressed through cranio-sacral integration.

Chapter 28

Cranial Nerve IX –
The Glosso-Pharyngeal Nerve

Principal functions

Sensory	to the pharynx, tongue and middle ear
Motor	to the stylopharyngeus muscle
Parasympathetic	to the parotid gland

Overview

Our glosso-pharyngeal nerves carry sensory impulses from various structures around the area of the throat, tongue and ears and consequently, in conjunction with cranial nerves X and XI, play an important role in enabling us to swallow and speak (Figure 28.1). Through their innervation of the parotid gland, they are the principal stimulators for the production of saliva and therefore aid in digestion and the various other functions of saliva.

They are predominantly *sensory*, but also carry a small *motor* component – also involved in swallowing – and a significant *parasympathetic* element (to the parotid gland). Their innervation of the tongue includes both somato-sensory functions (pain, temperature and touch) and the special sense of taste (particularly bitter and sour taste) – but only from the posterior third of the tongue.

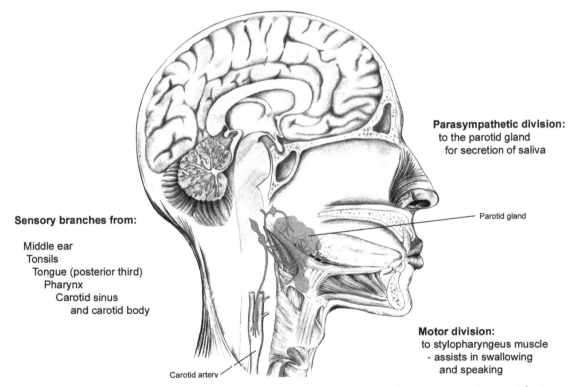

Parasympathetic division:
to the parotid gland
for secretion of saliva

Parotid gland

Sensory branches from:

Middle ear
Tonsils
Tongue (posterior third)
Pharynx
Carotid sinus
and carotid body

Carotid artery

Motor division:
to stylopharyngeus muscle
- assists in swallowing
and speaking

28.1   *The glosso-pharyngeal nerve (Cr IX) serves sensory, motor and parasympathetic functions, primarily around the throat and tongue*

Function

Sensory

The various sensory branches receive sensation from:

- the pharynx, tonsils and palate
- the middle ear cavity and auditory tubes (Eustachian tubes)
- the skin behind the ears
- the meninges of the posterior cranial fossa
- the tongue
- the carotid sinus and carotid body.

Motor

There is a tiny motor component, supplying just one small muscle – the stylopharyngeus muscle, which raises and opens the pharynx during swallowing and speaking.

Parasympathetic

The parasympathetic supply to the parotid gland stimulates the secretion of saliva.

Pathway

The glosso-pharyngeal nerve emerges from the anterolateral medulla, passing down immediately through the *jugular foramen* (together with the vagus (Cr X) and accessory (Cr XI) nerves) (Figure 28.2).

It has *two sensory ganglia* (superior and inferior) located within the jugular foramen. These are the sites of synapse for the various sensory divisions of the nerve.

At or below the inferior ganglion, it gives off several branches:

- the tympanic nerve – sensory and parasympathetic
- the nerve to stylopharyngeus – motor

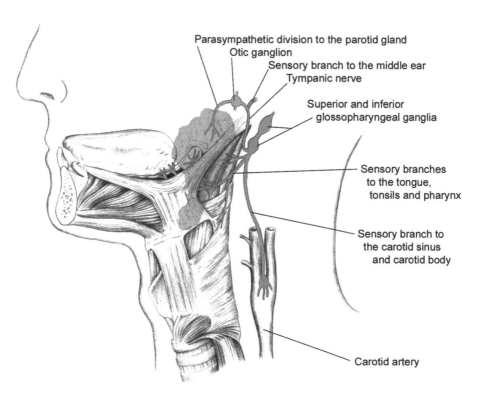

Parasympathetic division to the parotid gland
Otic ganglion
Sensory branch to the middle ear
Tympanic nerve
Superior and inferior glossopharyngeal ganglia
Sensory branches to the tongue, tonsils and pharynx
Sensory branch to the carotid sinus and carotid body
Carotid artery

28.2   The glosso-pharyngeal nerve and its branches

- a tonsilar branch – sensory
- a carotid branch – visceral afferent
- a branch to the tongue – taste from the posterior third of the tongue
- lingual branches – pain, temperature and touch from the posterior tongue
- branches to the pharynx and palate – sensory.

The *tympanic nerve* carries two types of fibre – sensory and parasympathetic:

- The *sensory fibres* receive sensation from the tympanic membrane, the middle ear, the auditory canal, and the mastoid air cells. The majority of pain from ear infections is transmitted via this nerve.[1]

- The *parasympathetic fibres* continue through the middle ear (as the lesser petrosal nerve), passing through the temporal bone, through the middle cranial fossa, and out via the foramen ovale to the *otic ganglion* (which hangs down from the mandibular nerve immediately below the foramen ovale). At the otic ganglion, these parasympathetic fibres synapse with postganglionic fibres to the parotid glands, stimulating secretion of saliva.

The *nerve to stylopharyngeus* is the only *motor* division, branching off to the stylopharyngeus muscle to assist in swallowing.

The *carotid branch* receives sensations relating to blood pressure, oxygen and carbon dioxide levels, and pH levels from baroreceptors and chemoreceptors in the carotid sinus and carotid body, located at the bifurcation of the common carotid artery, and influencing breathing and blood pressure (Figure 28.2).

The *pharyngeal branches, tonsilar branches* and *lingual branches* carry sensory information (pain, temperature and touch) from the pharynx, tonsils, and the posterior third of the tongue.

The *taste fibres* to the tongue travel separately from the other sensory fibres to the tongue, but travel initially along the same pathway as the pharyngeal branches.

The branches to the pharynx and palate contribute to the pharyngeal plexus together with the vagus nerve, and work in close cooperation with the vagus nerve (Cr X) and spinal accessory nerve (Cr XI) – both of which provide motor function to these same areas. When swallowing, the glosso-pharyngeal nerve provides the sensory input (together with the vagus), while the vagus and accessory nerves respond to this sensory input with appropriate motor function.

Clinical considerations

Disturbances to the glosso-pharyngeal nerve may interfere with swallowing, speaking, saliva secretion, and sensations of touch and taste (especially bitter and sour) from the posterior third of the tongue.

Chapter 29

Cranial Nerve X – The Vagus Nerve

Principal functions

Parasympathetic	to the thoracic and abdominal viscera – including the heart, respiratory tract, digestive tract
Sensory	from the viscera
Sensory	general sensation from the pharynx, larynx and palate
Sensory	taste and touch from the epiglottis
Motor	to muscles of the pharynx, larynx and palate

Overview

The vagus nerve is one of the most significant nerves in the body. It is the longest and most widespread of the cranial nerves. The name *vagus* means 'wanderer' and it lives up to its name by wandering extensively through the body, weaving its way through the thorax and abdomen, and diverging along many other nerve pathways. It travels from the medulla down to the lower abdomen, supplying a great many different structures from the cranium and throat through the thoracic and abdominal viscera as far down as the first half of the colon (Figure 29.1).

It is most commonly thought of in relation to its parasympathetic supply to the viscera – heart, lungs, digestive organs – but it also serves other significant roles, including sensory and motor functions. In fact, 80–90 per cent of its fibres are sensory,[1] carrying sensation from the viscera to the brain, including sensations of pain, hunger, the progress of digestion, and the state of the organs.

It is involved in speech, swallowing, cardiac function, respiratory function and digestive tract function. It regulates heart beat, the smooth muscles of the lungs which maintain breathing, and digestive system secretions and motility.

Vagus nerve disturbances are very common and may be responsible for a multitude of health issues, including asthma, digestive disorders and cardio-vascular conditions. They may be particularly relevant in persistent ill health with multiple symptoms, chronic fatigue, autism and many other debilitating conditions.

Because the vagus nerve is distributed so widely through the body, serving multiple functions and supplying many different organs and structures, its effects can be very widespread. It has connections and associations with many other neurological structures, extending its influence to areas beyond its evident supply, so that it affects and is affected by a wide range of influences, both physical and psycho-emotional, including mood and social interactions.

Recent research suggests that the vagus nerve has a wider range of functions and implications than has hitherto been recognized, and has led to the development of Dr Stephen Porges' Polyvagal Theory,[2] with significant clinical implications, particularly in relation to autism, hyperactivity, anxiety and chronic fatigue.

Pathway

Overview

The vagus nerve emerges bilaterally from the anterolateral medulla:

* passing down immediately through the *jugular foramen* (together with the glosso-pharyngeal and spinal accessory nerves and the internal jugular vein)
* providing various sensory and motor branches to the meninges, epiglottis, pharynx, larynx, palate and other structures of the throat
* then continuing down through the neck within the carotid sheath (together with the carotid artery and internal jugular vein)

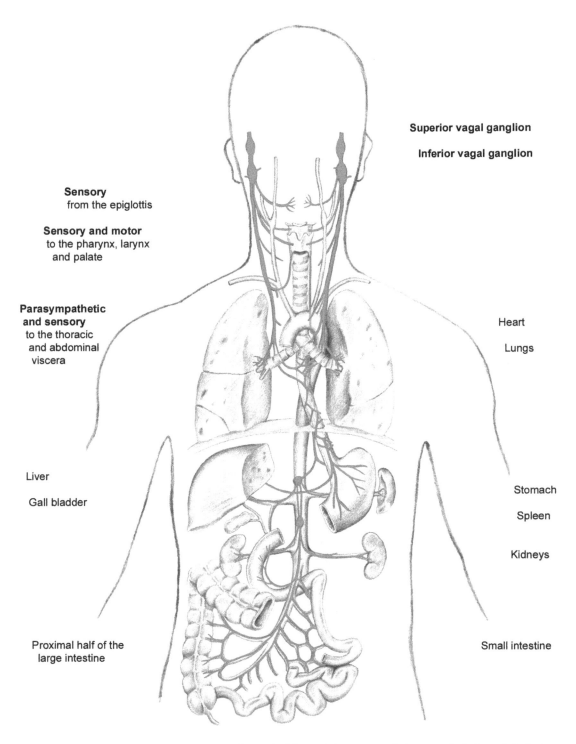

Superior vagal ganglion

Inferior vagal ganglion

Sensory
from the epiglottis

Sensory and motor
to the pharynx, larynx
and palate

**Parasympathetic
and sensory**
to the thoracic
and abdominal
viscera

Heart

Lungs

Liver

Gall bladder

Stomach

Spleen

Kidneys

Proximal half of the
large intestine

Small intestine

29.1   The vagus nerve is the longest and most widespread of the cranial nerves, wandering extensively through the body

- giving off branches to most of the organs of the thorax and abdomen
- passing through the diaphragm via the oesophageal opening
- providing parasympathetic supply to the viscera, and receiving sensation from the viscera, down to and including the first half of the colon (but excluding the adrenal glands).

Ganglia

It has two sensory ganglia:

- The *superior vagal ganglion* is located within the jugular foramen and is the site of synapse for the somatic sensory fibres from the pharynx, larynx, palate, epiglottis, ears and meninges.
- The *inferior vagal ganglion* is located just below the jugular foramen and is the site of synapse for the sensory fibres from the viscera.

Branches in the neck and throat

In the neck and throat, the vagus nerve gives off the following branches:

- a *meningeal branch – sensory* to the meninges of the posterior fossa
- an *auricular branch – sensory* to the external auditory canal and tympanic membrane
- a *nerve to the epiglottis* – a sensory branch receiving sensations of taste and touch from the epiglottis – a small flap of tissue which opens and closes the entrance to the trachea in order to ensure that food and drink pass into the oesophagus rather than the trachea
- *parasympathetic branches* to the mucous membranes of the pharynx and larynx for mucus secretion
- *motor branches* to various muscles of the throat, palate and tongue, including levator veli palatini and salpingo-pharyngeus, which assist in opening the Eustachian tube and may therefore be involved in middle ear infections
- two *pharyngeal branches – motor* to the soft palate and pharynx, contributing to swallowing and speech

- a *superior laryngeal branch – motor* to the muscles of the larynx
- three *superior cervical cardiac branches* providing *parasympathetic* supply to the heart
- several *inferior cervical cardiac branches* also providing *parasympathetic* supply to the heart
- a *recurrent laryngeal branch – motor* to the larynx.

The motor branches to the pharynx, larynx and palate are essential for swallowing and speaking, and operate in conjunction with (assisted by) the accessory nerve (Cr XI).

Recurrent laryngeal nerve

There are two branches to the larynx on each side – the *superior laryngeal nerve* and the *recurrent laryngeal nerve* ('recurrent' meaning coming back). The first branch very sensibly travels directly to the larynx. The second branch is known as the recurrent laryngeal nerve because it takes an interesting detour to the larynx, travelling down the throat and neck into the thorax, hooking under the right subclavian artery (on the right side) and under the aortic arch (on the left side) as they emerge from the heart, before returning all the way up the neck again to the larynx (Figure 29.2).

Why does it take this convoluted journey? It would be much easier for the nerve to run directly to the larynx on its way down. The reason for the detour is that we have evolved from more primitive animals. In fish, the equivalent nerves pass straight to the equivalent organs (the gills) passing beside the equivalent arteries – a straightforward and direct path. As mammals evolved, we developed necks which grew steadily longer. The subclavian artery and aortic arch remained in the thorax, the larynx ended up in the throat. The recurrent laryngeal nerve had to grow longer with each step of the evolutionary process in order to accommodate these evolving structural changes and maintain its pathway under the subclavian artery and aortic arch and back to the larynx.

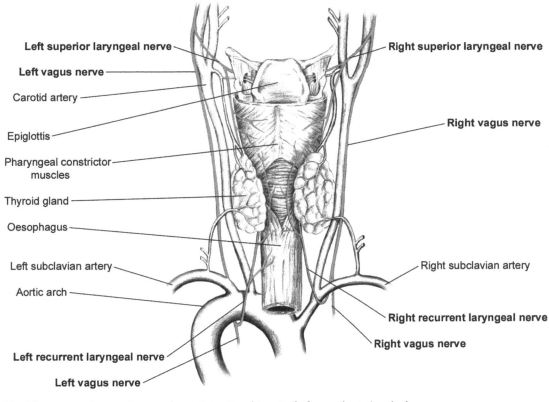

29.2 The recurrent laryngeal nerve takes an interesting detour to the larynx (posterior view)

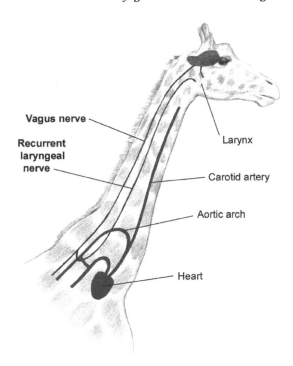

29.3 In an adult giraffe, the recurrent laryngeal nerve takes a detour of 15 feet in order to travel a distance of two inches

In humans, this involves a detour of around five inches for a journey that could be just half an inch. In an adult giraffe, this involves a detour of 15 feet in order to travel a distance of two inches (Figure 29.3).

The recurrent laryngeal nerves provide motor supply to the muscles of the larynx and are involved in speaking. Both left and right recurrent laryngeal nerves travel up between the trachea and the oesophagus, passing very close to the thyroid gland, so speech could potentially be affected by a thyroid tumour, by thyroid surgery, or by restrictions in the structures of the throat and neck.

Carotid sheath

In the neck, the vagus nerve travels within the carotid sheath, together with the carotid artery and the internal jugular vein. The carotid sheath is a fascial tube, intimately connected with the rest of the body fascia above and below. Fascial restrictions throughout the body may exert pulls on the carotid sheath, leading to constriction and disturbance of all three structures within the sheath, with widespread repercussions on arterial supply to the head, venous drainage from the head, and all the many functions of the vagus nerve. Identification of restrictions within the carotid sheath, whether due to local neck injury or transmitted from elsewhere in the body, and appropriate release of fascial tension and restriction, including fascial unwinding of the neck, can be crucial in relieving many obscure and multisymptomatic conditions.

Pathway in the thorax and abdomen

The main trunk of the vagus continues down through the body bilaterally, containing a mass of parasympathetic fibres travelling down to the viscera, together with an even larger mass of sensory fibres carrying sensations back from the viscera.

Each vagus nerve gives off branches to the thoracic viscera – the heart and the lungs – travelling through the cardiac plexus and pulmonary plexus (without synapse).

Within the thorax, the two sides start to differentiate, the left and right vagus nerves following different distributions and intermingling. The whole vagal complex gradually twists, so that the left vagus runs anteriorly and the right vagus runs posteriorly. There is then an intermingling of fibres just above the diaphragm, so that the vagus passes through the oesophageal hiatus as an anterior trunk (passing anterior to the oesophagus) and a posterior trunk (passing posterior to the oesophagus) – each trunk containing fibres from both left and right vagus.

The posterior vagal trunk then passes through the coeliac plexus (without synapse).

These combined trunks supply the abdominal viscera – stomach, spleen, pancreas, liver, gall bladder, small intestine, kidneys, and the proximal half of the large intestine.

Innervation of the colon

The innervation of the large intestine is clinically significant, because the vagus only supplies the first half, the remaining distal portion of the large intestine being supplied by the pelvic splanchnic nerves (S2, S3, S4) from the sacrum. This has implications for the diagnosis and treatment of conditions affecting the colon. Conditions affecting the ascending colon (on the right side of the abdomen), such as ilio-caecal valve dysfunction, may involve the vagus nerve (and might be traced back to the jugular foramen or the medulla). Conditions affecting the descending colon (on the left side of the abdomen), including left-sided irritable bowel syndrome (IBS), would not involve the vagus but would receive their nerve supply from the sacrum (and could therefore be affected by injuries, compressions and disturbance to the sacrum).

Also, because the two trunks intermingle, vagal influence within the abdomen on one side of the body would not be specifically attributable to the vagal nerve origin on the same side, but might be traced to the jugular foramen (or other regions of the nerve pathway) on either side.

Vital functions

The vagus nerve is involved in maintaining our survival and our everyday function from moment to moment. With its supply to the heart, lungs and viscera, its function is vital to life. It may potentially be involved in a range of heart conditions, respiratory disorders including asthma, and a wide variety of visceral dysfunctions, including colic in babies, peptic ulcers, irritable bowel syndrome, Crohn's disease, indigestion, diarrhoea, constipation, and many other conditions. Whilst damage could occur anywhere along its pathway, its most susceptible site of functional disturbance is at its emergence from the brainstem in the posterior cranial fossa around the foramen magnum, and most significantly within the jugular foramen, which as we have seen previously (see *Cranio-Sacral Integration – Foundation*) is a particularly vulnerable site.

Jugular foramen

Time and time again, the jugular foramen is found to be the source of a multitude of widespread symptoms and general debilitation, often misdiagnosed, undiagnosed, or mistaken for other conditions.

Passing through it are the internal jugular vein, the glosso-pharyngeal nerve, the vagus nerve and the spinal accessory nerve.

Compression of the jugular foramina, located between the occiput and the temporal bones as an expansion of the occipitomastoid suture, is very common, arising from birth trauma, childhood falls, head injuries, neck injuries, suboccipital tension, cervical tension, whole-body imbalances, and muscular pulls especially through the sterno-cleido-mastoid muscles. Disturbance anywhere in the system may reflect into the jugular foramina, with consequent repercussions on the vagus and the other structures passing through the foramen.

Compression of the internal jugular vein creates back pressure in the cranium and disturbance of fluid flow throughout the cranium, with multiple potential symptoms, as well as compression of the three cranial nerves within the foramen.

Compression of the vagus nerve can again induce widespread symptoms including asthma and other respiratory disturbances, palpitations and various cardiac symptoms and conditions, widespread digestive disturbance and disease, and the various repercussions on development and personality described under polyvagal theory.

Compression of the spinal accessory nerve may lead to torticollis, creating a cycle of disturbance throughout the occipitomastoid and upper cervical area, increasing and perpetuating compression of the jugular foramen, with aggravation of any vagal or venous disturbances.

The jugular foramina (along with the suboccipital region as a whole) are highly significant, potentially responsible for a very wide range of disturbances and disorders, many of which involve the vagus nerve.

Understanding the vagus – its functions, its distribution, its sites of vulnerability, the conditions that may be related to vagal dysfunction and its psycho-emotional associations – is of substantial significance to health and in the effective application of cranio-sacral integration.

Clinical considerations

Vagus nerve function can be disrupted through five principal means:

- injury or restriction to the efferent supply anywhere along its extensive pathway
- sensory feedback from the viscera and other sources

- disturbance within the brain and brainstem
- toxicity
- psycho-emotional factors, including sympathetic overstimulation, and ANS imbalance.

From a cranio-sacral perspective we need to identify and address all five possibilities.

Restriction to the efferent supply

This may involve:

- compressive and other traumatic forces imposed upon the brainstem and cranial base
- inflammation, sclerosis, and contraction within the posterior cranial fossa around the brainstem
- impingement within the carotid sheath
- disturbance elsewhere along its pathway, including the sympathetic plexi and the diaphragm.

Compressive forces

Compressive forces commonly arise from birth trauma, causing bony restriction, aggravated by muscular and membranous tension and contraction due to the shock effects of birth. Various traumatic forces may also be imposed by head and neck injuries. These forces may directly affect the brainstem, vagal nuclei and vagal nerve roots, or impinge upon the nerve within its surrounding structures including the cranial base, jugular foramina, foramen magnum, suboccipital and cervical regions.

Inflammation

Inflammation may be due to current or past meningitis, meningisms, lower level infections, or other inflammatory conditions affecting the membranes and tissues within the posterior crania fossa, cranial base and suboccipital regions, causing persistent tension, sclerosis, contraction, and irritation of the nerve.

Carotid sheath

The nerve could be impinged upon in the neck by tension and contraction within the carotid sheath (within which the carotid artery and internal jugular vein may also be affected). Fascial restrictions affecting the carotid sheath could be due to neck injury, neck tension, or fascial pulls from elsewhere.

Plexi

The nerve may be overstimulated as it passes through the cardiac, pulmonary and coeliac plexi, or through the oesophageal aperture of the diaphragm.

Sensory feedback

The vagus can be affected by sensory stimuli from many sources – visual, auditory, emotional, physical, visceral.

A common cause of vagal overstimulation is digestive disturbance feeding back from the gastro-intestinal tract through the sensory pathways of the vagus, bearing in mind that 80–90 per cent of the vagus nerve fibres are afferent:

> Any GIT distress can put pressure on the vagus and irritate it.[3]

> Symptoms of irritable bowel syndrome are thought to cause activation of the vagus nerve.[4]

> Activation of the vagus nerve occurs commonly in the setting of gastro-intestinal illness, or in response to other stimuli including pain from any cause.[5]

Toxins

Botox is known to close down the vagus, and mercury (present in amalgam and in various vaccines) blocks the action of acetyl choline (the neurotransmitter for the vagus). Various other toxins may also affect the nerve.

Psycho-emotional factors

Vagal disturbances will have emotional consequences as well as physical. The vagus provides a two-way communication system (motor function and sensory feedback) between the organs and the brain, independent of the spinal cord, and therefore plays a significant part in function and emotion – a point first noted by Charles Darwin in *The Expression of Emotions in Man and Animals* (1872).[6]

The vagal system makes a multitude of connections associated with facial expression, speech, hearing, eye contact, emotional wellbeing, communication and social interaction. Vagal function therefore influences our mood, emotional expression and social interactions, and our mood, emotional expression and social interactions influence our vagal function. Studies have found that higher vagal tone is associated with greater closeness to others and more altruistic behaviour.

Compensation for sympathetic stimulation

The vagus is also profoundly influenced by stress and sympathetic overstimulation, with consequent autonomic nervous system imbalance. Dysfunction may be due to persistent excessive sympathetic overstimulation leading to a corresponding parasympathetic overcompensation. Stress stimulates the sympathetic nervous system to override the parasympathetic system, leading to conflict – a tug of war – between sympathetic and parasympathetic, resulting in exhaustion and depletion of both divisions, with multiple symptoms of exhaustion and widespread dysfunction. The sympathetic stimulation could arise from birth trauma, other traumatic experiences, injury or stress.

Vagal disturbances may occur at any age and, particularly with birth trauma or early meningitis or other inflammatory conditions, may lead to a severely debilitated state in a baby or child, often unexplained and undiagnosed, potentially leading to severe developmental difficulties, including autism.

Microbiome

The vagus nerve is also able to read the gut microbiome and initiate a response to modulate inflammation based on whether or not it detects pathogenic or non-pathogenic organisms.[7]

The microbiome is the collective genome of all the microbes in the body – healthy and unhealthy. The microbiota is the totality of all the microbes in the body. (The two terms microbiome and microbiota are often used interchangeably.) The human microbiome or microbiota consists of around 100 trillion microbial cells.[8] Microbes outnumber the cells of the body by 10 to 1. They include bacteria, fungi and viruses.

In healthy individuals, the microbiota provide a wide range of metabolic functions which humans lack.[9] In unhealthy individuals, altered microbiota are associated with disease. Microbes are not an enemy to be eliminated or counteracted. They have evolved together with the body as an interactive symbiotic relationship, necessary for the development of the immune system, and for other aspects of development. It is known that germ-free animals possess an undeveloped immune system. Pathogens can disturb this symbiotic coexistence, leading to immune system dysregulation and susceptibility to disease.

Variations in the microbiome are associated with various diseases, whether through depletion of healthy microbes, or increase in unhealthy microbes. They play a part in various conditions, including autoimmune disease, obesity, schizophrenia, depression, anxiety, autism and chronic fatigue.

When an infant is born, their gut is quickly populated by commensal bacteria which affect their immune response. The immune system is able to recognize bacteria that are harmful to the host and combat them, while allowing helpful bacteria to flourish and carry out their functions.[10]

The presence of healthy bacteria in the gut creates a positive feedback loop through the vagus nerve, increasing its tone.[11] The presence of pathogens stimulates the vagus to modulate the inflammatory response. The gut microbiome will therefore influence inflammation, and the corresponding stimulation of the vagus can affect mood and stress levels.

Vagal symptoms

Initial overstimulation of vagal function (vagotonia) may eventually lead to vagal exhaustion with reduced function in the long term. Patients may also compensate for a vagal condition (feeling tired, listless and unwell) by increasing sympathetic stimulation in their day-to-day life in an attempt to override the vagal symptoms, leading to depletion of both components.

Overactive vagus

Vagotonia (overactive vagus) is an autonomic nervous system imbalance towards the parasympathetic division. Typical symptoms include hypotension (low blood pressure), bradycardia (slow heart rate), cold hands and feet, cold and clammy skin, and severe fatigue. It is also likely to involve digestive dysfunction characterized by overactivity of the gastro-intestinal tract, including pain, stomach cramps and intestinal spasms, and in the longer term may lead to peptic ulcers (due to persistent excessive acid production). It can also affect bladder control. It may sometimes lead to fainting (vasovagal syncope).

Underactive vagus

An underactive vagus leads to gastroparesis (reduced activity of the stomach). Typical symptoms include nausea, heartburn, abdominal pain, stomach spasms and, if persistent, may lead to weight loss. There may also be increased heart rate, arrhythmias, shortness of breath, and difficulties with swallowing and speech.

Recognizing vagal symptoms

Digestive disturbances (and other symptoms) could be due to an overactive or underactive vagus.

Vagal nerve disorders can also disturb the awareness of hunger and digestion through the sensory pathway, leaving the patient unable to recognize whether digestion is finished, and whether or not they are hungry.

Of course patients will not always experience all these symptoms. They may only experience a vague unidentifiable mixture of symptoms, easily mistaken for many other conditions (and often misdiagnosed). Patients will often spend many years going from doctor to doctor, receiving a wide variety of diagnoses such as postviral syndrome or chronic fatigue, and trying many different therapies and lifestyle changes.

Vagal disturbance can be difficult to identify, partly because the multiple symptoms are so widespread and non-specific, also because many of the typical symptoms – tiredness, fatigue, exhaustion, digestive disturbances and various others – are very common symptoms which could be attributable to many other causes, including stress.

Recognizing the vagal symptoms, while at the same time identifying causative factors including physical disturbances in those typical areas of the body where the vagus is commonly compromised, and psycho-emotional factors due to trauma or stress, may be the key to accurate diagnosis and appropriate treatment and is fundamental to resolution of any vagal condition. Appropriate cranio-sacral treatment is also likely to be beneficial for general health and function whatever the circumstances, and may prove beneficial in many cases of chronic fatigue and other conditions with multiple symptoms.

Vagus nerve imbalances

Maintaining balanced vagal nerve function is crucial to health because the vagus nerve plays such a vital part in regulating so many aspects of our physiology. Vagus nerve disturbances can be responsible for a wide range of dysfunctions – both transient episodes and, more significantly, in persistent ill health and debilitation, influencing not only our physical health but also our psycho-emotional state.

A healthy level of vagal tone enables the fluent function of many of our body systems, lowering blood pressure and heart rate, reducing risk of stroke and cardiovascular disease, improving digestion, enhancing blood sugar regulation, stomach acid secretion and digestive enzyme production, and reducing sympathetic stimulation. Balanced vagal tone is also associated with better mood, lower levels of anxiety and a more balanced response to stress.[12]

Low vagal tone is associated with cardiovascular conditions and strokes, depression, diabetes, chronic fatigue, cognitive impairment, and much higher rates of inflammatory conditions, including rheumatoid arthritis, inflammatory bowel disease, endometriosis, autoimmune thyroid conditions, lupus and many others.[13]

A shift towards a more parasympathetic or vagal state can be encouraged through a wide range of activities which either reduce sympathetic stimulation or enhance parasympathetic stimulation. These include relaxation – physical, mental and emotional, through yoga, meditation, social interaction, cranio-sacral integration, or any other means – eating, drinking hot soothing drinks (but not caffeine), warmth, hot weather, sitting by a fire, and taking a hot bath or shower.

Feeling cold stimulates sympathetic responses of peripheral vasoconstriction and pilo-erector muscle activation. Warmth is not only relaxing and comfortable in itself, but also counteracts this aspect of sympathetic activity.

There are also various specific techniques for vagal nerve stimulation.

Vagal nerve stimulation (VNS)

Where vagal tone is depleted, stimulating the vagus can be significant in restoring balance and healthy function.

Stimulating the vagus can reduce inflammatory conditions throughout the body, enhance immune function, reduce blood pressure and heart rate, improve digestive function, reduce food sensitivities and chronic digestive disturbance, enhance function of the liver, gall bladder and kidneys, reduce anxiety and depression, assist with chronic fatigue conditions, and influence mood, memory, sleep and emotional wellbeing.[14]

Stimulating the vagus nerve counteracts sympathetic nerve activity and therefore reduces stress, through the release of anti-stress enzymes and hormones including acetylcholine, prolactin, vasopressin and oxytocin.[15]

Research shows positive effects of vagal nerve stimulation for a variety of conditions, including anxiety disorders, heart disease, leaky gut, obsessive compulsive disorder (OCD), Alzheimer's, memory and mood disorders, migraines, fibromyalgia, obesity, tinnitus, alcohol addiction, autism, bulimia, severe mental diseases, multiple sclerosis and chronic heart failure.[16]

Medical use of VNS

The medical application of VNS involves implanting an electronic device in the chest which stimulates the vagus by sending repeated shocks to the vagus nerve. This has been used in the treatment of various conditions including rheumatoid arthritis, epilepsy and depression.[17]

Natural VNS

There are many ways of stimulating the vagus through natural means, including deep breathing, relaxation, submerging the tongue, and cold water face immersion. These can be used to relieve stress in the moment or, more significantly, can be utilized on a regular basis in chronic health disturbance in order to enhance vagal function. Establishing appropriate lifestyle factors through relaxation, mindfulness, a healthy diet, probiotics and social interaction can also play a very significant part in vagal function.

Deep breathing is clearly helpful at times of stress, but is even more significant for those with chronic debilitation. A few deep breaths may be beneficial, but far more productive is the establishment of a regular daily practice of mindfulness of the breath, thereby developing an unconscious habit pattern of deeper breathing 24 hours a day with consequent benefits to the vagal system.

Since *relaxation* plays a significant part in vagal function, meditation, yoga and other similar daily practices can be helpful. Research also shows that a positive outlook and a happy, kind, caring nature and a socially interactive personality are beneficial to vagal function.[18]

Submerging the tongue also stimulates the vagus.[19] This can be carried out by filling your mouth with warm water and holding it there for three minutes while breathing deeply (through your nose of course).

Cold water face immersion is one of the simplest and most effective means of VNS, readily applied in everyday life, with immediate reduction of anxiety, panic, stress, and sympathetic stimulation, also reducing inflammation throughout the body, and enhancing mood. For chronic conditions, regular application of cold water face immersion can enable improved vagal nerve function.

This process operates through the dive reflex.[20] It is most evident in aquatic mammals such as seals, otters and dolphins and also in diving birds such as penguins, enabling them to spend much longer under water by reducing oxygen consumption. In humans it is particularly significant in babies up to six months old. If a baby falls into water or is submerged under water, he or she is able to maintain respiration for a prolonged period through the dive reflex.[21]

The neurological response for the dive reflex is mediated through the trigeminal nerve (Cr V), which receives sensations of cold from the face and transmits messages to the vagus, which reduces heart rate and peripheral vasoconstriction in order to conserve oxygen. In doing this, it stimulates the whole parasympathetic nervous system, calming the system and restoring greater balance to the autonomic nervous system.[22]

Cold water face immersion is easy to apply in everyday life, whether to relieve stress in the moment or as a regular daily habit to counter chronic ill-health conditions brought on by vagal dysfunction. It can be carried out by immersing the face from forehead to chin in a basin of cold water for between thirty seconds and one minute while holding the breath. This can be carried out repeatedly as required. Simply splashing the face with cold water can be helpful to some extent, and making a habit of washing your face with cold water can have beneficial effects. It can also be effective to use an ice pack.

Parasympathetic function can also be influenced through the parasympathetic component of the oculo-motor nerve (Cr III) by applying a very soft gentle contact to the eyeballs.

One of the most significant influences on vagal function is our attitude and social interaction. Maintaining a positive outlook, a happy, kind, caring nature and a socially interactive lifestyle can have a profoundly beneficial influence.

Underlying cause

Such applications of VNS may be beneficial for relieving symptoms and enhancing function, particularly in cases of chronic ill health due to vagal disturbance, but from a cranio-sacral perspective, the principal aim is to release the underlying source of the vagal disturbance rather than merely stimulating a depleted vagus.

Cranio-sacral integration is likely to be beneficial in balancing the vagal system as a matter of course through the natural process of whole-person integration, but will be more specifically effective through the identification and addressing of specific causative factors that are disturbing the vagus.

Working with the vagus

The vagus may be disturbed by all the many factors described above – by birth trauma, compressive forces, structural injuries, meningeal inflammation, fascial restrictions, by feedback from the viscera, by sympathetic overstimulation, by toxins.

Working with the vagus therefore involves:

- recognizing the vagal symptom picture
- identifying the underlying causes to vagal disturbance – structural, inflammatory, digestive, emotional, traumatic, perinatal, etc.
- releasing restrictions (bony, membranous) around and within the brainstem
- release of the carotid sheath through treating the neck and through fascial unwinding
- reducing overstimulation of the cardiac, pulmonary and coeliac plexi via the heart centre and solar plexus centre
- working with the viscera – in order to relieve visceral symptoms such as spasms, pain, constipation, diarrhoea and poor digestion, to address underlying causes of digestive disturbance, and to reduce inappropriate sensory feedback from the viscera to the vagus
- settling the sympathetic nervous system
- reducing stress factors, managing lifestyle
- eliminating toxins
- overall cranio-sacral integration.

Patients with vagal dysfunction are often very depleted and may have been so for many years. With so many different factors involved, both in terms of symptoms and possible causative factors, a necessary part of the approach is general health care and support in conjunction with cranio-sacral treatment:

- In children this will be helped by establishing a calm, quiet supportive environment, reducing overstimulation, and establishing a healthy diet.
- In adults, relaxation, yoga, meditation, mindfulness, a healthy diet, stress reduction, and regular relaxation routines will be beneficial.

Cranio-sacral integration can play a very significant part in enabling this – identifying the relevant causative factors, addressing the relevant physical disturbances, establishing the necessary calm, peaceful state, and enabling overall integration of the whole person.

Polyvagal theory[23]

According to Dr Stephen Porges' polyvagal theory, the vagus nerve, formerly considered to be one functional unit, can now be seen to have two divisions, separate in structure, distribution and function, and arising from different nuclei in the medulla:

- an old vagus, concerned with primitive survival strategies, found in primitive vertebrates
- a new vagus, utilizing more sophisticated strategies, which has evolved in mammals.

The old vagus, also known as the dorsal vagus, arises from the dorsal motor nucleus, carries unmyelinated fibres and therefore responds more slowly, and regulates primitive vegetative function.

The new vagus, also known as the ventral vagus, arises from the nucleus ambiguus, carries myelinated fibres, enabling quicker transmission and therefore responding faster, and has more links to the body's communication systems.

This means that the autonomic nervous system, conventionally regarded as a two-division system (sympathetic and parasympathetic, either balancing each other or in conflict with each other and carrying out basic survival strategies), can now be perceived as having three levels of activity – one sympathetic and two parasympathetic – enabling different responses, which take precedence over each other according to circumstances:

- The new parasympathetic division enables a more sophisticated response to circumstances (particularly adverse circumstances) using communication strategies where possible – speech, facial expressions, eye contact, listening – as a means of dealing with the situation.

- Where this is not effective or appropriate, the system will turn to sympathetic responses of fight and flight, as the next step in the defence mechanism.
- Where this becomes impossible, the system resorts to the old primitive parasympathetic division, leading to a freeze response, in order to protect itself.

Appropriate responses to challenging circumstances

Because of its vagal connections, utilizing the active process of communication and social interaction is not only the most effective way of dealing with challenging circumstances, but also stimulates the ventral vagus to calm the system neurogenically, including the heart and other viscera, and reduces the destructive effects of sympathetic stimulus throughout the body, making us more metabolically efficient. When we deal with situations through this approach, we not only resolve conflicts, but also feel physiologically better inside.

Ideally, the response to demanding circumstances, threats and challenges will progress through those three levels of response, engaging through communication where possible and only resorting to the other levels where necessary.

However, patients with a disturbed vagus may be unable to activate the ventral vagus response effectively, and may therefore automatically go into fight–flight or freeze response. This may apply to those with autism, hyperactivity, bipolar disease or anxiety.

In a healthy state, the individual will respond to circumstances through the ventral vagal level of communication.

In hyperactivity, the nervous system is in an overstimulated state of constant sympathetic stimulation, easily activated, reacting to stimuli with further reaction, unable to process responses through communication.

In autism, the nervous system's inability to process information means that the level of stimulation is such that the system becomes overwhelmed and withdraws into a dorsal vagal level of freeze state.

Autism and vagal dysfunction

Autistic children often exhibit reduced facial expression, avoidance of eye contact, auditory hypersensitivity, disturbed digestive and other visceral responses, minimal communication, and withdrawal.

Normal levels of stimulus from the environment may be instigating exaggerated physiological reactions in the nervous system, heart, lungs and abdominal viscera. They are neurologically unable to process responses to circumstances in the environment around them, so their system becomes overloaded, they feel bombarded by overstimulation, they feel physiologically unsafe, and they either panic or withdraw.

Someone with a disturbed vagus nerve may therefore feel unsafe in ordinary everyday circumstances which others would consider safe. This is not a conscious cerebral decision, but an unconscious neurobiological reaction. Their neurological physiological response is to feel threatened. Their instinctive tendency is to see everyone as threatening, and to see neutral events as dangerous rather than pleasant.

The condition is physiological, not behavioural. If it is due to vagal dysfunction, it may render their nervous system physiologically unable to calm them and unable to activate a more sophisticated response. Once physiologically calmed, they will tend to perceive the world more neutrally and be able to engage more readily.

Addressing the underlying vagal dysfunction

With autistic children, it is not generally helpful to confront them through disciplined behavioural strategies or rational demands. It is necessary to address the underlying vagal dysfunction, both through appropriate external influences on vagal function, and through appropriate internal release of disturbances to vagal function.

Sometimes, parents can feel upset, disappointed, angry or rejected by their child's lack of response and communication, and may try to address the situation with an increased intensity of communication in order to elicit a response. This of course tends to make the situation worse.

In order to enable a more positive response, it is necessary to create a calm, quiet environment, eliminating distractions and disturbances, soothing and settling them, talking softly, not imposing demands such as eye contact or verbal interaction, allowing them simply to be there. This can engender feelings of safety, so that survival strategies of panic and withdrawal are not activated. The child can then feel safe and unchallenged, and can start to relax and open up as their internal physiological state changes and responds.

Creating a calmer, quieter state is not merely restful, reducing sympathetic activity. It is specifically altering the vagal response, inducing a physiological calming state on the heart, viscera and the whole body.

Porges (a psychologist) uses appropriate external stimulation to influence the vagal response – soothing, calming, creating a peaceful environment, and utilizing specific sounds – and reports very positive responses in autistic children.

Cranio-sacral integration does of course also create a calm, quiet environment, and also more specifically treats the physical body to release physiological disturbances which are compromising the vagus nerve, in order to restore balanced vagal function from within.

Cranio-sacral integration for autism

A significant aspect in treating autistic children involves establishing a quiet, peaceful environment, creating an atmosphere within which they can feel physiologically safe, taking care not to create any alarm or to stimulate sympathetic reactions that might take them into fight–flight or freeze, being undemanding of eye contact or verbal communication or any other interactions from them.

A cranio-sacral session is therefore ideal – a quiet, peaceful space where they can feel safe, with no demands to talk or respond in any way. This in itself will be therapeutic, but cranio-sacral integration can of course provide much more than that. Within that therapeutic environment, the therapist can then address any underlying vagal disturbance, through overall cranio-sacral integration, with attention to the specific areas relevant to vagal dysfunction – viscera, cranial base, brainstem or elsewhere along the vagal nerve distribution in accordance with the needs of the individual, along with any underlying traumatic causes of disturbance.

Working with the abdominal viscera can play a significant part in addressing vagal dysfunction. Relieving the spasm and tension in the viscera significantly reduces irritation of the vagus nerve, leading to a calmer state and improved vagal function. Initially the abdomen may be very sensitive and some children may find any contact overstimulating. So it is necessary to work gently at first. As the situation progresses, it becomes possible to work more deeply and fully and this can be very profoundly effective.

Faye's Story

Faye was five years old when she first came to see me. 'See me' is not really an appropriate expression, as she would never look at me directly, always looking away, hiding her face, occupying her attention elsewhere. Faye was autistic.

On her first visit, she was very shy and a little apprehensive, but as soon as she felt the magical feeling of engagement with her cranio-sacral system, her face changed, her body softened, and she settled comfortably into the treatment, welcoming the positive responses which she could feel spreading through her body.

She clearly enjoyed coming for treatment. Her mother reported that she always looked forward to her sessions. When she arrived, she was always eager to climb onto the couch of her own accord and get started and she welcomed my contact. Sometimes her little hands would move my hands to a different area of the body where she felt she needed treatment.

She had been receiving speech and language therapy for about a year, but was not yet talking, and she was also receiving other support, but progress had been slow. Her digestive function was very disturbed, with severe constipation. She was very easily alarmed by any sudden unexpected noise, which could leave her unsettled for hours or even days. She was fearful of many ordinary situations. Her communication was very limited, mostly to her mother, and generally consisting of just a few noises and pointing at things.

Initially there was a multitude of issues to address – severe contraction in her abdomen, digestive system and solar plexus, extreme tightness in her chest, neck and shoulders, and a very tight contracted head, especially in the temporal area, particularly on the left side. There was a great deal to do, and there were plenty of reasons to explain her condition.

Faye was very amenable to treatment. These various areas responded well – slowly but surely – and within a few weeks she was making significant progress. Her bowels and digestive system had settled completely. She was much calmer, no longer alarmed. Her speech and language therapist reported dramatic progress following her first cranio-sacral session and ever since. Her range of sounds and even words was expanding steadily.

Occasionally I would see out of the corner of my eye that she was looking at me, but as soon as I met her gaze and smiled, she would immediately turn away, giggle, and hide her face – but this was significant progress.

After a few months, Faye had progressed hugely. Week by week, her mother reported remarkable advances in her behaviour. She was talking. She had started mainstream school and her support teacher was amazed at her progress – observing how she was always exceptionally good the day after her cranio-sacral sessions. By now she would look me in the eyes – at least briefly – smile, and even say hello.

Her cranio-sacral system also felt hugely different. All the tension in her abdomen and solar plexus had disappeared completely. Her chest and thorax had softened significantly. Her head no longer felt tight.

Her left temporal area remained persistently restricted, even as the other areas softened, but eventually even this released and was accompanied by a significant leap in her speech and general progress.

One area, however, remained very resistant, and that was the area around her brainstem, foramen magnum, and posterior cranial fossa, where there was an intense contraction. It had been evident from the start, and it was changing, but only very gradually. Many of Faye's symptoms were typical of vagus nerve dysfunction, and the restrictions around her medulla and the roots of the vagus were undoubtedly highly significant. As that area steadily released, her progress again moved forward substantially.

By the age of seven, Faye was doing so well that she stopped coming for treatment – she was talking, communicating, playing contentedly with other children, progressing well at school. There were still aspects that weren't quite what would have been expected of a seven-year-old, but she had made enormous progress.

Chapter 30

Cranial Nerve XI – The Accessory Nerve (Spinal Accessory Nerve)

Principal functions

Motor	to sterno-cleido-mastoid and trapezius muscles
Motor	to the pharynx, larynx, palate (assisting the vagus)

Overview

The accessory nerve is clinically very significant and one of the cranial nerves which arises most commonly in everyday cranio-sacral practice. This is primarily because of its involvement in a three-way interaction with the sterno-cleido-mastoid muscle and the jugular foramen which can perpetuate jugular foramen compression and vagal impingement, along with all the many widespread ramifications described in the previous chapter (Chapter 29).

Through this same mechanism, it is particularly susceptible to compression from birth trauma and head and neck injuries, with consequent tension in the sterno-cleido-mastoid muscles leading to deeply ingrained imbalances in the cranial base and the upper cervical area, affecting the temporal bones and the balance of the cranium as a whole, with all the many repercussions on overall health, including the various dental and whole-body patterns described in the chapters on dentistry.

The significant feature here is its pathway through the jugular foramen and the upper cervical spine.

Two divisions

The accessory nerve has two divisions (Figures 30.1 and 30.2):

- The spinal division provides motor supply to the sterno-cleido-mastoid and trapezius muscles.
- The cranial division provides motor supply to the pharynx, larynx and palate (assisting the vagus in these functions).

The accessory nerve is also known as the spinal accessory nerve because, unlike any other cranial nerve, it has some of its roots in the spine (rather than in the brainstem).

Its two divisions are almost completely independent of each other, in their pathways and in their functions, as if they were two separate nerves, except that they come together briefly as they pass through the jugular foramen.

Spinal division

The spinal division, as its name suggests, arises from the spine – specifically the cervical spine at vertebral levels C1,2,3,4 (Figure 30.2). But instead of passing straight out from the spine to its destination (like spinal nerves):

- its four roots join together as a single trunk
- this single trunk passes up *inside* the vertebral canal within the dural membrane
- it enters the cranium through the foramen magnum
- here it briefly joins the cranial division
- it then immediately turns to pass back out of the cranium again through the jugular foramen (together with the glosso-pharyngeal and vagus nerves)
- to provide motor supply to the sterno-cleido-mastoid and trapezius muscles.

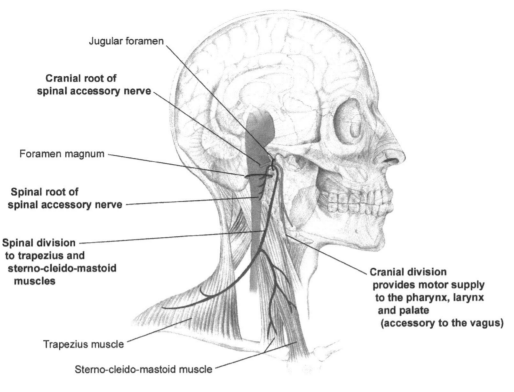

Jugular foramen

Cranial root of spinal accessory nerve

Foramen magnum

Spinal root of spinal accessory nerve

Spinal division to trapezius and sterno-cleido-mastoid muscles

Trapezius muscle

Sterno-cleido-mastoid muscle

Cranial division provides motor supply to the pharynx, larynx and palate (accessory to the vagus)

30.1 *The accessory nerve (Cr XI) has two divisions – a spinal division and a cranial division*

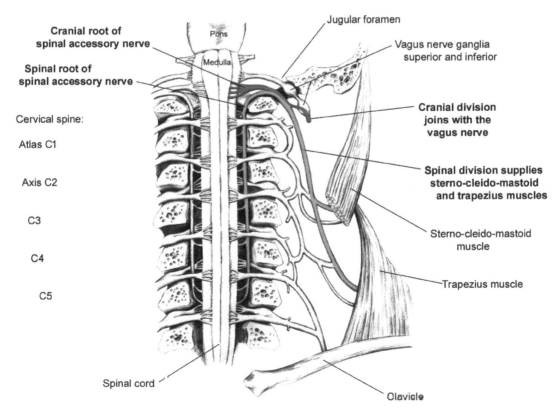

Cranial root of spinal accessory nerve

Pons

Spinal root of spinal accessory nerve

Medulla

Cervical spine:

Atlas C1

Axis C2

C3

C4

C5

Spinal cord

Jugular foramen

Vagus nerve ganglia superior and inferior

Cranial division joins with the vagus nerve

Spinal division supplies sterno-cleido-mastoid and trapezius muscles

Sterno-cleido-mastoid muscle

Trapezius muscle

Clavicle

30.2 *The spinal division provides motor supply to the sterno-cleido-mastoid and trapezius. The cranial division is accessory to the vagus*

Cranial division

The cranial division can be considered as an extra group of fibres belonging to the vagus nerve, and its function reflects this, since it is indeed 'accessory to' (in other words, assisting) the vagus in its motor functions to the pharynx, larynx and palate.

The fibres of the cranial division:

- arise from the medulla
- join the spinal division briefly
- pass out through the jugular foramen (with cranial nerves IX and X)
- separate from the spinal division
- then merge with fibres of the vagus for the latter part of their pathway, travelling to the same destinations in the pharynx, larynx and palate, performing the same functions as the vagus, and becoming virtually indistinguishable from each other.

Clinical considerations

The spinal portion of the spinal accessory nerve is particularly relevant in clinical practice.

Vicious circles

The sterno-cleido-mastoid muscle attaches on both the occipital (posterior) and temporal (anterior) sides of the occipitomastoid suture, so tension in the muscle will tend to compress the occipitomastoid suture and jugular foramen.

The tripartite inter-relationship between the spinal accessory nerve, the sterno-cleido-mastoid muscle and the jugular foramen is crucial:

- Restriction of the jugular foramen can lead to compression of the spinal accessory nerve.
- Compression of the spinal accessory nerve may in turn lead to tension in the sterno-cleido-mastoid muscle.
- Tension in the sterno-cleido-mastoid muscle further compresses the jugular foramen – leading to further compression of the accessory nerve, leading to further tension in the sterno-cleido-mastoid muscle, and so on ad infinitum.

In other words, each element of the cycle perpetuates a vicious circle of tripartite compression, over-stimulation, and spasm.

Birth trauma

Tension and contraction in the sterno-cleido-mastoid and trapezius muscles is very common. In some cases, this may be attributable to stress and psycho-emotional tension held in the neck and shoulders, especially when it is bilateral and symmetrical.

When it occurs as a unilateral pattern, it is most commonly attributable to birth trauma – a trauma which may establish patterns of disturbed health for life.

When a baby is born through the birth canal, the birth process involves a significant twisting of the head and neck as they negotiate the shape of the pelvic inlet and outlet. Combined with the compressive forces of the birth process, this frequently leaves some degree of twist embedded in the base of the skull and neck, compressing the occipitomastoid suture and jugular foramen either unilaterally or bilaterally, the twist often extending throughout the body. In many cases, this twist can be quite clearly evident, and in some cases it may manifest as infant torticollis. Even when there is no obvious external indication of torticollis, some evidence of this pattern may be imprinted into the base of the skull and throughout the body, and the same pattern is also clearly palpable in many adults, with underlying restrictions of the occipitomastoid suture and jugular foramen, compression of the accessory nerve and vagus nerve, and restriction of venous drainage through the internal jugular vein.

In a baby or young child, the restricted blood flow could affect brain development; and throughout life the compression of the jugular foramen may lead to symptoms of headache, migraine, neck pain, and all the many symptoms and dysfunctions throughout the body described in relation to the jugular foramen in the previous chapter regarding vagus nerve function.

Torticollis

Many cases of infant torticollis are attributable to this cause. Severe infant torticollis is often treated by surgery to lengthen the sterno-cleido-mastoid muscle, without any recognition of birth trauma, or this tripartite interaction, or the other imbalances in the cranium and neck. Although this may straighten the neck to some extent, it does not address the many other repercussions of the condition. Appropriate cranio-sacral integration at an early age can resolve the torticollis *and* resolve the other underlying torsions, imbalances and compressions, not only relieving the baby of its discomfort and asymmetry, but also enabling the restoration of a more balanced underlying state from which the baby's whole future can benefit, avoiding the possible consequences of various other discomforts and dysfunctions that could arise from that underlying imbalance and restriction – and of course abrogating the need for an operation.

The spinal accessory nerve may also be involved in adult torticollis (wry neck), in which patients experience severe spasm, pain and immobility in the neck, with the neck twisted to one side. This may be particularly likely if there is an underlying susceptibility due to a birth pattern involving a compressed jugular foramen. Appropriate cranio-sacral integration is generally very effective, involving a combination of gentle fascial unwinding of the neck and subtle engagement with the underlying patterns, with particular attention to the accessory nerve, the jugular foramen, the occipitomastoid suture and the upper cervical spine.

Autism

Even when the pattern of tension in the sterno-cleido-mastoid and trapezius muscles is bilateral, it may also be due to birth trauma, creating a pattern of tension and rigidity in the neck which can in turn affect not only the surrounding muscles and vertebral segments, but again affecting the vagus, with all its ramifications in relation to polyvagal theory. In treating autistic children, I have often encountered an extreme rigidity in the upper cervical and cranial base area, which appears to be contributing substantially to their autistic tendencies. Their symptoms will often improve steadily as the rigidity in the neck and the pressure on both vagus nerves is released. The vagus nerve can of course also be affected

by many other factors, and autism can arise from many other sources, so this is by no means the causative factor in all cases of autism.

Cervical spine

As well as receiving nerve supply via the spinal accessory nerve, the sterno-cleido-mastoid and trapezius muscles also receive direct innervation from the upper cervical spine (sterno-cleido-mastoid from C2, trapezius from C3,4), the spinal nerves emerging from the spine at their respective intervertebral foramina as usual and passing directly to the muscles. The fibres of the spinal accessory nerve join with these cervical nerves on their pathway to the muscles. Disturbances of the upper cervical spine will also therefore have repercussions on these muscles and on this whole vicious circle, and the upper cervical vertebrae also need to be considered in conjunction with the jugular foramen, occipitomastoid suture and accessory nerve.

Psycho-emotional contribution to the vicious circle

Furthermore, where the tension in the sterno-cleido-mastoid and trapezius muscles is due to psycho-emotional tension and stress, this additional psycho-emotional element may also feed into the vicious circle, initiating or perpetuating the whole pattern as a four-part cycle.

The interaction of compression at the cranial base, disturbed vagal and other function, and psycho-emotional disturbance is another three-part cycle which is very common. A baby or child who is hyperactive, ADHD, or considered to have a behavioural disorder may well be suffering from cranial base compression involving the various factors described above, and may consequently be very unresponsive to psychological support or behavioural training. If untreated, this pattern of behaviour may continue through childhood, teenage years and adulthood, establishing patterns of dysfunction, difficulty, and disturbed behaviour throughout life. Cranio-sacral integration, particularly at an early age, may often bring about a dramatic change in function and behaviour, potentially transforming that child's whole future.

Chapter 31

Cranial Nerve XII – The Hypoglossal Nerve

Principal functions

Motor	to the tongue

Overview

Your hypoglossal nerves enable you to stick your tongue out, move it from side to side and up and down and all around, using the various intrinsic and extrinsic muscles of the tongue. (*Hypo* is Greek for under, *glossus* is Greek for tongue.)

It is a purely motor nerve, mainly supplying the muscles of the tongue, with a small contribution to the suprahyoid muscles of the throat (Figure 31.1).

Pathway

The hypoglossal nerve:

- emerges from the lower medulla anterolaterally

- passes directly into the *hypoglossal canal*, in the condylar portion of the occiput, within the medial wall of the foramen magnum

- emerges at the inferior surface of the base of the cranium, immediately anterior to the *occipital condyles*

- then passes forward below the angle of the mandible, to provide motor supply to the extrinsic muscles of the tongue including genioglossus, geniohyoid, hyoglossus and styloglossus (but excluding palatoglossus which is innervated by the vagus) and to the intrinsic muscles of the tongue (Figure 31.2).

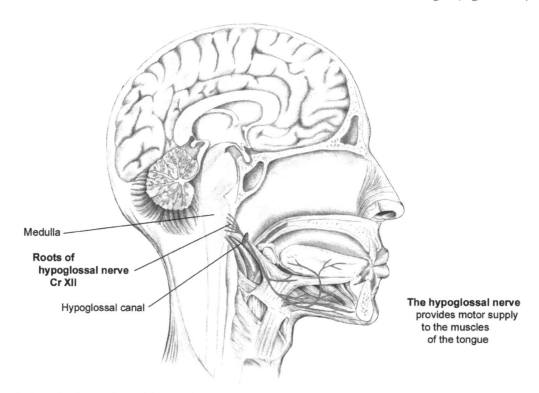

Medulla

Roots of hypoglossal nerve Cr XII

Hypoglossal canal

The hypoglossal nerve provides motor supply to the muscles of the tongue

31.1 *The hypoglossal nerve (Cr XII) is a purely motor nerve supplying the muscles of the tongue*

It also provides a small branch to the ansa cervicalis (a cervical nerve loop) which, together with cervical nerves from C1,2,3,4, provides motor supply to the suprahyoid muscles of the throat.

Clinical considerations

Occipital condyles

Because the hypoglossal nerve emerges from the cranium very close to the occipital condyles, it may be affected by distortions, imbalances and compressions of the condylar area. Distortions of the condyles are again a common consequence of the twisting and compressive pattern of the birth process.

In any baby or child (or adult) with impaired tongue movement it is advisable to check the occipital condyles and the suboccipital region, tracing the hypoglossal nerve along its pathway and ensuring the release of any restrictions or impingements on the nerve. A pattern imposed at birth may also manifest later in life if any underlying condylar imbalance is aggravated by subsequent tensions or injuries which may accumulate in the suboccipital area.

Tongue tie

This would *not* of course apply to tongue-tie conditions involving the frenulum, which are *not* neurological, and which need to be identified and addressed appropriately (as described in Chapter 5).

Suprahyoid muscles

The hypoglossal nerve passes through various muscles of the throat along its pathway, and tensions in these muscles may impinge upon the nerve. Release of the suprahyoid muscles and other soft tissues of the throat, particularly just below the mandible, may be appropriate.

Speech and language

Some speech and language difficulties may be the result of hypoglossal nerve compression, and appropriate measures need to be taken to identify the source of the difficulty – whether cerebral, neurological, structural, muscular, motor function, sensory, auditory or psychological.

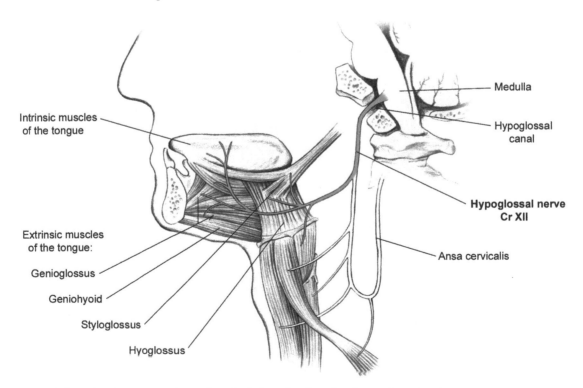

31.2   The hypoglossal nerve exits the cranium via the hypoglossal canal and passes forward to the tongue

Sensory innervation of the tongue (*not* the hypoglossal nerve)

Sensory innervation of the tongue does *not* involve the hypoglossal nerve, which is purely motor.

Sensory supply to the tongue, for both taste and touch, is provided by four different cranial nerves, and while on the subject of the tongue, this provides a useful opportunity to summarize that sensory supply (see below).

	Taste	*Touch, temperature and pain*
Anterior two-thirds	Facial nerve (Chorda tympani)	Trigeminal nerve (Lingual branch of mandibular division)
Posterior third	Glosso-pharyngeal nerve	Glosso-pharyngeal nerve
Epiglottis	Vagus nerve (Internal laryngeal branch)	Vagus nerve (Internal laryngeal branch)

Chapter 32

Autonomic Nervous System Disturbances in the Face and Head

Hyper-reactivity

In the 1960s and 1970s, physiologist Irvin Korr carried out extensive research into the effects of sympathetic stimulation, and demonstrated that increased sympathetic stimulus anywhere in the body increases the excitability of neural junctions and tissue reactions.[1] In other words, sympathetic stimulation not only carries out recognized sympathetic functions, but also increases the reactivity of other nerves (including motor and sensory somatic nerve pathways) and can therefore exaggerate all physiological responses, triggering increased physiological reactivity to any stimuli. *All tissues subjected to sympathetic overstimulation are in a heightened state of alert, liable to overreact.*

This has implications throughout the body, since there is sympathetic innervation to all parts. In relation to the face, it may manifest as exaggerated reaction to irritants, dust, particles, pollen and spicy foods, increased irritability of tissues causing itching, sneezing and inflammatory response, disturbed glandular secretions, enhanced sensations of taste, smell and hearing, and increased pain sensation.

Increased sympathetic stimulation may therefore contribute to any number of conditions affecting the face, including hay fever, rhinitis, sinusitis, allergic responses, hypersensitivity, acne, skin conditions, excess mucus secretion, ear infection, hearing loss, tinnitus, hyperacusis, labyrinthitis, visual disturbances, dry eye, vascular disturbances, migraine, headache, tension in the head, tightness of the intracranial membranes, tooth sensitivity, jaw pain, TMJ syndrome, trigeminal neuralgia, asthma – the list is endless.

Local or systemic

Increased sympathetic activity may arise as a result of local structural disturbance anywhere

along its pathway. Alternatively, it may be due to stress factors and underlying trauma.

Local symptoms may manifest in a particular area due to specific structural or physiological disturbances in that area. *Generalized symptoms* as a result of persistent stress or underlying trauma may manifest as a wide range of exaggerated physiological reactions and dysfunctions.

Underlying trauma includes birth trauma, childhood injuries, abuse, shock, car accidents, injuries, traumatic incidents of any kind – all of which may establish an underlying state of persistent systemic sympathetic overstimulation. This in turn may predispose to hypersensitivity, hyperactivity, agitation, reactivity to stimuli, and the whole range of symptoms and conditions associated with sympatheticotonia.

In patients with *widespread symptoms* and hypersensitivity, where there is an underlying increased level of sympathetic overstimulation predisposing to multiple symptoms – for which the cause of the susceptibility might conventionally be regarded as unknown or inexplicable – the first priority is to address the underlying trauma in the system through overall cranio-sacral integration, thereby reducing the sympathetic overdrive rather than merely targeting local structures and symptoms. This in itself may often be enough to eliminate the symptoms and perhaps transform the quality of life.

For specific *local symptoms* within that wider picture, or where the sympathetic overstimulation appears to be limited to a local area, it is also relevant to identify the cause of local disturbance and local increased sympathetic stimulation – such as a neck injury, a head injury, a nerve compression, a blow to the face, or any restriction to cranio-sacral mobility specifically affecting that area, or affecting the sympathetic nerve supply to that area.

Many conditions are frequently attributed to stress – irritable bowel syndrome, migraine, tinnitus, etc. – but it is necessary to question why the stress is manifesting as that specific condition in that particular part of the body, rather than as any of the many other conditions commonly attributed to stress. The implication is that there is some local disturbance which is rendering that specific area more susceptible. Stress may be raising the level of sympathetic stimulation throughout the body, but may manifest in a particular area or as a particular symptom as a result of an additional local disturbance.

In each case, it is necessary to evaluate whether the cause of the sympathetic overstimulation is local, systemic, or both – rather than merely attributing the condition to stress, or merely treating locally.

The autonomic nervous system plays a crucial role in our health, a role which is often inadequately acknowledged or understood. Both divisions, sympathetic and parasympathetic, play a major part in maintaining homeostasis throughout the body.

Sympathetic understanding

There is sympathetic innervation to every part of the body. Sympathetic nerve supply is vital to survival. However, excessive sympathetic stimulation, whether local or general, leads to dysfunction. It can have specific detrimental effects on physiological activity and is potentially highly destructive.

Excessive sympathetic stimulation reduces arterial supply to the cortex of the brain, reduces healing, contributes to hypertension, inhibits bone growth, inhibits pituitary and pineal function, facilitates spinal cord segments, and contributes to atherosclerosis, thereby predisposing to stroke and heart attack.[2] Sympathetic stimulation also reduces blood supply to the gastro-intestinal tract, leading to digestive disturbances, and to other organs including the heart and lungs, contributing to asthma and cardiac conditions. The meninges and fascia receive a particularly rich sympathetic supply and are therefore liable to widespread contraction and tension in response to trauma, shock and stress. Skin problems may also be due to disturbed sympathetic supply. In other words,

persistent sympathetic overstimulation is steadily destroying the body.

Sympathetic stimulation also tends to maintain its own vicious cycles, each stimulus generating further sympathetic responses:

> Once overactive and hypertonic, the sympathetic system often seems to generate its own stress and then responds to it with further activity.[3]

Consequently, a local disturbance or a facilitated segment[4] may lead to more widespread sympathetic stimulation throughout the body. Sympathetic activity generates agitation, agitation generates further sympathetic activity. Sympathetic excitement stimulates the release of adrenalin and noradrenalin, generating further sympathetic stimulation in an ever-perpetuating cycle – like young children at a birthday party becoming increasingly overexcited by each other's excitement.

Furthermore, within the sympathetic distribution, there is a ratio of 32 postganglionic fibres to each preganglionic fibre[5] – so the effects of stimulation of a single preganglionic fibre can immediately be multiplied many times, like the rapid spread of a rumour.

Acknowledging and identifying the effects of sympathetic overstimulation can be fundamental to resolving many disturbances to health, both through reduction of overall levels of sympathetic stimulation arising from stress, and through tracing and addressing the source of local structural disturbances along neurological pathways.

In relation to sympathetic distribution to the face and head, particularly relevant areas include the superior cervical sympathetic ganglion (SCSG), where sympathetic neurons synapse on their way to the head; the upper thoracic spine, where sympathetic fibres emerge from the spinal cord; and the whole sympathetic pathway through the neck and through the carotid canal. It also includes the local distribution of branches throughout the cranium and face to the eyes, ears, nose, sinuses and other regions, according to individual circumstances, including the pterygopalatine ganglia and other autonomic ganglia. As so often, the suboccipital region is crucial, and the many restrictions which accumulate there – from birth compression, head and neck injuries, imbalances from elsewhere in the body, postural disturbances and psycho-emotional tension – can play a significant part in maintaining and perpetuating sympathetic overstimulation in the head and face.

Parasympathetic overview

Parasympathetic distribution is more specific than sympathetic distribution, generally directed to specific organs in order to enable particular functions. Its role can still be very significant in many conditions. It has specific distribution to targets within the eyes, nose, mouth, sinuses, face and throat, including the lacrimal glands, the salivary glands, and the mucous glands of the nose, mouth and sinuses. It can therefore be involved in many of the conditions mentioned above, particularly disturbances of glandular secretions. It can again be affected by structural restrictions and impingement of nerve pathways as well as psycho-emotional factors and general health depletion.

Combined pathways

Autonomic nerve fibres follow their own distribution, but also often travel with cranial nerves for some parts of their pathway, 'hitching a ride' along the same pathway for convenience.

Parasympathetic fibres follow much of their pathway in association with a specific cranial nerve (cranial nerve III, cranial nerve VII, cranial nerve IX or cranial nerve X).

Sympathetic and parasympathetic fibres often travel together along the same pathways for parts of their journey when both are travelling to the same targets, in the same direction, or in the same region.

Various named nerves (e.g. chorda tympani, lingual nerve, short ciliary nerves, long ciliary nerves, vidian nerve) contain a combination of sympathetic, parasympathetic and sensory fibres which have joined together for that small portion of their pathway.

Sympathetic fibres also travel in association with most arteries – since every artery needs sympathetic innervation – and form sympathetic plexi at various locations (carotid plexus, tympanic plexus).

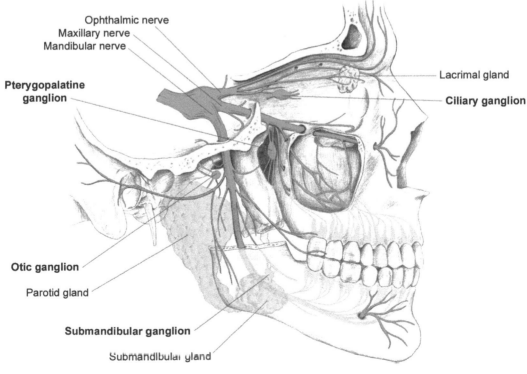

Ophthalmic nerve
Maxillary nerve
Mandibular nerve

Pterygopalatine ganglion

Lacrimal gland

Ciliary ganglion

Otic ganglion

Parotid gland

Submandibular ganglion

Submandibular gland

32.1   There are four pairs of parasympathetic ganglia related to the face

Ganglia

There are four pairs of autonomic ganglia related to the face – ciliary, otic, pterygopalatine and submandibular (Figure 32.1). These are *parasympathetic* ganglia within which parasympathetic pathways synapse before passing to their final destination.

Sympathetic fibres often pass through these ganglia together with the parasympathetic fibres, but do *not* synapse there. Similarly, sensory fibres may also pass through the ganglia (without synapse) simply for convenience of distribution.

Ciliary ganglia

The ciliary ganglia are associated with the eyes. They are located in the posterior portion of the orbits, between the optic nerve and the lateral rectus muscle. Preganglionic parasympathetic fibres travelling with cranial nerve III (the oculo-motor nerve) synapse here. Postganglionic fibres continue as the short ciliary nerves to supply the ciliary muscles and iris muscles of the eyeball.

The ganglia (and the short ciliary nerves) also carry sympathetic and sensory fibres.

Otic ganglia

The otic ganglia are located below the foramen ovale on each side, between the mandibular nerve (laterally) and the cartilaginous portion of the Eustachian tube (medially). They are the site of synapse for parasympathetic fibres travelling with cranial nerve IX (the glosso-pharyngeal nerve) passing to the parotid gland and the mucous membranes of the posterior tongue and the pharyngeal wall.

Sympathetic and sensory fibres also pass through the ganglion without synapse.

Pterygopalatine ganglia

The pterygopalatine ganglia (also known as the sphenopalatine ganglia) are located in the pterygopalatine fossa on each side, a space bounded by the lateral pterygoid processes of the sphenoid, the palatine bones, and the maxillae. They hang down from the maxillary nerve ('suspended like a traffic light from an overhead cable', as Sutherland described them[6]) beneath the apex of the orbit, with the sphenoid body superiorly, the pterygoid processes posteriorly, the vertical component of the palatine bones medially, and the maxillae anteriorly (Figure 32.2).

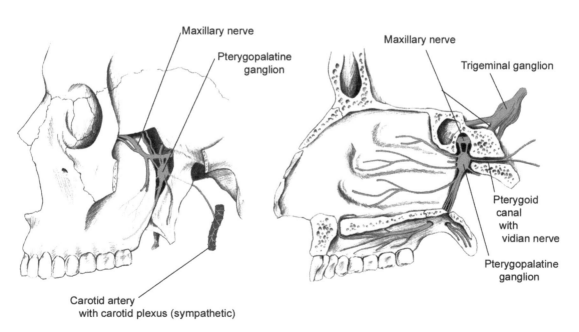

32.2 Parasympathetic and sympathetic fibres passing through the pterygopalatine ganglion play a significant part in disturbances of the face

They receive preganglionic fibres from the parasympathetic division of cranial nerve VII (the facial nerve). Postganglionic fibres supply the glands of the face, including the lacrimal and nasal glands, along with the mucous membranes and glands of the nasal cavity, the maxillary, ethmoidal and sphenoidal sinuses, the tonsils, the palate, the upper lip and gums and the upper part of the pharynx.

The ganglia also carry sympathetic and sensory fibres which pass through without synapse.

Submandibular ganglia

The submandibular ganglia (also known as the submaxillary ganglia) are located on the medial side of the mandible on each side, close to the junction of the ramus and body, just above the submandibular glands.

They also receive preganglionic parasympathetic fibres from cranial nerve VII (facial nerve). After synapsing in the ganglion, the postganglionic fibres supply the submandibular and sublingual glands, enabling the secretion of saliva and mucus from both glands, and mucus from the mucous membranes of the mouth.

Sympathetic and sensory fibres also pass through the ganglion without synapse.

Parasympathetic distribution

Parasympathetic fibres travel predominantly in association with four cranial nerves (cranial nerves III, VII, IX and X). The parasympathetic fibres emerge from their own separate nuclei in the brainstem, and follow much of their pathway with their respective cranial nerve, before branching off along separate pathways, travelling with other nerves to their various destinations (Figure 32.3).

Parasympathetic fibres synapse in a terminal ganglion (as described above) close to their target organ, the postganglionic fibres continuing the short distance to their final destination.

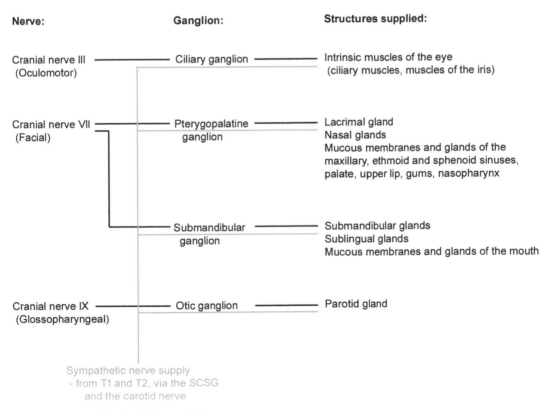

32.3 Parasympathetic distribution to the face

Oculo-motor nerve (Cr III)

Parasympathetic fibres travelling with the oculo-motor nerve (Cr III) enter the orbit through the superior orbital fissure (along with the inferior branch of Cr III). They then branch off to the ciliary ganglion in the posterior orbit where they synapse and continue as the short ciliary nerves, entering the eyeball to supply the ciliary muscles (for lens accommodation) and the muscles of the iris (for pupil constriction).

Disturbance to this parasympathetic distribution will therefore affect lens accommodation and pupil constriction, and may occur in conjunction with disturbance to the extrinsic muscles of the eye supplied by the oculo-motor nerve.

Facial nerve (Cr VII)

Parasympathetic fibres travelling with the facial nerve (Cr VII) enter the facial canal along with the facial nerve. However, they do not follow the facial nerve all the way to its emergence at the stylomastoid foramen. Instead, they diverge from the main trunk, either at the geniculum (first branch) or between the geniculum and the stylomastoid foramen (second branch).

The parasympathetic fibres travelling with Cr VII arise from the superior salivatory nucleus in the pons. Initially they travel under the name 'nervus intermedius' through the facial canal as far as the geniculate ganglion. The fibres then separate into two divisions.

First division

Some of the preganglionic fibres exit from the facial canal at the geniculate ganglion and travel through their own bony canal as the 'greater petrosal nerve', emerging into the middle cranial fossa, passing down through the foramen lacerum, where they join with sympathetic fibres (from the deep petrosal nerve) and travel forward together as the 'vidian nerve', passing through the pterygoid canal (at the base of the medial pterygoid plate within the floor of the sphenoid body) to emerge into the pterygopalatine fossa. After synapsing at the pterygopalatine ganglion, they are distributed to the lacrimal glands, nasal glands and other structures as described above (under pterygopalatine ganglia).

Second division

Other preganglionic fibres continue down the facial canal, exit the facial canal just above the stylomastoid foramen and branch off through a small bony canal as part of the 'chorda tympani nerve' (together with the sensory branch of the facial nerve to the tongue) and subsequently with the 'lingual nerve' (a sensory branch of the mandibular division of the trigeminal nerve), where they are joined by sympathetic fibres before travelling to the submandibular ganglion to be distributed as described above (under submandibular ganglia).

The chorda tympani nerve (including the parasympathetic fibres) passes through the middle ear, and may therefore be affected by middle ear infections, affecting taste and glandular secretions.

The lingual nerve is a branch of the mandibular division of the trigeminal nerve (Cr V-3), which receives general sensation from the anterior tongue. It also carries fibres from the facial nerve, receiving taste information from the anterior two thirds of the tongue (previously travelling as the chorda tympani) and parasympathetic fibres to the submandibular and sublingual glands (also previously travelling as the chorda tympani).

Disorders involving facial secretions – dry eyes, excessive lacrimation, reduced or excessive secretions of mucus in the nose and sinuses and mucus and saliva in the mouth – may involve disturbance of either or both of these divisions of parasympathetic distribution associated with the facial nerve. A particularly vulnerable area is the pterygopalatine ganglion.

(*Note:* These parasympathetic fibres, although travelling initially with the facial nerve, do *not* pass out through the stylomastoid foramen, nor do they pass through the parotid gland, so they would not be affected by injury or disturbance in either of these areas – both of which are potential sites of disturbance for the motor branches of the facial nerve.)

Glosso-pharyngeal nerve (Cr IX)

The parasympathetic division of the glosso-pharyngeal nerve (Cr IX) branches off from the main trunk as part of the tympanic nerve (which also carries sensory fibres to the tympanic membrane, the middle ear and the auditory canal). The tympanic nerve separates from the main glosso-pharyngeal trunk within the jugular foramen at the inferior glosso-pharyngeal ganglion. It then passes through its own tiny bony canal through the temporal bone from the jugular foramen to the tympanic cavity (the middle ear). The sensory fibres terminate here.

The parasympathetic fibres pass through the middle ear, continuing as the lesser petrosal nerve. The lesser petrosal nerve re-enters the cranial cavity through its own bony canal, exits the cranium again, either at the foramen ovale or through the spheno-temporal suture, and from there passes to the otic ganglion (just below the foramen ovale) where it synapses. The postganglionic parasympathetic fibres travel on to supply the parotid gland for secretion of saliva and mucus and also supply the mucus cells of the posterior tongue and pharyngeal wall.

Disturbance may therefore affect saliva secretion.

Saliva

Saliva is 99.5 per cent water, the other 0.5 per cent consisting of digestive enzymes, mucus, electrolytes, glycoproteins, and antimicrobial compounds. It is produced primarily by the submandibular glands (70%, a mixture of serous and mucous secretions), also by the parotid glands (20%, mainly serous), and in smaller quantities by the sublingual glands (5%, mainly mucous). There are also around 1000 minor salivary glands distributed throughout the oral cavity, mostly producing mucus.

Saliva serves various functions. It is essential to initiating the process of digestion of both carbohydrates and fats, through the enzymes amylase (also known as ptyalin) and salivary lipase. It also aids digestion by lubricating food, rendering it easier to swallow and digest.

Its lubricant function is also significant in forming a protective layer over the mucosa, protecting it from damage and disease. Saliva plays a significant part in oral hygiene, protecting the teeth from decay by washing away particles, breaking down food particles trapped between and within teeth, and through its antimicrobial properties. Inadequate saliva production increases the occurrence of dental caries, gum disease and other oral problems.

Saliva also plays a role in the sense of taste, by providing the medium through which chemicals can be transmitted to the taste buds and through its digestive enzymes and proteins. Inadequate saliva production can lead to decreased sense of taste or a metallic taste in the mouth.

Cranio-sacral integration may be helpful in treating inadequate salivary production by working directly on the salivary glands and through ensuring adequate unrestricted nerve supply, via the parasympathetic components of cranial nerves VII and IX, and also through their sympathetic supply.

In other species, saliva can also serve various other functions. Some mammals lick their wounds to promote healing. Many swifts use saliva to build nests. Some snakes use it to carry venom.

Vagus nerve (Cr X)

The vagus nerve (Cr X) is the most substantial parasympathetic nerve in the body. However, it does not serve parasympathetic functions in the face and head. Its distribution and function have been described in Chapter 29.

Addressing parasympathetic disturbance

In addressing any disturbance of parasympathetic supply to the face, the first priority, as always, is overall integration of the face, cranium, and the system as a whole. Within this context, it is necessary to consider the nerve pathways relevant to the circumstances, including their origins, bony relations, associated foramina, location of ganglia, membranous attachments and other connections, using whatever cranial and facial contacts may be appropriate according to the individual situation.

A common site of disturbance to the parasympathetic distribution is the pterygopalatine ganglion.

Within the context of overall integration of the face, relevant contacts for addressing disturbances of the pterygopalatine ganglion include contacts for the palatines, maxillae, vomer and sphenoid. It is also possible to take up specific contact at the pterygopalatine fossa (although overall integration of the palatines, sphenoid and the face and cranium as a whole are more likely to be relevant).

Contact for the pterygopalatine fossa and pterygopalatine ganglion

Stand beside the head on the opposite side of the patient. Take up contact on the spheno-frontal area. Once engaged, ask the patient to open their mouth, and insert the index finger up as far as it will reach medial to the mandible and lateral to the maxilla on the opposite side, with the pad of the finger facing medially towards the lateral pterygoid plate and the pterygopalatine fossa (Figure 32.4).

Sympathetic distribution

Sympathetic innervation originates from the hypothalamus, and preganglionic fibres pass down within the spinal cord before emerging at T1 and T2.

All sympathetic supply to the head emerges bilaterally from the spinal cord in the upper thorax at vertebral levels T1 and T2, and travels up the neck within the sympathetic chain, synapsing at the superior cervical sympathetic ganglion (SCSG) on each side.

Postganglionic sympathetic fibres continue upwards as the carotid nerve, travelling through the carotid canal together with the internal carotid artery into the base of the cranium. On the surface of the carotid artery, the carotid nerve divides into a network of fibres as the carotid plexus. On emerging from the superior opening of the carotid canal into the cranium (at the foramen lacerum) the carotid nerve passes up through the cavernous sinus, giving off numerous branches, widely distributed throughout the head and face. Sympathetic fibres travel with

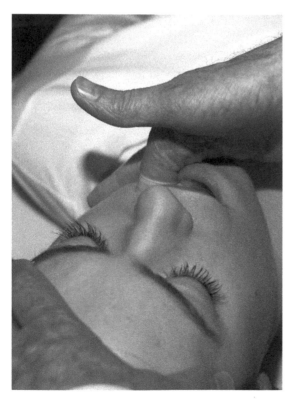
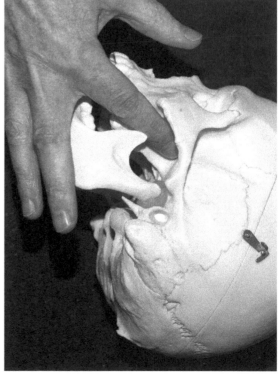

32.4   Contact for the pterygopalatine fossa and ganglion

most of the cranial nerves, joining their pathways briefly or for more substantial sections of their pathways, branching off in order to travel to the eyes, ears, nose, glands, arteries, and all parts of the cranium. Sympathetic fibres also join together with parasympathetic pathways and pass through the various parasympathetic ganglia.

One of the most common areas of sympathetic disturbance is the suboccipital region, particularly affecting the superior cervical sympathetic ganglion. Each superior cervical sympathetic ganglion is approximately one inch long, located on the anterior surface of the transverse processes of cervical vertebrae C1,2,3,4 on each side. It lies between the carotid artery and the jugular vein, medial and posterior to the ramus of the mandible.

It can be disturbed by compressions, injuries, restrictions and imbalances around the suboccipital region, upper cervical spine and the muscles of the neck, and by tension in the neck and contraction in the suboccipital area. Activation of the superior cervical sympathetic ganglion may lead to widespread sympathetic stimulation in the eyes, the ears, the nose, the sinuses, the pineal gland, the pituitary gland and throughout the head, stimulating contraction of the intracranial membranes, and potentially reducing arterial supply to the brain and throughout the face and cranium. Sympathetic fibres from the SCSG (and from all three sympathetic ganglia in the neck) also travel to the heart via the cardiac plexus, and to other structures outside the head and face, further emphasizing the significance of this crucial area.

Sympathetic disturbance in the eyes

Within the orbit, sympathetic fibres pass through the ciliary ganglion, joining with the parasympathetic fibres to continue as the short ciliary nerves to the eyeball, where they supply the muscles of the iris for pupil dilation. Increased sympathetic stimulation may lead to overdilated pupils and consequent photophobia (oversensitivity to light).

Sympathetic overstimulation inhibits lacrimal secretion and also causes vasoconstriction of arteries. Many symptoms affecting the eyes – photophobia, tired eyes, dry eyes, susceptibility to infection and other symptoms – may be attributable to excessive sympathetic stimulation.

Sympathetic supply to the eyes also assists in raising the upper eyelid through its innervation of the superior tarsal muscles – smooth muscles of the eyelid (with sympathetic nerve supply) – which act in conjunction with the levator palpebrae superioris muscles (supplied by the oculo-motor nerve Cr III).

If both pupils are dilated and photophobic, stress factors or suboccipital restriction may be the more likely cause. However, if only one pupil is dilated, particularly if this is accompanied by a drooping eyelid (ptosis), then damage to Cr III (responsible for pupil constriction and motor supply to the levator palpebrae superioris muscle) might be indicated, requiring more detailed investigation and treatment. If one pupil is constricted, in combination with unilateral ptosis and unilateral increased lacrimation, this would suggest loss or decrease of sympathetic supply on that side (Horner's syndrome).

Sympathetic disturbance in the ears

Sympathetic innervation travels to the ears from the carotid plexus. Within the middle ear it forms the tympanic plexus on the medial wall of the tympanic cavity (together with parasympathetic and sensory fibres of the glosso-pharyngeal nerve), where excessive sympathetic stimulation may contribute to tinnitus and hyperacusis and other disturbances of the ear.

In view of the increased reactivity of all nerves and tissues brought about by sympathetic overstimulation, disturbance of sympathetic supply is also likely to increase susceptibility to ear infections, earache, and various other conditions affecting the ears.

Sympathetic disturbance in the nose, mouth, sinuses and face

Sympathetic overstimulation in the nose, mouth, sinuses and face may inhibit secretions, leading to dryness and irritability of the mucous membranes. Once again, the increased reactivity brought about by excessive sympathetic supply is likely to increase hypersensitivity to irritants and allergens, contributing to dry nose, dry mouth, dry skin, hay fever, sinusitis and other disturbances.

Many of the sympathetic fibres to the nose, mouth, sinuses and face travel with the parasympathetic fibres associated with the facial nerve, passing through the pterygoid canal as the vidian nerve. These fibres then pass through the pterygopalatine ganglion before being distributed throughout the face, again highlighting the significance of the pterygopalatine ganglion. Other sympathetic fibres travel along somatic sensory and motor nerve pathways.

Migraine and headache

Sympathetic disturbances to the head are a significant factor in migraine, contributing to vascular disturbances, and may also be involved in many other forms of headache.

Addressing sympathetic disturbance

Once again, in addressing any condition reflecting disturbance of sympathetic supply to the face, the first priority is to consider the whole person – identifying whether the sympathetic disturbance is systemic, local, or both; and also whether it is stress-related, the result of a local structural restriction, or both.

Overall cranio-sacral integration of the system is likely to reduce sympathetic stimulation significantly, and if the causes are stress-related or trauma-related this may be the principal requirement.

Within that context, it will be relevant to identify specific disturbance to the sympathetic pathway, most commonly at the superior cervical sympathetic ganglion, subocciput and upper thoracic spine, but potentially anywhere along its pathway, identifiable according to the nature of the symptoms, and most significantly through cranio-sacral palpation.

Because sympathetic distribution is so widespread and ubiquitous, overall integration of the head and face, resolving any restrictions or imbalances and restoring full mobility and fluency, is likely to be more significant than tracing detailed pathways, and may therefore, as always, be the most effective therapeutic approach. However, specific local restrictions also need to be identified and addressed.

Summary

- In every patient with indications of sympathetic overstimulation, it is essential to assess the overall level of stress and trauma.
- If the system as a whole is overstimulated, overall integration including psycho-emotional factors may be the principal requirement.
- If the head and face are specifically affected, then within the context of overall integration it is relevant to assess and address the superior cervical sympathetic ganglion, the subocciput, the neck, and the whole sympathetic pathway to the head and face.
- If the symptoms are more local, for example eye, ear or sinus, then within the context of overall integration it may be helpful to explore specific local disturbances – bony restrictions, muscular and fascial tensions, mucous and vascular congestion, and any disturbance to the free fluent mobility of the area.

Sympathetic supply is fundamental to all parts of the body. Overstimulation causes excessive physiological reactivity of all tissues and nerves, and consequent dysfunction.

There is a multitude of sympathetic branches to every part of the face and head, passing through most foramina and along many different pathways. Informed awareness is helpful in tracing and identifying specific areas of restriction but, in view of the complexity of distribution, ultimately it is overall integration of the system as a whole – allowing the cranio-sacral system, in its infinite wisdom, to perform its own inherent treatment process – that will be most significant.

Sympathetic innervation plays a crucial and underestimated part in function and dysfunction. A great deal of unnecessary and ineffective medication is prescribed and treatment carried out to suppress symptoms which are due to sympathetic overstimulation. Understanding the sympathetic nervous system and its supply to the face, both in relation to stress factors and in terms of neuroanatomy and distribution, can abrogate the need for much of this unnecessary medical treatment, and can resolve many persistent conditions. As always, the key is overall cranio-sacral integration – of the face, the head and the whole person.

Chapter 33

The Cranial Nerves – An Abbreviated Summary for Quick Reference

I. Olfactory

Sensory	Smell

- travels from the olfactory mucosa of the Nose
- passes up through the Cribriform Plate of the ethmoid
- synapses in the Olfactory Bulb
- travels back along the Olfactory Tract
- to the Forebrain

II. Optic

Sensory	Vision

- visual images are received by the Retina
- they are transmitted from the back of the eyeball along the Optic Nerve
- passing through the Optic Canal
- the two optic nerves meet at the Optic Chiasma (in front of the pituitary gland)
  - the medial fibres decussate, the lateral fibres do not decussate
- the fibres continue as the Optic Tract to the thalamus
- they then continue as the Optic Radiation
- spreading out to the visual cortex in the Occipital lobe

III. Oculo-motor, IV. Trochlear, VI. Abducent

Nerve	Type	Function
Cr III Oculo-motor	Motor Parasympathetic	Eye movement Pupil constriction, Lens accommodation
Cr IV Trochlear	Motor	Eye movement
Cr VI Abducent	Motor	Eye movement

- the three nerves emerge from the brainstem (midbrain/pons)
- they travel forward together along the floor of the middle cranial fossa, on each side of the sphenoid body
- pass through the cavernous sinus
- enter the orbit through the Superior Orbital Fissure
- branch out in various directions

Cr VI (Abducent)	Supplies Lateral Rectus muscle	Abducts the eye
Cr IV (Trochlear)	Supplies Superior Oblique muscle	Directs the eye down and out
Cr III (Oculo-motor)	Supplies the other extrinsic muscles: Superior Rectus, Inferior Rectus, Medial Rectus, Inferior Oblique,	Other eye movements
	Levator Palpebrae Superioris.	Raises the upper eyelid
	Carries Parasympathetic fibres branching off into the eyeball	Pupil constriction and Lens accommodation

V. Trigeminal

Sensory	Sensation from the face
Motor	Movement of the muscles of mastication

Three sensory divisions

- Ophthalmic, Maxillary, Mandibular
- all emerging from the pons via the Trigeminal Ganglion

Ophthalmic division

Sensory from the forehead, etc.:

- travels with Cr III, IV, VI
- travels along the floor of the middle cranial fossa, on each side of the sphenoid body
- passes through the cavernous sinus
- enters the orbit through the Superior Orbital Fissure
- divides into three branches: Lacrimal, Nasociliary, Frontal
- the main Frontal branch emerges at the Supraoribital Foramen/Notch

Maxillary division

Sensory from the cheeks, upper teeth, etc.:

- passes down through the Foramen Rotundum
- enters the orbit through the Inferior Orbital Fissure
- gives off Alveolar branches to the upper teeth
- the main nerve travels along a groove/tunnel in the floor of the orbit
- emerges at the Infraorbital Foramen

Mandibular division

Sensory from the lower jaw, lower teeth, temporal area, ear, etc.:

- passes down through the Foramen Ovale
- gives off a recurrent meningeal branch which turns upward to pass through the Foramen Spinosum to the meninges
- enters the Mandibular Foramen (in the medial wall of the ramus of the mandible)
- travels through the mandible
- giving off Alveolar branches to the lower teeth
- emerges at the Mental Foramen

Motor division

(The Motor division is generally described as part of the Mandibular division, but in view of its distinct functions, it is helpful to look at it separately.)

Movement of the muscles of mastication:

- passes down through the Foramen Ovale (together with the sensory component of the Mandibular division)
- supplies the Muscles of Mastication (and other muscles)

VII. Facial

Motor	Movement of the muscles of the face
Sensory	Taste from the anterior tongue, etc.
Parasympathetic	Secretion from the glands of the face (lacrimal, nasal, sublingual, submandibular – NOT parotid)

- emerges from the pons
- enters the Internal Auditory Meatus (together with Cr VIII)
- travels through the Temporal Bone within the Facial Canal
- within the canal, it gives off a sensory branch to the tongue and two parasympathetic branches to the glands of the face

- the main motor branch emerges at the Stylomastoid Foramen
- travels forward through the Parotid Gland (NOT supplying it)
- and branches out to the muscles of the face

VIII. Vestibulo-Cochlear (formerly known as the Auditory nerve)

Sensory	Hearing and Equilibrium

- travels from the Inner Ear (within the Temporal Bone)

- passes through the Internal Auditory Meatus (together with Cr VII)
- to the Pons

IX. Glosso-Pharyngeal

Sensory	Sensation from the tongue and pharynx
Motor	Movement of one small muscle (Stylopharyngeus)
Parasympathetic	Secretion of Saliva from the Parotid Gland

- emerges from the Medulla
- passes out through the Jugular Foramen (together with Cr X and Cr XI)
- gives off a parasympathetic branch to the Parotid Gland

- sends sensory branches to the pharynx, larynx, palate, tongue and ear

V

33

X. Vagus

Parasympathetic	to most of the thoracic and abdominal viscera
Sensory	from the viscera, throat, epiglottis, etc.
Motor	to the pharynx, larynx, palate, tongue

- emerges from the Medulla
- passes out through the Jugular Foramen (with Cr IX and Cr XI)
- gives off motor branches to the pharynx and larynx, and a sensory branch to the epiglottis
- the main trunk passes down the neck within the Carotid Sheath on each side (together with the Carotid artery and Internal Jugular vein)
- to supply the Thoracic Viscera
- the left and right vagus then intermingle, forming an anterior and posterior vagus
- these continue down through the Oesophageal opening
- to most of the Abdominal Viscera
- as far as the first half of the Large Intestine (Colon)

XI. Accessory (Spinal Accessory)

Two divisions:

Division	Type	Function
Spinal division	Motor	to Sterno-Cleido-Mastoid and Trapezius muscles
Cranial division	Motor	assisting the Vagus to the pharynx, larynx, palate

Spinal division

- arises from the cervical spine C1, 2, 3, 4
- passes up through the Foramen Magnum
- joins the Cranial division
- passes out through the Jugular Foramen (with Cr IX and Cr X)
- separates from the Cranial division
- provides motor supply to the Sterno-Cleido-Mastoid and Trapezius muscles

Cranial division

- emerges from the Medulla
- joins the Spinal division
- passes out through the Jugular Foramen (with Cr IX and X)
- separates from the Spinal division
- merges with the Vagus
- provides additional motor supply to the pharynx, larynx, etc. (assisting the Vagus)

XII. Hypoglossal

Motor	Movement of the tongue

- emerges from the Medulla
- passes through the Hypoglossal Canal (within the wall of the Foramen Magnum)
- travels forward to supply the muscles of the tongue

Part VI

The Eyes

Chapter 34

The Eyes

Sylvia was suffering from intense pain behind her right eye. She had been suffering for years, with accompanying symptoms of severe headache, neck pain, tightness in the right side of her head, poor memory, and difficulty concentrating. Her ability to work was seriously affected, and she was struggling to keep her job. She had seen several doctors and specialists, all of whom said that there was nothing wrong and that it was psychosomatic. She was living on pain killers.

Her symptoms were the classic indications of the chronic after-effects of meningitis. She had indeed had meningitis twenty years previously, which was when the symptoms had started, but all her doctors insisted that the symptoms had nothing to do with the meningitis and that she was simply stressed or malingering – a concept with which she could not identify at all.

Taking up contact on Sylvia's head, it was clearly evident that the right side of her head was extremely tight – typical of the severe contraction of the meninges – and pulling down into the right side of her neck. The first treatment brought substantial relief and Sylvia felt better than she had done in years. It took a few further sessions to clear the restriction completely, since the condition had been there for so long, but in due course Sylvia was completely symptom-free and feeling healthier than she could ever remember.

One of the more common but often unrecognized causes of persistent pain in the eyes is the chronic after-effects of meningitis or meningism.[1] In some cases there may be a clear diagnosis of meningitis in the history. Often, there has been no specific diagnosis, just a milder, perhaps unremarkable, cold or ear infection which has led to inflammation and consequent sclerosis of the meninges. But the typical contracted quality in the tissues is very distinctive and can be clearly palpated cranio-sacrally.

Introduction

Our eyes are an integral part of everyday function, in constant use throughout most of our waking life, crucial to carrying out most of our day-to-day activities, structures which we certainly wish to preserve in optimal health insofar as possible, yet easily taken for granted – until their function becomes disturbed.

They are complex structures, so complex that they used to be regarded as evidence against evolution, too complicated to have evolved naturally, but in fact a remarkable example of the power of evolution.

They are also very delicate structures, which need to be looked after with great care, susceptible to a wide range of diseases and dysfunctions.

Symptoms affecting the eyes include squint, astigmatism, persistent pain, recurrent infection, dry eye, excessive lacrimal secretions, blocked lacrimal ducts, photosensitivity, pressure, eye strain, myopia, hyperopia, poor vision, deteriorating vision, loss of sight, and various visual disturbances.

They can be subject to direct injury, which may damage the eye itself, or distort the orbit and associated structures, leading to disturbed function.

They may be affected as part of a wider symptom picture, as in diabetes, rheumatoid disease or Bell's palsy. There are also numerous pathologies associated with the eyes, such as glaucoma, to which it is essential to be alert, since several of these can lead rapidly to blindness. They will be addressed below.

Complex structures

There are a great many structures involved in the eye – seven different bones contributing to each orbit, six extrinsic muscles, various intrinsic muscles, six cranial nerves, sympathetic and parasympathetic nerve supply, lacrimal glands, arterial supply, venous drainage, and the eyeball itself – and therefore plenty of potential causes of dysfunction. The eyes are readily susceptible to infection and disturbance. The overall balance of the cranium and the face inevitably influences their function, and so therefore does the balance of the cranio-sacral system as a whole.

They are particularly susceptible to membranous tensions, whether from meningitis or from psycho-emotional pressure, partly due to potential impingement on the many cranial nerve and vascular pathways which supply them, but also because of the inherent structure of the eye. The eye is not a separate organ. It is an extension of the brain; and the sclera – the membrane enveloping the eyeball – is therefore an adapted extension of the dural membrane, connected via the optic nerve pathway to the rest of the intracranial membranes. Membranous tensions can therefore be directly transmitted to the eyeball – one reason why the effects of meningitis may be so keenly felt in the eyes.

Another common cause of discomfort in the eyes is disturbance of the sympathetic nerve supply – whether due to contraction of the meninges or through direct sympathetic supply to the eyes themselves. This may be due to injury and structural restriction of the sympathetic pathway, particularly in the upper cervical, upper thoracic and suboccipital areas. It may also be due to stress and psycho-emotional factors – whether due to current stresses or past trauma. Photosensitivity, reactivity to flash photography, sensitivity to car headlights and other bright lights, eye strain from persistent use of computer monitors – potentially leading to headache and migraine – and other sensations of weakness in the eyes may be indications of sympathetic disturbance.

Cranio-sacral integration often brings a sense of ease to the eyes and a greater clarity of vision, even when the treatment is not specifically directed at the eyes, as a result of the release of tensions and restrictions throughout the system which have been affecting the eyes. It can also play a significant part in addressing specific conditions affecting the eyes.

Causes of disturbance

The causes of disturbance to the eyes include all the usual factors – birth patterns, genetic patterns, head and neck injuries, facial injuries, whole-body imbalances, infections, pathologies, distortion of the orbit or the cranium, compression of foramina, contraction of membranes, impingement of nerve supply, blood vessels and lymphatic drainage. These disturbances can, as always, originate anywhere in the body.

ANATOMY OF THE EYE

- Bones
- Foramina
- Muscles
- Membranes
- Nerve supply
- Arterial supply
- Venous drainage
- The eyeball

Bones

There are seven different bones which contribute to each orbit (Figure 34.1):

- the frontal bone – forms the roof and superior rim of the orbit
- the maxilla – forms the floor, medial rim and anteromedial rim
- the zygoma – forms the lateral wall, lateral floor, and anterolateral rim
- the sphenoid:
  - the greater wing – forms the posterior portion of the lateral wall
  - the lesser wing – forms the posterior portion of the roof
  - the body – forms the posterior portion of the medial wall
- the ethmoid – forms the medial wall
- the lacrimal bone – forms the anterior portion of the medial wall
- the palatine bone – the orbital plate of each palatine bone forms a tiny portion of the floor, just below the optic canal.

VI

34

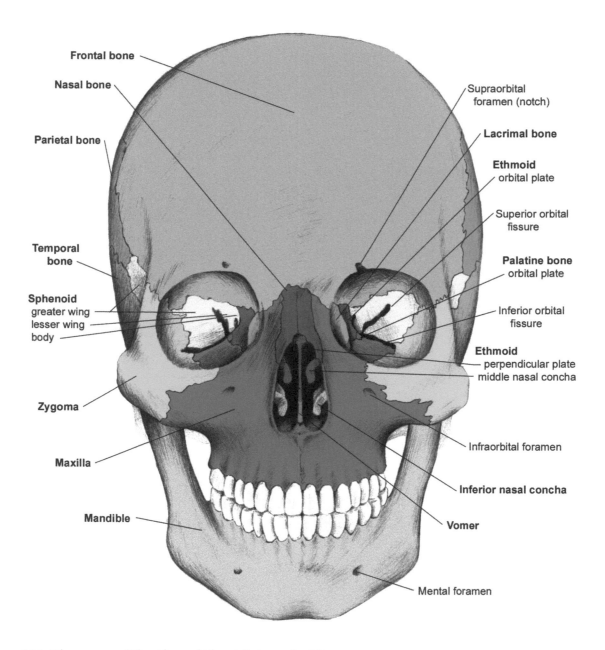

34.1   There are seven different bones which contribute to each orbit

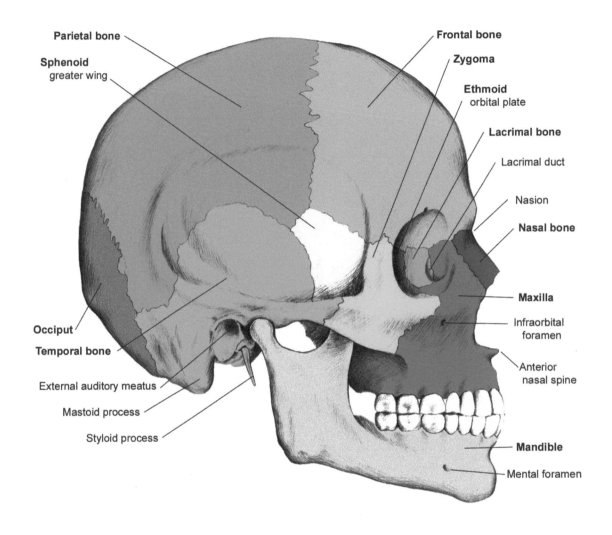

Parietal bone

Sphenoid
greater wing

Occiput

Temporal bone

External auditory meatus

Mastoid process

Styloid process

Frontal bone

Zygoma

Ethmoid
orbital plate

Lacrimal bone

Lacrimal duct

Nasion

Nasal bone

Maxilla

Infraorbital
foramen

Anterior
nasal spine

Mandible

Mental foramen

34.2   The orbit and cranium – Lateral view

VI

34

The sphenoid is of particular significance, not only because it plays such a central role in the balance of the cranium as a whole, articulating with every other bone of the cranium and several bones of the face and orbit. It also forms a substantial portion of the back of the orbit through its body, greater wings and lesser wings. Several of the cranial nerves, blood vessels and other structures supplying the eyes and orbit travel in close relation to the sphenoid throughout their pathway and pass through foramina and fissures within the sphenoid, within which they may be compressed. These include cranial nerves II, III, IV, V and VI, and the ophthalmic artery and ophthalmic vein (Figure 34.3).

Disturbances of the occiput and suboccipital area are also particularly relevant. The visual cortex – where visual images are processed and interpreted – is located within the occipital lobe of the brain. Injury or restriction to the occiput or upper cervical spine may impact directly on the visual cortex, or restrict the arterial blood supply to the occipital lobe through the basilar and vertebral arteries. Venous drainage may also be affected through the confluence of sinuses, the transverse sinuses, sigmoid sinuses and down through the jugular foramina, potentially leading to venous back pressure throughout the intracranial venous system. The visual disturbances associated with migraine (and in fact the whole propensity to migraine) can often be related to vascular disturbance resulting from injury or compression at the occiput and suboccipital region. The sympathetic pathway to the head and eyes also passes through this area.

Foramina

The many nerves and blood vessels supplying the eye and orbit pass through various foramina in order to reach their destination (Figures 34.3 and 34.4). These are areas of potential distortion and compression and can play a significant part in the function of the eyes.

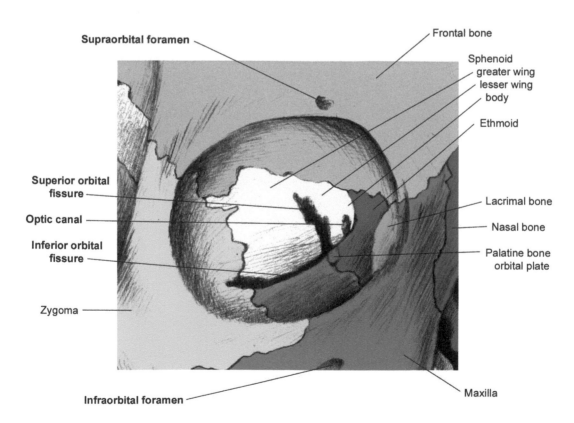

34.3 The many nerves and blood vessels supplying the eye and orbit pass through various foramina in order to reach their destination

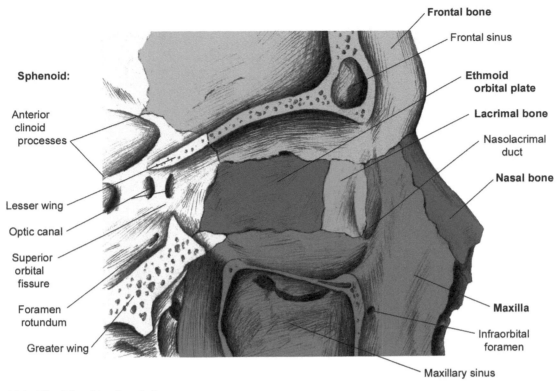

Frontal bone
Frontal sinus
Ethmoid orbital plate
Lacrimal bone
Nasolacrimal duct
Nasal bone
Maxilla
Infraorbital foramen
Maxillary sinus

Sphenoid:
Anterior clinoid processes
Lesser wing
Optic canal
Superior orbital fissure
Foramen rotundum
Greater wing

34.4   The right orbit – lateral view

The *optic canal* passes between the body and the lesser wing of the sphenoid, carrying the optic nerve (cranial nerve II) and the ophthalmic artery.

The *superior orbital fissure* lies between the lesser and greater wings of the sphenoid and carries cranial nerves III, IV and VI (oculomotor, trochlear and abducent), the ophthalmic branch of cranial nerve V (trigeminal) and the ophthalmic vein, all of which may be susceptible to compression of the fissure or disturbances of the sphenoid.

The *inferior orbital fissure* is located between the greater wing of the sphenoid and the horizontal portion of the maxilla, and allows entry of the maxillary branch of the trigeminal nerve (Cr V-2) into and along the floor of the orbit.

The *supraorbital foramen* (or supraorbital notch) is located within the superior rim of the orbit, carrying the frontal nerve, a branch of the ophthalmic division of the trigeminal nerve (Cr V-1) which emerges to the surface of the face at this point, receiving sensory input from the forehead and frontal region of the face. It can be a painful trigger spot in trigeminal neuralgia, and sensitive in headaches and migraine. Pressure on this spot can also sometimes bring relief of local pain.

The *infraorbital foramen* is located within the maxilla, inferior to the orbit. It is the point of exit for the maxillary division of the trigeminal nerve (Cr V-2), receiving sensation from the maxillary region of the face.

Muscles

The muscles of the eyes comprise two groups:

- The extrinsic muscles – which attach to the external surface of the eyeball and move the eye in order to direct the gaze (Figures 34.5–34.7).

- The intrinsic muscles – located within the eyeball, regulating pupil size and lens accommodation (Figure 34.8).

VI

34

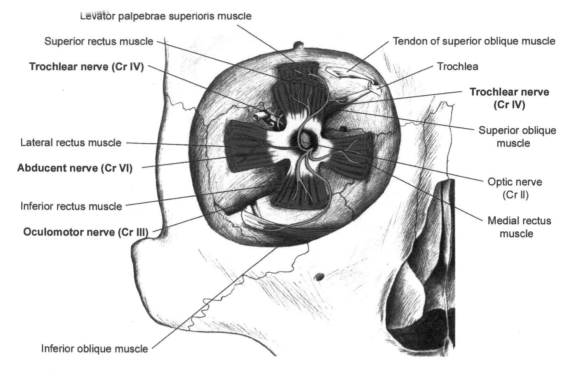

Levator palpebrae superioris muscle

Superior rectus muscle

Trochlear nerve (Cr IV)

Lateral rectus muscle

Abducent nerve (Cr VI)

Inferior rectus muscle

Oculomotor nerve (Cr III)

Inferior oblique muscle

Tendon of superior oblique muscle

Trochlea

Trochlear nerve (Cr IV)

Superior oblique muscle

Optic nerve (Cr II)

Medial rectus muscle

34.5   The extrinsic muscles move the eyeball in order to direct the gaze

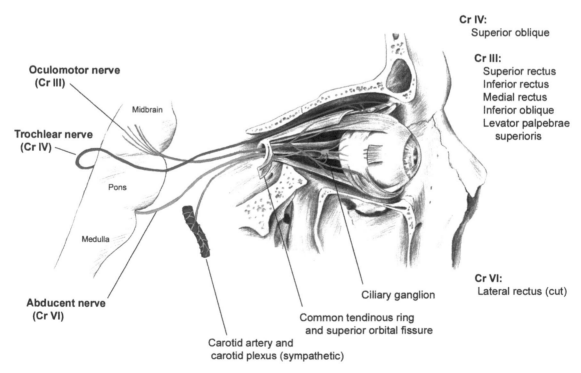

Oculomotor nerve (Cr III)

Midbrain

Trochlear nerve (Cr IV)

Pons

Medulla

Abducent nerve (Cr VI)

Ciliary ganglion

Common tendinous ring and superior orbital fissure

Carotid artery and carotid plexus (sympathetic)

Cr IV:
Superior oblique

Cr III:
Superior rectus
Inferior rectus
Medial rectus
Inferior oblique
Levator palpebrae superioris

Cr VI:
Lateral rectus (cut)

34.6   The extrinsic muscles of the eye are supplied by cranial nerves III, IV and VI

Extrinsic muscles

The extrinsic muscles (together with their innervations and functions) are:

Muscle	Innervation	Function
Superior Rectus	Cranial Nerve III	directs the gaze upwards
Inferior Rectus	Cranial Nerve III	directs the gaze downwards
Medial Rectus	Cranial Nerve III	directs the gaze medially
Lateral Rectus	Cranial Nerve VI	directs the gaze laterally (abducts the eye)
Superior Oblique	Cranial Nerve IV	directs the gaze down and out
Inferior Oblique	Cranial Nerve III	directs the gaze up and out

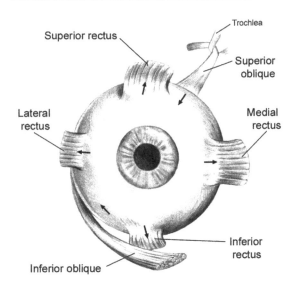

34.7 Movements of the eyeball (right eye)

These muscles are often involved in strabismus (squint) and associated diplopia (double vision) which may arise from a disturbance in the muscle itself, or within its nerve supply, or due to a distortion of the orbit, or to asymmetrical pulls exerted through the cranio-sacral system.

Also within the orbit is the *levator palpebrae superioris* muscle, which raises the upper eyelid, receiving its innervation from cranial nerve III. The upper eyelid has a dual muscular action, since it is also raised by the superior tarsal muscle, smooth muscle innervated by sympathetic nerve supply.

Most of the extrinsic muscles emanate from the *common tendinous ring* – a ring of fibrous tissue at the back of the orbit, attaching to the sphenoid body, greater wing and lesser wing, and continuous with the dura of the middle cranial fossa – through which some of the cranial nerves (Cr II, III and VI) pass on their way into the orbit.

The muscles which emanate from the common tendinous ring are:

*   superior rectus
*   inferior rectus
*   medial rectus
*   lateral rectus
*   superior oblique.

The levator palpebrae superioris attaches indirectly through the tendon of the superior rectus.

The superior oblique muscle is also associated with the frontal bone, since it passes through a cartilaginous *trochlea* (Latin for pulley) attaching to the periosteum of the frontal bone in the medial roof of the orbit, in order to gain a position (or direction of pull) through which it can exert its desired effect on the eyeball of directing the gaze down and out. This muscle passes up to the trochlea (medial to the eyeball) where its tendon passes through the pulley, and doubles back on itself in order to attach onto the superior-lateral surface of the eyeball, thereby drawing the top of the eyeball medially in order to direct the gaze down and out.

The inferior oblique muscle attaches to the maxilla in the floor of the orbit.

Intrinsic muscles

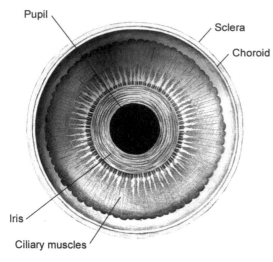

34.8 *The intrinsic muscles comprise the muscles of the iris and the ciliary muscles*

The *intrinsic* muscles (Figure 34.8) comprise:

- the *muscles of the iris*, which regulate pupil size in response to light. They are innervated by:
  - parasympathetic fibres travelling with Cr III – for pupil constriction
  - sympathetic nerve supply – for pupil dilation
- the *muscles of the lens* (the ciliary muscles) which adjust the shape of the lens for near and distant focus. They are innervated by:
  - parasympathetic fibres travelling with Cr III (via the short ciliary nerves).

Pupil dilation is enabled through sympathetic nerve supply, which is why excessive sympathetic stimulation may lead to photosensitivity.

Pupil constriction is enabled through parasympathetic nerve supply, travelling with Cr III. A persistently dilated pupil could be an indication of damage to Cr III preventing constriction.

The ciliary muscles are arranged concentrically around the perimeter of the lens, attaching to the lens via suspensory ligaments. The iris muscles are positioned slightly anterior to the lens, suspensory ligaments, and ciliary muscles.

Membranes

Contraction, constriction or sclerosis of the membranes which envelop the brain – the dura, arachnoid, and pia mater – perhaps due to meningitis, meningisms, inflammation, membranous tension, bony displacements or psycho-emotional tension – may exert pulls which reflect into the eyeball itself, contracting and constricting the scleral membrane which surrounds and envelops the eyeball or disturbing the function of the nerves and blood vessels supplying and draining the eye and the orbit.

As mentioned above, the sclera – the white membrane enveloping the eyeball – together with its transparent corneal portion, are adapted extensions of the dura mater, and are continuous with the intra-cranial dural membrane. They are therefore susceptible to disturbance from membranous tensions.

The cranial nerves are continuous with the dura through their epineural sheaths and, together with the blood vessels supplying the eye and orbit, are in intimate contact with the dural membrane through much of their pathway to the orbit. Membranous constrictions and contractions can therefore exert pulls and constrictions on all of these neurological and vascular structures with consequent ramifications on the function of the eye. The tentorium cerebelli is of particular significance because it is penetrated by cranial nerves III, IV and VI.

Nerve supply

The eyes and orbits are supplied by six cranial nerves (II, III, IV, V, VI, VII) and by sympathetic and parasympathetic nerve supply (Figure 34.9):

- Cranial nerve II (optic nerve) receives and relays visual impulses from the retina.
- Cranial nerve III (oculo-motor nerve) provides motor supply to the superior rectus, inferior rectus, medial rectus, inferior oblique and levator palpebrae superioris muscles. It also carries parasympathetic fibres.
- Cranial nerve IV (trochlea nerve) provides motor supply to the superior oblique muscle.
- Cranial nerve VI (abducent nerve) provides motor supply to the lateral rectus muscle.

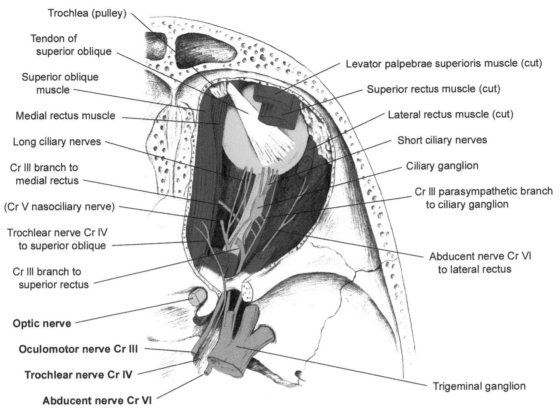

Trochlea (pulley)
Tendon of superior oblique
Superior oblique muscle
Medial rectus muscle
Long ciliary nerves
Cr III branch to medial rectus
(Cr V nasociliary nerve)
Trochlear nerve Cr IV to superior oblique
Cr III branch to superior rectus
Optic nerve
Oculomotor nerve Cr III
Trochlear nerve Cr IV
Abducent nerve Cr VI

Levator palpebrae superioris muscle (cut)
Superior rectus muscle (cut)
Lateral rectus muscle (cut)
Short ciliary nerves
Ciliary ganglion
Cr III parasympathetic branch to ciliary ganglion
Abducent nerve Cr VI to lateral rectus
Trigeminal ganglion

34.9   The eyes and orbits are supplied by six cranial nerves

- Cranial nerve V (trigeminal nerve) – the ophthalmic branch carries sensation from the orbit and its environs.
  - Parasympathetic innervation travelling with cranial nerve III (oculo-motor nerve) supplies the intrinsic muscles of the eye, passing to:
    ○ the muscles of the iris – enabling constriction of the pupil
    ○ the ciliary muscles of the lens – adjusting the lens for near and far vision.
  - Parasympathetic innervation travelling with cranial nerve VII (facial nerve) supplies the lacrimal gland, enabling secretion of tears.
  - Sympathetic innervation, passing up from the carotid plexus, supplies:
    ○ the intrinsic muscles of the iris – dilating the pupil
    ○ the superior tarsal muscle which assists in raising the upper eyelid (in conjunction with the levator palpebrae superioris muscle innervated by Cr III)

○ the arteries of the orbit (and the rest of the cranium) – inducing vasoconstriction.

Nerve pathways

Cranial Nerve II – Optic

Fibres from the rod and cone cells of the retina aggregate at the back of the eyeball to form the optic nerve. The *optic nerve* (containing approximately one million nerve fibres for each eye) travels posteriorly from the back of the eyeball through the optic canal (between the body of the sphenoid and the lesser wing of the sphenoid), emerging medial to the anterior clinoid process, anterior to the pituitary gland. Here, the two optic nerves come together as the *optic chiasma.*

Within the optic chiasma, medial fibres from each optic nerve decussate (cross over to the opposite side). Lateral fibres continue along the same side. The combined fibres which emerge from the chiasma posteriorly (lateral fibres from the same side and medial fibres from the

VI

34

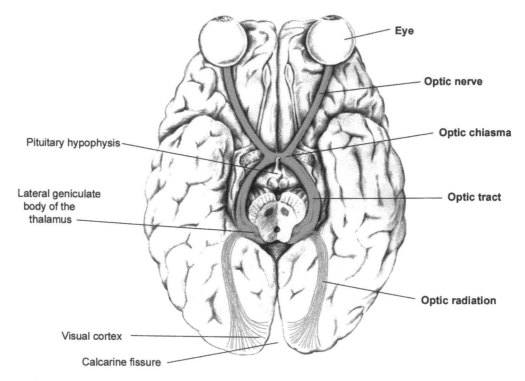

34.10 The optic pathway travels from the retina of each eyes, via the optic nerves, optic chiasma, optic tracts and optic radiation, to the visual cortex within the occipital lobes

opposite side) continue on each side as the *optic tract*, communicating with the lateral geniculate body of the thalamus and then continuing as the *optic radiation* to the visual cortex, located within the calcarine fissure of the occipital lobe (Figure 34.10).

Further details of all the cranial nerves are included in Chapters 22–31.

Cranial Nerves III, IV and VI

Cranial nerves III (oculo-motor), IV (trochlear) and VI (abducent) travel together from the midbrain to the orbit (Figures 34.6 and 34.9):

- Cranial nerve III emerges from the anterolateral midbrain.
- Cranial nerve IV emerges from the posterolateral midbrain (the only cranial nerve to emerge from the posterior aspect of the brainstem).
- Cranial nerve VI emerges from the anterior pons.

The three nerves travel together along the floor of the middle cranial fossa, on each side of the sphenoid body. They penetrate the posterior wall of the cavernous sinus (cranial nerves III and IV passing close to the lateral wall of the cavernous sinus, cranial nerve VI passing more medially). After travelling through the cavernous sinus, they emerge together from the anterior wall of the cavernous sinus and pass into the orbit together through the superior orbital fissure:

- Cranial nerve VI enters the orbit through the medial part of the fissure and passes through the common tendinous ring directly to the lateral rectus muscle.
- Cranial nerve IV enters through the lateral part of the fissure and travels medially across the back of the orbit, above and behind the common tendinous ring, to the superior oblique muscle.
- Cranial nerve III enters through the middle of the fissure, passes through the common tendinous ring, and gives off branches to the superior rectus, inferior rectus, medial rectus, inferior oblique, and levator palpebrae superioris muscles, also carrying parasympathetic fibres to the intrinsic muscles of the eye for pupil constriction and lens accommodation.

Ophthalmic division of the trigeminal nerve (Cr V-1)

The ophthalmic division of the trigeminal nerve (Cr V-1) travels along the floor of the middle cranial fossa together with cranial nerves III, IV and VI, passes through the cavernous sinus, enters the orbit through the superior orbital fissure and gives off a lacrimal branch, a nasociliary branch and a frontal branch. These three branches carry sensory supply from the various structures of the orbit:

- The lacrimal nerve carries sensory input from the lacrimal gland (sensory, *not* secretory), the conjunctiva and the upper eyelid.

- The nasociliary nerve carries sensory input from the cornea, the iris, the ciliary muscles and the pupil dilator muscles, and gives off branches which penetrate into the nasal cavity and pass to the frontal, ethmoidal and sphenoidal sinuses.

- The frontal nerve carries sensory input from the upper eyelid, the frontal sinus and the forehead and emerges to the surface through the supraorbital notch.

The maxillary division of the trigeminal nerve (Cr V)

The maxillary division of the trigeminal nerve (Cr V) exits the cranium at the foramen rotundum (behind the apex of the orbit), then immediately turns forward to enter the orbit through the inferior orbital fissure, passing forward along a groove in the floor of the orbit within the maxilla. The groove then deepens to become a tunnel, penetrating the floor of the orbit as the nerve proceeds anteriorly to its emergence onto the surface of the face at the infraorbital foramen. It does not play any part in the function of the eye, but it receives sensation from the area immediately below the eye, and may be affected by disturbances to the eye or orbit.

Parasympathetic nerve supply

Parasympathetic supply to the *intrinsic muscles* travels with *cranial nerve III*. The parasympathetic fibres diverge from the inferior branch of the oculo-motor nerve and enter the *ciliary ganglion* where they synapse. They are joined by sympathetic fibres. Both parasympathetic and sympathetic fibres then travel together as the short ciliary nerves which penetrate the surface of the eyeball in order to reach the intrinsic muscles.

Parasympathetic supply to the *lacrimal gland* (enabling secretion) travels with *cranial nerve VII* (facial), synapsing in the *pterygopalatine ganglion*, travelling on to join the lacrimal nerve (a sensory branch of the ophthalmic division of the trigeminal nerve Cr V-1). The seventh cranial nerve (the facial) is the nerve involved in Bell's palsy, and lacrimal gland secretions may therefore be affected when the palsy is due to proximal facial nerve damage. However, the parasympathetic fibres separate from the main trunk of the facial nerve within the facial canal of the temporal bone, at the geniculum, travelling independently to the lacrimal gland, and will not therefore be affected by facial nerve damage distal to this separation. This can prove relevant clinically in tracing and addressing the source of lacrimal gland disturbance, or in tracing the site of injury in Bell's palsy.

Isabelle was constantly irritated to the point of distraction by her painful, dry left eye. She was using ointment and drops every day, but this only partially relieved her symptoms. She had other indications of Bell's palsy, but it was her eye which troubled her most. The symptoms had started following an operation for an acoustic neuroma (on the vestibulo-cochlear nerve Cr VIII). As with Vera in Chapter 26, the operation had damaged her facial nerve, causing Bell's palsy – the two nerves travelling in close proximity through the internal auditory meatus. As so often in such cases, the extent of the nerve damage was such that a complete resolution was not possible, but cranio-sacral integration reduced her symptoms significantly, both in the eye and with the other vestiges of Bell's palsy, making life far more comfortable.

Sympathetic nerve supply

The sympathetic pathway to the eyes originates in the upper thoracic spine at the first and second thoracic vertebral levels, travels up through the neck, synapsing at the superior cervical sympathetic ganglion, enters the cranium through the carotid canal as the *carotid nerve* and *carotid plexus* (together with the carotid artery)

VI

34

and continues up through the cavernous sinus (together with the carotid artery). Sympathetic supply is then distributed throughout the cranium.

The branches to the orbit include fibres to the intrinsic muscles of the iris travelling via the ciliary ganglion for pupil dilation, other fibres passing to the upper eyelid, the membranes of the conjunctiva, the eyelids, and the arteries within and around the orbit. Injury or restriction anywhere along this pathway may affect the eyes and is particularly prevalent in the upper cervical and suboccipital regions, predisposing to photosensitivity and other symptoms.

The *ciliary ganglion* is located in the posterior part of the orbit. It is the site of synapse for parasympathetic fibres travelling to the eyeball. Sympathetic fibres and sensory (trigeminal) fibres also pass through, without synapse.

The *short ciliary nerves* are that portion of the combined nerve pathway which passes from the ciliary ganglion to the eyeball, containing parasympathetic fibres to the intrinsic muscles, together with sympathetic fibres and some sensory (trigeminal) fibres. They pierce the sclera, pass forward in delicate grooves on the inner surface of the sclera, and are distributed to the ciliary muscles, iris and cornea.

The *long ciliary nerves* are sensory branches of the ophthalmic division of the trigeminal nerve to the eyeball and cornea, also carrying sympathetic fibres to the pupil dilator muscles of the iris.

Arterial supply

Ophthalmic artery

Arterial supply to the eye is provided by the *ophthalmic artery*, which emanates from the carotid artery. The carotid artery passes up through the carotid canal and continues up through the cavernous sinus. The ophthalmic artery diverges from the carotid artery and passes through the optic canal (together with the optic nerve Cr II) before dividing to supply the structures within the orbit (Figure 34.11).

The *central artery of the retina* branches off from the ophthalmic artery, penetrates the optic nerve and passes along the central core of the optic nerve to supply the retina (Figure 34.12).

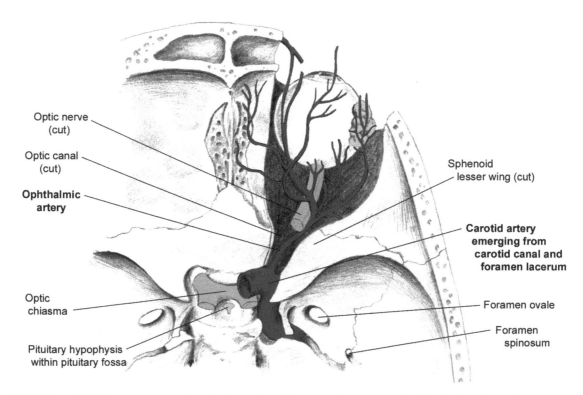

Optic nerve (cut)

Optic canal (cut)

Ophthalmic artery

Optic chiasma

Pituitary hypophysis within pituitary fossa

Sphenoid lesser wing (cut)

Carotid artery emerging from carotid canal and foramen lacerum

Foramen ovale

Foramen spinosum

34.11 The ophthalmic artery emanates from the internal carotid artery and passes into the orbit via the optic canal

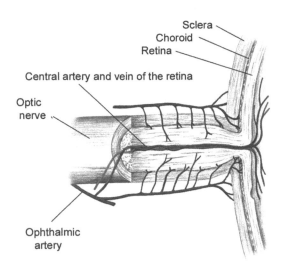

Sclera
Choroid
Retina
Central artery and vein of the retina
Optic nerve
Ophthalmic artery

34.12 The central artery of the retina travels within the central core of the optic nerve to supply the retina

Vertebral arteries

The vertebral arteries (Figure 34.13) also contribute a major arterial supply to the intracranial structures, passing up through the vertebral foramina of the cervical spine (from vertebral levels C6 to C1), following a tortuous S-bend between the atlas and occiput (where they are prone to compression), entering the cranium through the foramen magnum, combining together to form the basilar artery, and joining the Circle of Willis, with important contributions to the arterial supply of the occipital lobe of the brain – the location of the visual cortex where visual sensations are received and interpreted.

Due to the location of the vertebral arteries in that vulnerable suboccipital region, they may be particularly involved in reduced arterial supply to the brain and cranium and to the occipital region in particular (vertebro-basilar insufficiency) due to restriction and compression in the suboccipital area. This may be due to trauma, injury, stress or postural tension (particularly common in the elderly), may adversely affect function, leading to poor concentration, poor memory, vagueness and dizziness, and may affect vision, either through effects on the visual cortex or through reduced arterial supply to the head and eyes. Reduced

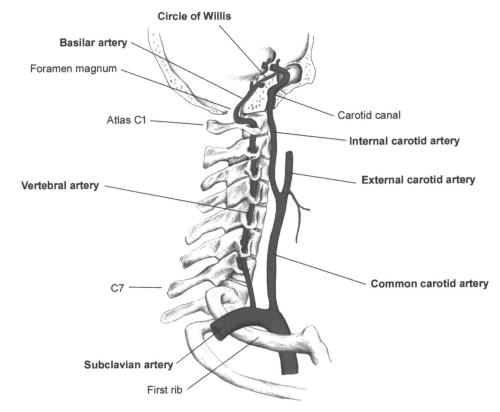

Circle of Willis
Basilar artery
Foramen magnum
Atlas C1
Carotid canal
Internal carotid artery
External carotid artery
Vertebral artery
Common carotid artery
C7
Subclavian artery
First rib

34.13 The vertebral and carotid arteries both play a part in providing arterial supply to the eyes and to the visual cortex

VI

34

venous drainage through this area (particularly through the jugular veins at the jugular foramina) may also affect eye function through venous congestion. Cranio-sacral integration can be very beneficial in addressing the restrictions in this area, through attention to the occiput, subocciput and other related structures, and including fascial unwinding of the neck.

Venous drainage

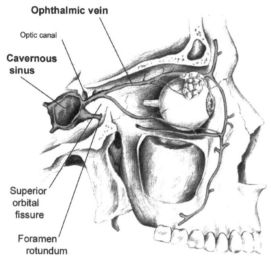

34.14 Venous drainage of the eye is primarily through the ophthalmic vein, passing out of the orbit through the superior orbital fissure into the cavernous sinus

Venous drainage of the eye is through the ophthalmic vein, passing out of the orbit through the superior orbital fissure (together with cranial nerves III, IV and VI and the ophthalmic branch of V), draining into the cavernous sinus on each side of the sphenoid body (Figure 34.14). From the cavernous sinus, drainage continues back via the superior and inferior petrosal sinuses to the sigmoid sinus, and out of the cranium via the internal jugular vein through the jugular foramen (on each side) down through the throat and neck to the heart.

The jugular foramen is therefore a key site for the drainage of the cranium and therefore for the drainage of the eyes, the foramen being readily restricted by suboccipital tensions and traumas and by restrictions of the occipitomastoid suture, whether due to birth trauma, head injuries,

cervical restrictions involving the upper cervical spine, or disturbances of the sterno-cleido-mastoid muscle and its nerve supply (the spinal accessory nerve (Cr XI) with its roots emerging from vertebral levels C1,2,3,4, and direct nerve supply from vertebral level C2).

The whole intracranial venous sinus system is dependent on drainage at the jugular foramen. Fluent intracranial venous drainage is relevant to the function of the eyes – whether affecting the visual cortex or the orbital structures – with potential disturbance to function through congestion and venous back pressure. The venous sinus system is in turn readily influenced by membranous tensions and restriction within the intracranial membranes and throughout the reciprocal tension membrane system. The cranio-sacral release of tensions and contractions within the intracranial membranes can bring substantial relief to the eyes.

The eyeball

The eyeball is an extension of the brain (Figure 34.15). Like other parts of the brain it is enveloped in three layers of membrane:

- The outer layer is the *sclera*, a white membrane continuous with the dural membranes of the cranium. It is partially visible as 'the whites of the eyes'. Anteriorly it is transparent, forming the cornea.

- The middle layer is the *choroid*, a vascular lining of the eyeball containing a rich blood supply of arterioles deriving from the central artery of the retina.

- The innermost layer is the *retina*, a light-sensitive structure which receives visual images. It contains many millions of photoreceptors (rods and cones) and ganglion cells whose nerve fibres unite posteriorly to form the optic nerve.

The main cavity of the eyeball is the *vitreous chamber*. It is filled with *vitreous humour*, a transparent gelatinous fluid, which maintains the shape of the eyeball. Anteriorly, it is separated from the aqueous humour by the lens and the ciliary body.

The *lens* is a flexible mass of transparent fibres, contained within a capsule, dividing the aqueous

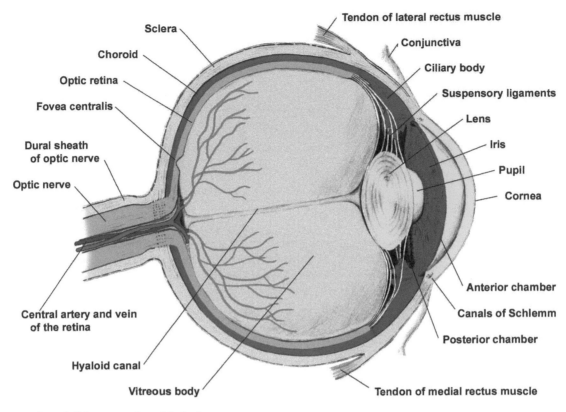

34.15 The eyeball is an extension of the brain

humour (anteriorly) from the vitreous humour (posteriorly). It is held in place by suspensory ligaments attaching to the ciliary body.

The *ciliary body* contains the ciliary muscles, arranged concentrically around the lens, and attaching to the lens via the *suspensory ligaments*. Contraction of these concentric muscles reduces the size of the circle, enabling the suspensory ligaments to slacken and the lens to become thicker, resulting in a closer focus. Relaxation of the ciliary muscles enlarges the circle, drawing the suspensory ligaments tight, making the lens thinner, resulting in a more distant focus. The ciliary muscles are innervated by parasympathetic supply travelling with cranial nerve III.

The lens consists of concentric layers of cells. With age, the lens hardens, becoming less malleable, so that the eyes become less able to adapt to near and far vision. It may also become more opaque, potentially leading to cataracts.

In front of the lens are two chambers – an *anterior* and a *posterior chamber* – separated from each other by the iris. The muscles of the iris surround the pupil and contract or relax in response to light. The anterior and posterior chambers contain aqueous humour, a thin watery lymph-like fluid. There is a continuous flow of aqueous humour, in order to maintain the integrity and clarity of the structures of the eye. This fluid is produced by the ciliary body, from which it flows into the posterior chamber, passing from the posterior chamber to the anterior chamber, and then draining via a trabecular network into the canals of Schlemm and into the venous system. The aqueous humour is recycled approximately every four hours.

The canals of Schlemm are small venous sinuses arranged in a circular formation around the perimeter of the anterior chamber, within the sclera, at the angle of the cornea and the iris. They may be susceptible to blockage due to particles of waste matter accumulating in the aqueous humour (dust particles and other residue, particularly following infection), reducing drainage of the eyeball and potentially contributing to glaucoma.

The *iris* is a vascular mass of connective tissue containing two rings of muscle which surround the pupil (Figure 34.8). Contraction of the circular muscles (the inner ring) reduces pupil size in response to bright light, mediated by parasympathetic innervation. Contraction of the radial muscles (the outer ring) dilates the pupil in response to sympathetic innervation. The iris is visible as the pigmented part of the eye.

Light enters the eye through the pupil and is focused by the lens onto the retina.

The *retina* is the innermost of the three membranous layers which envelop the eyeball. It contains many millions of photoreceptors (rods and cones) and ganglion cells whose nerve fibres unite posteriorly to form the optic nerve.

The *rods* are the photoreceptors responsible for light and dark vision. There are approximately 125 million rods in each retina, distributed widely around the retina.

The *cones* are the photoreceptors responsible for colour vision. There are approximately 7 million cones in each retina, concentrated centrally around the fovea centralis.

The *macula* is a small yellow spot in the centre of the retina, two millimetres lateral to the optic disc. Centrally, it contains the fovea centralis.

The *fovea centralis* is the point of most acute vision located in the centre of the macula. It contains many closely packed cones, and no rods.

The *optic disc* is the point of convergence of fibres from the ganglion cells of the retina as they unite to form the optic nerve. It forms a small *blind spot* at the back of the retina. The nerve fibres uniting at the optic disc penetrate the sclera to form the optic nerve.

The *central artery of the retina* is a branch of the ophthalmic artery which travels through the centre of the optic nerve to enter the retina at the optic disc, dividing into branches to supply the retina. It is accompanied by the *central vein of the retina*, draining into the ophthalmic vein or directly into the cavernous sinus.

The *hyaloid canal* is a small transparent membranous canal running through the vitreous body from the optic disc to the lens. In the foetus, the hyaloid canal contains the hyaloid artery, a continuation of the central artery of the retina, which supplies blood to the developing lens. After birth, the hyaloid canal contains lymph, and its purpose is to facilitate changes in the volume of the lens.

The *eyelid* consists of protective folds of tissue containing the eyelashes (cilia), meibomian (sebaceous) glands, sweat glands, and muscle. The upper eyelid is raised by the levator palpebrae superioris muscle (supplied by motor fibres from cranial nerve III). The upper eyelid is also raised by the superior tarsal muscle (innervated by sympathetic nerve supply). The posterior surface of the eyelid is lined with conjunctiva.

The *conjunctiva* is a folded mucous membrane forming the lining of the eyelids and also folding down over the covered surface of the cornea.

The *lacrimal gland* is located on the superior lateral aspect of the eyeball (Figure 34.16). It secretes tears which wash across the eyeball towards the inferior medial aspect of the eye. Lacrimal secretions (tears) drain via the lacrimal canaliculi into the *nasolacrimal duct* (lacrimal duct) located in the inferior medial corner of the eye, carrying tears into the nasal cavity through a bony canal formed by the maxillae, the lacrimal bone and the inferior nasal concha.

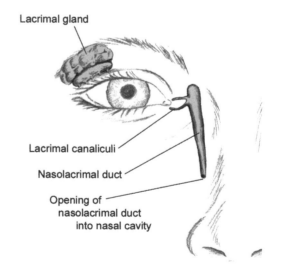

Lacrimal gland

Lacrimal canaliculi

Nasolacrimal duct

Opening of nasolacrimal duct into nasal cavity

34.16 Lacrimal secretions from the lacrimal gland drain via the nasolacrimal duct into the nasal cavity

Conditions affecting the eyes

The eyes are susceptible to various pathologies, some of which can lead rapidly to blindness, so it is essential to be aware of potential indications of pathology. Some of the more significant pathologies are described below.

Systemic disease

Diabetes, both Type 1 (IDD, early onset) and Type 2 (NIDD, late onset), leads to vascular disease which may affect the blood vessels of the eyes, leading to a deterioration of vision, either gradual or sudden, along with an increased tendency to cataract, glaucoma and retinal detachment. It is the most common cause of blindness in the Western world.

Hypertension may lead to vascular disease, with repercussions on the eyes.

Multiple sclerosis may lead to *demyelination* of the optic nerve, causing progressive blindness. This may often be the first area affected by the disease and the first indication of the presence of multiple sclerosis. However, the eyes may also be totally unaffected by the disease.

Various other systemic diseases may involve the eyes, including rheumatoid disease, ankylosing spondylitis, Reiter's syndrome, Sjögren's syndrome, sarcoidosis, Graves' disease (thyroiditis) and various genetic conditions.

In *meningitis*, the acute phase often involves extreme photophobia, a symptom which, in conjunction with other indications of meningitis, may act as an alert to the presence of meningitis and a need for immediate medical attention. The chronic consequences of meningitis often involve persistent severe pain in the eyes together with photophobia, severe headache and neck pain – a condition which is highly responsive to effective cranio-sacral integration.

Local disease

Glaucoma arises due to increased pressure within the eyeball as a result of disturbed flow of aqueous humour. It can lead to retinal damage and blindness if untreated. It affects 2 per cent of the population over the age of 40.[2] It is a condition which needs immediate medical attention and is routinely checked for by ophthalmic opticians. It involves an imbalance of secretion of aqueous humour by the ciliary body relative to drainage from the anterior chamber via the trabecular meshwork into the canals of Schlemm.

Glaucoma is usually symptomless in its early stages and therefore difficult to detect. The first sign may be a slight loss of peripheral vision. Although there are many other possible (and less serious) causes of discomfort in the eyes, any patient suffering persistent sensations of pressure in the eyeball should be checked for glaucoma by an ophthalmic optician. Once glaucoma (and any other pathology) has been eliminated as a possible cause, other possible factors can be investigated and potentially addressed through cranio-sacral integration. Early treatment through cranio-sacral integration may prevent the development of glaucoma and abrogate the need for an operation, but the situation always needs to be monitored carefully.

Cataract involves opacity of the lens, leading to gradual deterioration of vision. It is the most common cause of blindness in the developing world and is also common in the Western world, affecting 15 per cent of the population over the age of 50.[3] The cause of cataracts is unknown,[4] but it is thought that changes in the protein structure of the lens over time may render the lens increasingly opaque. This tendency can be aggravated by conditions such as diabetes mellitus and hypertension.[5] It may initially be noticed as stable motes, multiple images, and halos around street lamps, with blurred or cloudy vision and patches of unclear vision, progressing to increasing opacity and blindness. It is unaffected by medication but can be very successfully treated through an operation to replace the lens.

Maintaining a healthy environment within and around the eyes and in general health may help to reduce susceptibility to cataracts, but once the lens has become opaque, there is no potential for this process to be reversed. The usual treatment is an operation to replace the lens with an artificial lens, a very common operation which is generally very successful, although operations do vary considerably, and patients can be left with persistent side effects, associated damage and varying qualities of vision. Whilst cranio-sacral integration would not be expected to help the

VI

34

cataract, it is always useful in order to assist with reintegration following any operation.

Detachment of the retina involves the separation of the neuroretinal layer from the retinal pigment epithelium, generally leading to immediate blindness in the affected eye. Immediate treatment to reattach the retina may restore sight, but prolonged separation leads to degeneration of the photoreceptor cells and permanent loss of sight. Detachment may occur spontaneously, may be triggered by exertion or trauma, or may be the result of degenerative changes in the retina leading to haemorrhage.

Strabismus (squint) is a condition in which the eyes do not look in the same direction. Squints are common, affecting 1 in 20 children,[6] usually developing before the age of five years. They may be constant or intermittent, congenital or acquired. Acquired squints may develop in response to some other visual defect (such as astigmatism). They may be accompanied by diplopia (double vision). The most common form is *convergent strabismus* in which the gaze is directed medially.

A baby's eyes will often wander independently, or appear cross-eyed when they are tired. This is normal for the first four months of life. If this tendency persists beyond four months, or if a squint is constant (fixed), then it requires attention.

If a squint is left untreated in young children, *lazy eye* (amblyopia) can develop. If the vision in one eye is poor, the brain ignores signals from that eye, and the affected eye functions less and less efficiently.

Amblyopia is a condition involving brain development rather than the eye itself, but may develop in response to a problem with the eye such as a squint. It is generally treated by using an eye patch covering the good eye to encourage the use and development of the weak eye and the corresponding development in brain function. A lazy eye can be treated up until about seven years of age – the age at which visual development is usually complete – and should be treated as soon as possible. The most common cause is a squint.

There is no known medical cause for squints. Conventional treatments include glasses, eye exercises, botulinum toxin injections into the eye muscles, or surgery to move the muscles.

From a cranio-sacral perspective, it is common to find imbalance and asymmetries in the structure of the orbit, or in the associated muscles and membranes, which may respond to cranio-sacral integration. These may often be associated with imbalances throughout the body, particularly associated with birth trauma. In the most common form, convergent strabismus, the obvious factors to consider are weakness in the lateral rectus muscle or the abducent nerve which supplies it, or possibly an overcontracted medial rectus muscle. But, as always, it is essential to restore the overall integration of the whole system. It is also essential to treat as early as possible, while the system is more adaptable, and before developmental patterns become ingrained.

Mark developed a fixed squint at an early age and was due to have an operation to correct it. His cranio-sacral system revealed a strong torsion pattern right the way down through the body to the sacrum and pelvis, a common but in this case quite severe birth pattern. Addressing the torsion, releasing the primary focus at the pelvis, and bringing his system into balanced integration eliminated the squint and abrogated the need for an operation.

Astigmatism is a common condition, usually congenital, in which the curvature of the cornea or lens is uneven, forming a more oval shape (like a rugby ball) instead of a perfectly rounded shape. This results in poor ability to focus and consequent blurred vision. It can lead to headaches, eye strain and tiredness, particularly after prolonged periods of reading or looking at computer screens. It is usually treated through corrective glasses or contact lenses which adjust the vision to compensate for the defect, or sometimes through surgery.

Irregular astigmatism is a less common variation in which the cornea is scarred or more unevenly distorted. It is more likely to be caused by an injury to the cornea. This form cannot be treated with glasses, and requires contact lenses.

There is no known cause for astigmatism, but as with any asymmetry or imbalance, it may respond to cranio-sacral integration.

Bobby was five years old and had been experiencing various difficulties with his vision for some time. He wore glasses and had been diagnosed with astigmatism among other disturbances. As cranio-sacral treatment progressed, his mother observed that he was noticing things more readily, seeing more clearly, and often not using his glasses. Although he was not due for a check-up for several months, she took him to the ophthalmologist who reported that his vision had improved significantly and that the astigmatism had disappeared. He immediately prescribed new glasses.

Tumours, both benign and malignant, may occur in the orbit, leading to disturbance in the function of the eye. A pituitary tumour may impinge on the optic chiasma, potentially manifesting initially as tunnel vision (loss of peripheral vision).

Inflammatory conditions

The eye is prone to a wide variety of infectious and inflammatory conditions.

One possible cause of infection is *toxocariasis*, a bacterial infection ingested (especially by children) by swallowing the ova of toxocara canis, a roundworm picked up from the faeces of dogs in parks and other public places. The larvae can migrate to various parts of the body including the retina and may cause blindness. There are approximately 10,000 identified cases annually in the United States, of which permanent loss of vision occurs in 700.[7] The condition is less common these days in England and Wales with only 30 cases between 2000 and 2010.

Conjunctivitis is an irritation of the conjunctiva causing a generalized redness of the eye. It may be caused by irritation, infection, allergy and other sensitivities. It is not serious in itself but may lead to complications.

Various other inflammatory conditions may affect different structures within the eye, including keratitis (affecting the cornea), blepharitis (affecting the eyelid), scleritis, uveitis, iritis, choroiditis, cyclitis (affecting the ciliary body) and optic neuritis. Infections and inflammation may arise from many different sources.

Persistent infectious or inflammatory conditions may be helped through cranio-sacral integration by encouraging the free mobility of surrounding structures with consequent free drainage and flow of fluids – enhancing the body's inherent ability to address such conditions.

Conditions such as conjunctivitis, a stye (inflammation of a sebaceous gland) and blockage of the nasociliary duct may also be assisted through naturopathic methods such as wiping the eye with cotton wool soaked in salt water. Wiping should be carried out from medial to lateral, using each piece of cotton wool for only one wipe and never using the same piece for both eyes.

In the case of a stye, hot compresses and other naturopathic approaches may also be helpful to encourage drainage and fluid flow.

Blockage of the nasolacrimal duct can be helped cranio-sacrally by encouraging the free mobility of the maxillae, the lacrimal bones, the inferior nasal conchae, and the orbit as a whole, along with overall integration of the face. Energy drives to the area may also be beneficial. Specific contact on the lacrimal bones can be taken up, either with a single finger on the affected side, or with finger and thumb engaging with both sides simultaneously. Even if only one lacrimal duct is affected, it is generally beneficial to take up contact with both sides, in order to engage more fully with the inherent forces and enable more comprehensive balancing of the surrounding area (Figure 34.17).

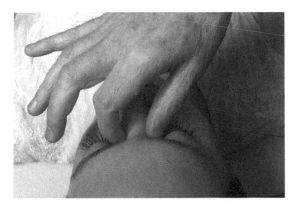

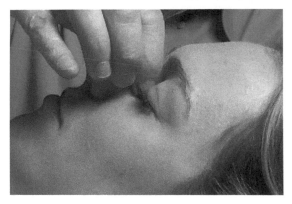

34.17 The lacrimal bones and lacrimal ducts are most effectively addressed through a bilateral contact

VI

34

Addressing conditions of the eye through cranio-sacral integration

It is not of course possible to resolve every condition affecting the eyes. Myopia (short-sightedness) and hyperopia (long-sightedness) may be influenced by the shape of the eyeball, which may in turn be influenced by the shape of the orbit. Restoring balance, shape and mobility to the orbit can therefore sometimes influence the development and progress of such conditions, particularly at an early age, but miracle cures are not to be expected. Where there is evident distortion of the cranium, face and orbit, perhaps due to birth trauma, treatment through cranio-sacral integration may become more relevant.

Many pathologies affecting the eyes will need, or will already be receiving, medical attention. This is crucial, but we can also recognize that general integration and mobilization may enable the body to deal more effectively with pathology, particularly in its early stages, and may help to prevent further recurrence. In particular, persistent or recurrent conditions which are not responding to medical treatment may well have an underlying cause that can be addressed through cranio-sacral integration; and maintaining a healthy balanced structure can help the body not only to address conditions, but also to prevent their development in the first place.

This is especially the case with persistent or recurrent infections, the presence of which suggests that structural blockage or congestion is preventing the body's natural resources of arterial supply, venous drainage, and lymphatic drainage from fighting off the infection, creating a susceptibility to recurrent episodes.

Maureen's left eye had troubled her for years. It was usually dry and sore and, although it was not serious, it was very irritating and frustrating. She had been putting drops in her eye every day for years and had tried various creams prescribed by her doctor, some of which brought brief temporary alleviation of the symptoms, but the condition was still always there every day. Engaging at her head showed a clear restriction of mobility in the left side of her head and face, continuing down through her neck into her thorax and left shoulder. She was not sure where this had come from but felt it may have been related to a car accident many years ago which had injured her neck, shoulder and back. It required several sessions of cranio-sacral integration to clear the underlying restrictions to mobility which extended down her left side. Addressing the restrictions in the neck, shoulder and back enabled the restoration of free mobility and fluent function of arterial, venous and lymphatic flow in the head and face, thereby restoring the body's inherent ability to deal with infection. Her eye symptoms cleared completely and permanently, after years of suffering.

In addressing eye infections, the first priority is to assess whether there is an acute condition requiring medication and referral, or whether the condition can be addressed naturopathically, through regular salt water bathing of the eye and other natural resources, along with cranio-sacral integration. Subsequently, the requirement is to ensure the free mobility of the face, head and neck, including the orbits and eyes, reintegrating bony, muscular, fascial, membranous, neurological and vascular structures, in order to optimize the body's resources, and taking into account that the restrictions to function may be arising from anywhere in the body. The body's natural defences against infection are mediated primarily through arterial supply, venous drainage and lymphatic drainage. Ensuring unrestricted flow of these fluid pathways through mobility of the underlying structure and function can maximize the body's ability to address the infection.

AN APPROACH TO TREATMENT OF THE EYES

Any approach to treatment of the eyes will vary according to individual circumstances, but certain principles can apply:

1. Check for any pathologies where appropriate, and ensure that they are being addressed.

2. Overall cranio-sacral integration, identifying and addressing restrictions and imbalances elsewhere, bringing the system as a whole into balance.

3. Within that context, we can consider all the structures and factors specific to the eyes which might be relevant to the needs of the individual, based on an understanding of the structure and function of the eyes described above:

   a. ensuring mobility and integration of all local structures

   b. unrestricted vascular and neurological pathways

   c. free expression of rhythmic motion and vitality

   d. overall integration of function throughout the matrix.

Relevant areas to address

Depending on the circumstances, relevant areas and factors to take into account might include:

- the upper thorax and heart centre
  - for the sympathetic outflow to the eyes, venous drainage back to the heart, and emotional stresses held there
- the neck and suboccipital region
  - for the sympathetic pathway, the superior cervical sympathetic ganglion, venous drainage through the jugular veins and jugular foramina, arterial supply through the vertebral arteries and basilar artery to the occipital lobe and the Circle of Willis
- the cranium as a whole
  - as an integral part of the whole person
  - as an integral part of the whole cranio-facial structure
  - with particular attention to the bones most directly involved with the eyes
    - the occiput – in relation to the visual cortex in the occipital lobe
    - the sphenoid – contributing to the orbit, containing the optic canal and the superior and inferior orbital fissures, and with so many vital structures relating to the eyes associated with it
    - the frontal bone, contributing to the orbit
- the face in general
  - both for overall integration of the orbit and face and to address specific findings
  - identifying patterns of restriction involving the face and perhaps extending down through the head, neck, thorax and beyond
  - giving attention to each of the facial structures which contribute to the orbit and eye including the maxillae, palatine bones, nasal bones, zygomata, lacrimal bones, ethmoid
- the membrane system
  - including the falx cerebri, falx cerebelli and tentorium cerebelli
  - addressing tensions throughout the membrane system
  - addressing meningeal restriction due to meningitis or meningisms
  - releasing tensions which may be causing constriction of neurological and vascular pathways including cranial nerve pathways that penetrate the tentorium
  - tracing specific pathways to the eyes along the cranial nerves through therapeutic attention
  - bearing in mind that the sclera is a continuation of the membrane system and will be directly affected by tension in the intracranial membranes and in the reciprocal tension membrane system as a whole
- the foramina leading to and from the eye
  - optic canal, supraorbital fissure, infraorbital fissure

- integration of the muscular structures of the eye and their nerve supply
  - extrinsic muscles, and cranial nerves III, IV, VI
- nerve supply
  - Cr II for disturbances of vision
  - Cr III, IV and VI to the extrinsic muscles – particularly in relation to squints
  - Cr V for sensory innervation
  - Cr VII for flaccidity and disturbance of the facial muscles around the eye, including Bell's palsy
  - the parasympathetic component of Cr VII
    › for dry eye and other associated symptoms, tracing its pathway from the facial canal to the eyeball via the pterygopalatine ganglion
    › also for disturbances of lacrimal secretion
  - the parasympathetic component of Cr III for pupil and lens disturbance
  - the sympathetic pathway
    › for photosensitivity, pupil dilation, tired eyes, weak eyes, tightness
    › the superior tarsal muscle of the eyelid
    › vasoconstriction of the arterial supply
    › in relation to sympathetically induced hyper-reactivity
  - the parasympathetic ganglia
    › the ciliary ganglion in relation to the parasympathetic component of Cr III, and the fluent function of the intrinsic muscles of the iris and lens
    › the pterygopalatine ganglion – in relation to disturbances of secretion
    › both ganglia also contain sympathetic fibres passing through (but not synapsing)
- arterial supply
  - arising from the carotid artery through the carotid canal
  - also arising from the vertebral arteries
  - taking into account the ophthalmic artery through the optic canal
- venous drainage
  - through the supraorbital fissure
  - the cavernous sinus
  - the whole venous sinus system through the cranium back to the jugular foramen and jugular vein
  - for venous back pressure
- the lacrimal gland, together with its nerve supply from the parasympathetic component of Cr VII
- the nasolacrimal duct – ensuring free mobility of the lacrimal bones, maxillae, and inferior nasal conchae, and free drainage of lacrimal secretions
- lymphatic drainage
- the eyeball itself, including
  - the sclera
  - the intrinsic muscles and their sympathetic and parasympathetic nerve supply
  - the canals of Schlemm.

As always, the objective is to create a healthy environment within which the eye can operate with optimal function, by integrating the whole matrix.

Cranio-sacral motion

The cranio-sacral motion of the orbits is noteworthy in that, during the *expansion* phase, the eyes appear to be *closing*, and during the *contraction* phase, they appear to be *opening* (Figure 34.18). Bearing in mind the movement of the surrounding structures, the reasons for this are readily understandable.

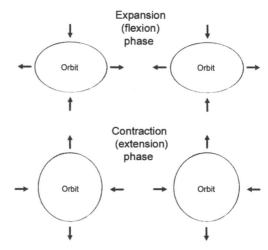

34.18 During cranio-sacral motion, the orbits widen and shorten during the expansion phase

As the frontal bone and sphenoid arc forward and down during the expansion phase, so the face structures (maxillae, palatines, vomer, ethmoid) are rising up to meet them. The eyes are therefore 'squashed' (vertically) between the frontal and the facial bones, squeezing the orbits out laterally during expansion. Consequently:

- During the *expansion phase* (flexion phase)
  - the orbits widen laterally (together with the temporal bones and zygomata)
  - while at the same time becoming smaller top to bottom (as if the eyes were closing).
- During the *contraction phase* (extension phase)
  - the orbits narrow side to side
  - while becoming larger top to bottom (as if the eyes were opening).

Contacts

Many standard cranio-sacral contacts will be appropriate to addressing the various areas and structures throughout the body, cranium and face, which might be contributing to dysfunction of the eyes. Various contacts will also be relevant for enabling balance and integration of the many bones and other structures contributing to the orbits. Within the context of overall cranio-sacral integration, we can also include contacts specific to the eyes.

Lateral contact on the eyes

Sitting at the top of the head, take up contact with all four finger tips at the lateral corners of the eyes bilaterally, engaging with the cranium as a whole and the orbits and eyes in particular. This can be a profoundly integrative contact for the eyes and their surrounding environment (Figure 34.19).

Orbital contact

Sitting at the top of the head, with the patient supine, place your elbows on the couch in such a position that your hands and fingers can hang loosely from your wrists, immediately over the eyes. Keep your wrists high so that your hands, fingers and thumbs can hang loosely without holding on to any unnecessary tension.

Allow the fingers and thumbs to drop gently through the energy field to alight very softly around the rim of the orbits (Figure 34.20).

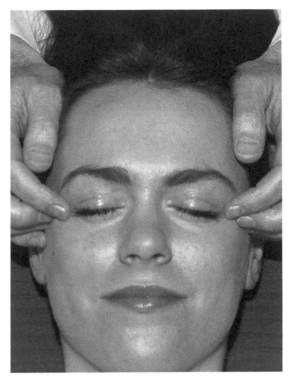

34.19 Engaging with the eyes through the lateral corners of the orbits

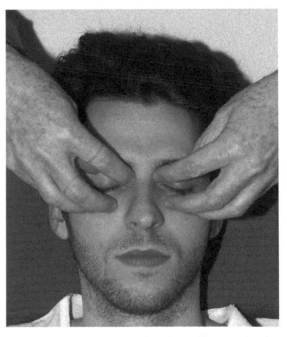

34.20 Contact for integrating the orbits – allow your hands and fingers to hang loosely from your wrists, in order to enable a very light contact

You can engage with the rhythmic motion as the orbits gently open (during the contraction phase) and close (during the expansion phase). You can observe the quality, symmetry and motion that arise, and observe the system finding its way to points of stillness and release. Perhaps the orbits, or one orbit in particular, might draw spontaneously and persistently into one phase of motion or the other, or you could ask yourself whether there is any tendency for the eyes to draw into one phase. You could allow them to follow into that preferred phase, observing the inherent treatment process evolving around the fulcrum of your contact, feeling the system drawing into stillness, releasing, reorganizing, settling back into neutral and establishing greater balance and integration.

The exact position of the fingers is not crucial, but a thorough comprehensive contact could involve:

- the index fingers at the medial corners of the orbits
- the ring and middle fingers along the lower rims of the orbits
- the little fingers in the lateral corners of the orbits
- the thumbs on the superior rims of the orbits.

Through this contact you can engage with the system, allowing the usual inherent treatment process to evolve, following the responses within the system, both local and general. You may notice differences between the two eyes or orbits. As you engage more deeply with the system, you could let your therapeutic attention survey through the structures of the orbit – bones, muscles, membranes, nerves, the eyeball – allowing your attention to identify focal points as appropriate. Your attention may be drawn to one eye in particular, either due to symptoms or palpatory findings.

Energy drive to the eye

Energy drives can be very powerful for the eyes, giving detailed attention to all the structures within the orbit and eyeball (Figure 34.21).

If one eye requires particular attention, either due to your palpatory findings or due to symptoms in that eye, you could direct an energy drive into the eye.

Keeping the same contact as before over the affected eye (or alternatively placing the palm of your hand over the eye), take your other hand to the back of the head, resting your index or middle finger under the head at the opposite pole of the head (directly across the cranium from the selected eye) – usually around or just behind the occipitomastoid area.

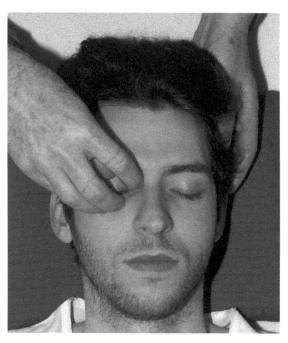

34.21 An energy drive to the eye can be very powerful, giving detailed attention to all the structures within the orbit and the eyeball

Once settled, direct your energy drive through the head to the target area and, as the effects of the energy drive develop, survey the various structures within the orbit and eyeball, identify areas of restriction, or structures requiring attention, feeling the effects of the energy drive dissolving restrictions and clearing the matrix.

As your attention projects through to the orbit, you can give detailed attention to all the structures described above – bones, sutures, foramina, muscles, the common tendinous ring, membranes, nerves, blood vessels, the lacrimal gland – visualizing along nerve pathways, visualizing into the depths of the eyeball, into the canals of Schlemm, the intrinsic muscles, the inner matrix of the eye. Observe any changes in quality, symmetry and motion as your attention moves from one structure to another. Identify any sites of tension or restriction, directing your attention and the power of the energy drive to that area, following the process through to completion.

Eyeball contact

This contact involves a very light contact with the *pads* of the thumbs, resting gently onto the eyeballs (through the closed eyelids) (Figure 34.22).

a.

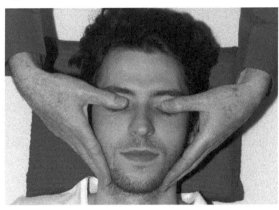

b.

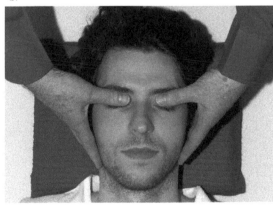

34.22 *The eyeball contact can be exceptionally profound, with significant connections to the autonomic nervous system and the brain. It requires a very delicate contact. (a) Practitioner sitting; (b) practitioner standing*

This contact may be carried out with the practitioner sitting or standing. The advantage of standing is that the arms can hang loosely from the shoulders, with no weight of the hands or arms resting onto the eyes.

In order for this contact to be most effective, it is essential that the thumbs are resting solely on the eyeball, not on the surrounding orbit. Many practitioners, particularly when sitting, allow their thumbs to rest on to the bony orbit, thereby negating or significantly reducing the beneficial effects of this contact.

Let your fingers rest lightly on the sides of the head, the exact location depending on relative size of head and hands, in order to stabilize and support the hands and to avoid weighing too heavily on the eyes.

Move your *wrists out laterally*, so that the *thumbs are pointing medially*. Again this is essential in order to avoid resting the thumbs on the bony orbit (Figure 34.22).

Allow the pads of the thumbs to come to rest very lightly and softly on the centres of the eyeballs (with the eyelids closed). The eyes are sensitive and the contact needs to be very light – but not hesitant or tentative. It is advisable to ask your patient if the contact is comfortable.

This contact is perfectly comfortable when carried out appropriately. However, any tendency to weigh too heavily on the eyeballs can cause discomfort. It is not advisable for any prospective practitioner to use this contact until they have developed a suitably soft, light, gentle, spacious contact. If the patient feels any pain or excessive pressure, the contact is too firm.

There can be a tendency for practitioners to feel so tentative about contacting an area as delicate as the eyes that they do not contact the eyes at all, holding their thumbs off the body and holding tension in their hands. Whilst it is of course perfectly possible to work off the body, the decision to do so should be guided by the patient's energy field, not by the practitioner's tentativeness. Remember that a tense or tentative contact *off* the body is likely to feel more invasive than a soft, relaxed contact *on* the body. Remember also that settling more deeply into a contact is generally perfectly comfortable, as long as the contact is introduced very gradually (and never suddenly or too quickly). Resting softly onto the eyes can enable a much more effective response – always ensuring that your patient is comfortable.

Having established an appropriate contact, follow the inherent treatment process as usual, observing the quality in the eyes, comparing the two sides, feeling the activity and movement

VI

34

within the cyeballs themselves and any pulls exerted by the extrinsic muscles, following each eyeball along its individual journey, observing that the eyes may move independently of each other, visualizing through the detailed anatomy. Allow responses to arise and feel the system gradually settling to deeper stillness.

This contact can be exceptionally profound. The contact on the eyes in itself engages with deep levels of the patient's being. But we are also making a very direct connection with the deeper core structures of the body.

Since the eyeball is an extension of the brain, we are in effect taking up contact on the brain itself. And since the sclera of the eyes is an extension of the dural membrane, when we rest our thumbs on the eyelids we are as close to contacting the membrane system as is possible externally, with just the eyelids between our thumbs and the membrane system. The responses within the system as a whole often reflect this deep level of engagement.

The contact on the eyelids also influences the autonomic nervous system, through the sympathetic supply to the superior tarsal muscle, and through the sympathetic and parasympathetic supply to the eyeballs. Patients may often feel their whole system softening and settling on a profound level in response to this contact – so long as the contact is soft and settling – and often report a particularly deep sense of engagement.

As always, these contacts for the eyes would be used as part of an integrated treatment, rather than in isolation, incorporating specific eye contacts along with a wide range of other cranial and facial contacts, in order to address individual circumstances as necessary, bringing the whole system into integrated balance as necessary, always maintaining a broad awareness of the whole person.

Part VII

The Ears

Chapter 35

The Ears

We met Fiona briefly in Chapter 1. Here is her story.

Fiona was in her late forties when she discovered cranio-sacral integration. She had suffered countless middle ear infections in childhood. Each time antibiotics had been prescribed, providing temporary relief. Each time the infection would recur soon afterwards. Grommets again provided only temporary relief. The condition persisted into adulthood, and with no apparent cure available, she put up with constant discomfort in her right ear, a continuous sense of blockage and congestion in the right side of her head, varying levels of pain, limited hearing, and a persistently uncomfortable and restricted quality of life. Her job involved international travel, but every flight was a nightmare, with excruciating ear pain, leading to numerous burst ear drums, particularly during flights, and eventually having to give up her job and avoid air travel.

The various doctors and specialists that she consulted acknowledged that her right Eustachian tube was blocked, but told her that there was no treatment for that. She explored various other therapies without success.

After more than 30 years of suffering persistent ear infections, burst ear drums, intense pain, avoiding air travel, and a multitude of ineffective treatments, she discovered cranio-sacral integration. After the first session she felt some unusual subtle movements in her blocked ear, but not much else. After the third treatment, the changes became more noticeable. During her fifth session, her ear popped and her whole experience of life changed dramatically. For the first time in her adult life, she could hear clearly. The world around her came alive. Her ear no longer felt uncomfortable, blocked and congested. She was able to fly. Life was transformed.

Ear conditions of one kind or another, particularly involving a long history of recurrent ear infections, congestion, hearing loss, repeated courses of antibiotics, and ineffective medical treatment, are a very common part of cranio-sacral practice. Cranio-sacral integration has proved to be consistently effective in relieving such conditions and transforming the patient's life experience. Fiona is just one of many similar cases.

Middle ear infections affect 90 per cent of the population,[1] potentially leading to more serious complications including meningitis and hearing loss. The ears are a very frequent source of disturbance and discomfort in all ages from newborn babies to the elderly. Conditions involving the ears include tinnitus, hearing loss, persistent and recurrent ear infection, glue ear, disturbance of balance, dizziness, vertigo, labyrinthitis, Ménière's disease, mastoiditis (infection of the mastoid air cells within the mastoid portion of the temporal bone), hyperacusis (heightened sensitivity to sound) and distorted auditory signals (perhaps as a result of cranial nerve dysfunction). Disturbances of the ears can also lead to speech and language difficulties, and potentially significant influences on quality of life.

Many of these conditions arise due to restricted mobility of the structures which house and surround the ears, leading to blockage, congestion, poor drainage of mucus and fluids, impingement, and consequent disturbed function.

Other factors to consider in relation to the ears include enlarged adenoids, referred pain from the teeth, a tooth abscess or cavitation, acoustic neuromas, nerve damage due to medication or surgery, and brain tumours.

Fundamental to the healthy function of the ears is structural balance and integrity. Imbalances may be local or distant, and particularly relevant are those which draw the temporal bones into asymmetry or restriction, or which restrict the cranial base. If the underlying structure is disturbed, the body's ability to maintain free drainage of the middle ear and fluid balance within the inner ear, and to combat infection through healthy immune function and other inherent self-healing mechanisms, can be compromised. Restoration of free fluent mobility through cranio-sacral integration can enable the body to address many of these disturbances.

Cranio-sacral integration is exceptionally effective at addressing persistent and recurrent ear infection and glue ear, particularly because of its unique ability to address the underlying cause. If a research programme were established to explore the clinical effectiveness of cranio-sacral integration, persistent and recurrent ear infection would be one of my first choices for research.

Structure

The *external ear* consists of the *auricle*, also known as the *pinna*, the lower portion of the auricle being the *ear lobe*. Apart from the visible portion of the external ear, the structures of the ear, including the organs of hearing and balance, are contained within the cavities and canals of the temporal bones. The ear has three main internal divisions (Figure 35.1):

- the external auditory canal
- the middle ear
- the inner ear.

The *external auditory canal*, approximately one inch long in an adult, is separated from the middle ear by the *tympanic membrane* (ear drum), forming a closed membrane which protects the middle ear from contact with the outside world and potential

infection. The outer opening of the canal is the *external auditory meatus* (also known as the external acoustic meatus).

The *middle ear* contains the three tiny ossicles (malleus, incus, stapes), the smallest bones in the body, through which vibrations are transmitted from the tympanic membrane to the inner ear (Figures 35.2 and 35.3). The Eustachian tube passes from the middle ear to the nasopharynx, enabling drainage of the middle ear to the back of the upper throat behind the nasal cavity. The middle ear is separated from the inner ear by the oval window, covered with a thin membrane.

The *inner ear* contains the organs of hearing and balance – the shell-shaped cochlea (hearing) and the semicircular canals of the vestibular mechanism (balance). The vestibular and cochlear divisions of the vestibulo-cochlear nerve (Cr VIII) travel together from the inner ear, transmitting sensory impulses from the cochlea and vestibular mechanisms respectively. The combined nerve passes out of the temporal bone and into the cranial cavity through the internal auditory meatus, passing into the brainstem at the pons (Figure 35.4).

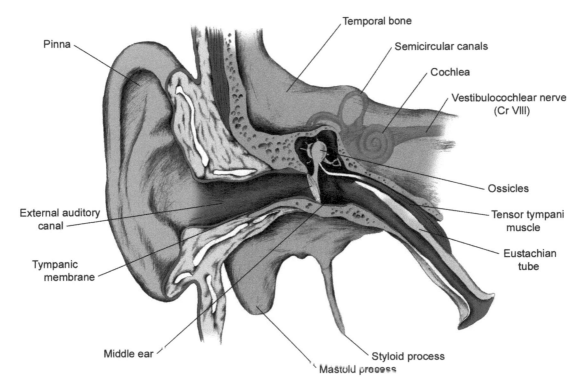

35.1 *The ear has three main internal divisions – the external auditory canal, the middle ear and the inner ear*

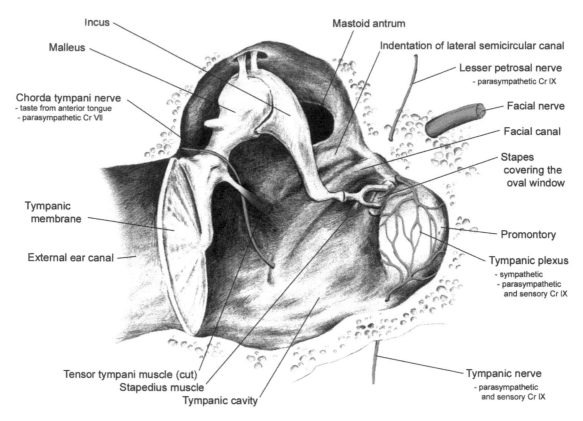

Incus

Malleus

Chorda tympani nerve
- taste from anterior tongue
- parasympathetic Cr VII

Tympanic membrane

External ear canal

Tensor tympani muscle (cut)
Stapedius muscle
Tympanic cavity

Mastoid antrum

Indentation of lateral semicircular canal

Lesser petrosal nerve
- parasympathetic Cr IX

Facial nerve

Facial canal

Stapes covering the oval window

Promontory

Tympanic plexus
- sympathetic
- parasympathetic and sensory Cr IX

Tympanic nerve
- parasympathetic and sensory Cr IX

35.2   The middle ear

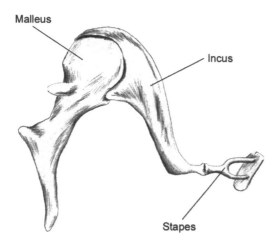

Malleus

Incus

Stapes

35.3   The tiny ossicles within the middle ear are the smallest bones of the body

Function

Hearing mechanism

Sound is gathered by the auricle and funnelled into the external auditory meatus, passing along the external auditory canal until it reaches the tympanic membrane, approximately one inch into the canal.

Vibration of the tympanic membrane passes to the ossicles and is transmitted via the malleus (hammer), incus (anvil) and stapes (stirrup) of the middle ear, through the oval window, into the cochlea of the inner ear.

Within the snail-shell-shaped cochlea, vibrations stimulate tiny sensory hair cells, converting the vibrations into neurological impulses to be transmitted along the *cochlear division of the vestibulo-cochlear nerve* to the brainstem.

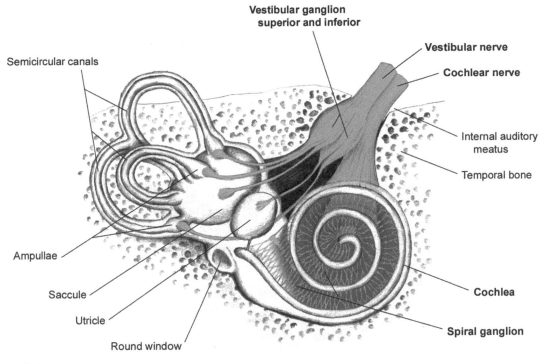

35.4   The inner ear

Vestibular mechanism

The vestibular mechanism consists of three *semicircular canals* together with the *utricle* and *saccule* containing fluid (*endolymph*) (Figure 35.4). Movement of the fluid stimulates the many thousands of tiny hair-like receptors on the inner surface of these structures, transmitting sensory impulses along the *vestibular division of the vestibulo-cochlear nerve* to the brainstem.

The semicircular canals transmit information regarding rotational movements of the head, with each canal set at a different angle in order to respond to different directions of motion. The utricle and saccule reflect gravity and linear acceleration of the head. Together they enable sensations of equilibrium, body position and gaze stability.

Nerve supply

Nerve supply to the organs of hearing and balance within the inner ear is via the vestibulo-cochlear nerve (Cr VIII), which has been described in Chapter 27 (Figure 35.5).

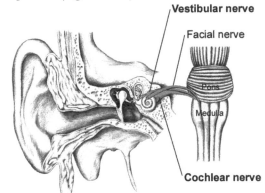

35.5   Nerve supply to the organs of hearing and balance within the inner ear is via the vestibulo-cochlear nerve (Cr VIII)

The facial nerve (Cr VII) within the facial canal forms an indentation into the middle ear cavity (Figure 35.2). It gives off a branch to the stapedius muscle. A further branch of the facial nerve, the chorda tympani, receiving taste sensation from the anterior tongue and providing parasympathetic supply to the submandibular and sublingual glands, also passes through the tympanic cavity (Figure 35.2).

The tympanic plexus, carrying sympathetic fibres, and also sensory and parasympathetic fibres from the glosso-pharyngeal nerve (Cr IX) via the tympanic nerve, is also located within the middle ear. The majority of pain from earache is transmitted via the tympanic nerve.[2]

Sensory input from various parts of the ear is also carried by other branches of the facial and glosso-pharyngeal nerves, and also by branches of the trigeminal and vagus nerves.

The Eustachian tube

The Eustachian tube is named after Bartolomeo Eustachi of Rome (c.1514–1574), one of the earliest anatomists. It is also known as the *auditory tube* or *pharyngo-tympanic* tube and connects the middle ear to the nasopharynx at the back of the nasal cavity on each side, enabling adjustment of the pressure within the ear and drainage of the middle ear (Figure 35.6).

The tube starts as a *bony canal* within the temporal bone which opens onto the inferior surface of the base of the cranium at the spheno-temporal suture, between the carotid canal (posteriorly) and foramen ovale (anteriorly) (Figure 35.8). It continues as a *cartilaginous 'incomplete tube'* (actually C-shaped in cross-section like an upside-down gutter) passing anteromedially and almost horizontally along the inferior surface of the spheno-temporal suture at the base of the skull (Figure 35.8). It terminates by emptying into the nasopharynx, close to the top of the medial pterygoid plate of the sphenoid, posterior and inferior to the inferior nasal concha, just below the roof of the pharynx and above the level of the palate (Figures 35.7 and 35.8).

a.

b.

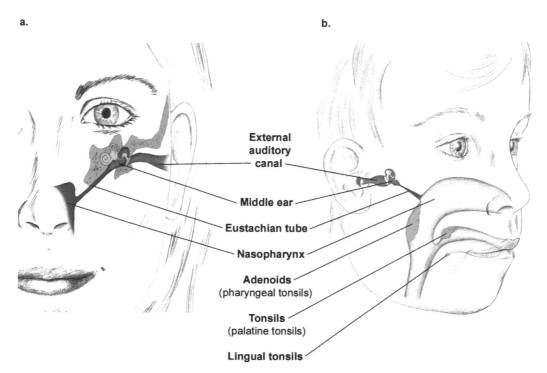

External auditory canal

Middle ear

Eustachian tube

Nasopharynx

Adenoids (pharyngeal tonsils)

Tonsils (palatine tonsils)

Lingual tonsils

35.6   The Eustachian tube passes from the middle ear to the nasopharynx, enabling drainage of the middle ear

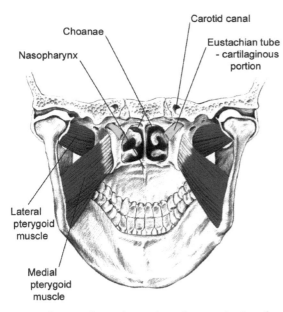

Choanae

Carotid canal

Nasopharynx

Eustachian tube - cartilaginous portion

Lateral pterygoid muscle

Medial pterygoid muscle

35.7   The Eustachian tube terminates by emptying into the nasopharynx, close to the top of the medial pterygoid plate of the sphenoid

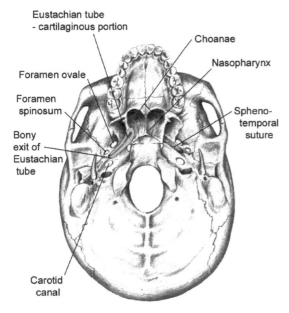

Eustachian tube - cartilaginous portion

Choanae

Foramen ovale

Nasopharynx

Foramen spinosum

Spheno-temporal suture

Bony exit of Eustachian tube

Carotid canal

35.8   The cartilaginous portion of the Eustachian tube passes anteromedially and almost horizontally along the inferior surface of the spheno-temporal suture at the base of the skull

The whole tube (bony and cartilaginous) is lined with a soft mucous membrane and remains closed except when swallowing, yawning, or blowing

forcefully. Swallowing activates the muscles which open the Eustachian tube. Swallowing therefore relieves pressure in the ear (as can be observed when travelling in an aeroplane), thereby equalizing the pressure inside the middle ear with the surrounding atmosphere. Pressure difference causes temporary hearing loss due to reduced mobility of the tympanic membrane and the ossicles. We swallow approximately 1800 times per day. This also encourages drainage of mucus and infectious organisms from the middle ear to the nasopharynx.

However, the Eustachian tube also enables infection from common colds and throat infections to pass up from the nasopharynx into the middle ear, leading to middle ear infection. The inner surface of the tube is lined with cilia, whose action tends to encourage the movement of mucus (and infectious organisms) away from the middle ear towards the nasopharynx, thus preventing infections from ascending into the middle ear. But this natural tendency may be overcome by adverse circumstances, including forceful nose-blowing and positional factors. Babies are particularly susceptible because their Eustachian tubes are shorter, relatively wider, and more horizontal, and because they spend much of their time in a horizontal position.

The Eustachian tube is 13mm long at birth, 18mm long in infants, and 36mm long in an adult. Two thirds of this length is the cartilaginous portion. By the age of seven, it is approximately the same length as in an adult. The angle of descent of the tube from middle ear to nasopharynx also changes with age, being angled at approximately 10 degrees to the horizontal in infants, increasing to 45 degrees in an adult. The narrowest point of the tube is at the junction of the bony and cartilaginous portions.

The muscles involved in opening and acting upon the Eustachian tube are levator veli palatini and salpingo-pharyngeus – both innervated by motor branches of the glosso-pharyngeal nerve (Cr IX) and the vagus nerve (Cr X) – and tensor veli palatini and tensor tympani, supplied by motor branches of the trigeminal nerve (Cr V).

The Eustachian tube opens during external rotation of the temporal bones and closes during internal rotation. Restriction of the temporal bones in internal rotation – a common pattern, particularly involving the occipitomastoid suture, whether due to birth trauma, injury, or tension – can therefore be instrumental in contributing to Eustachian tube dysfunction and persistent middle ear infection.

Due to the proximity of the adenoids (pharyngeal tonsils) to the opening of the Eustachian tube in the roof of the nasopharynx, enlarged adenoids may contribute to restricted drainage of the middle ear and consequent middle ear infections (Figure 35.6).

Mastoid air cells

The mastoid air cells form a honeycomb of air spaces within the mastoid process of the temporal bone, posterior to the middle ear, to which they connect via the mastoid antrum, with potential for middle ear infections to spread into the mastoid air cells (Figure 35.9). *Mastoiditis* is a potential complication of middle ear infections. Since the walls of the air cells are very thin, there is the additional possible complication that infection may spread from the mastoid air cells into the cranial cavity, leading to meningitis or encephalitis.

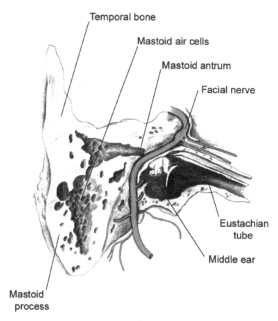

Temporal bone

Mastoid air cells

Mastoid antrum

Facial nerve

Eustachian tube

Middle ear

Mastoid process

35.9 The mastoid air cells connect to the middle ear via the mastoid antrum, with potential for middle ear infections to spread into the mastoid air cells

Ear infections

Otitis media

Middle ear infections (otitis media) occur primarily as a result of an infectious organism passing up from the nose and throat into the middle ear via the Eustachian tube. The infectious cause is most commonly a virus[3] from a cold or throat infection, but can also be bacterial.

It can occur as an acute episode – acute otitis media (AOM) – or can develop into a chronic condition of otitis media with effusion (OME), commonly known as glue ear. It affects 90 per cent of the population, mostly during childhood, and is one of the most common conditions for which medical treatment is requested in children.

Young children are more susceptible, partly because their Eustachian tubes are shorter and partly because their immune systems are less developed (a significant factor in immune system development is exposure to infections), and in the case of babies because they spend much of their time lying horizontal. Other factors which contribute to the susceptibility include passive smoking,[4] use of a dummy (pacifier), and early exposure to other children at day care and playgroups. There is a reduced susceptibility in children who are exclusively breastfeed for at least six to twelve months, since breastfeeding enhances immunity.[5]

Burst ear drum

In some cases, the tympanic membrane may rupture (a burst ear drum), allowing the release of pus into the external ear canal. Whilst this may appear (and smell) unpleasant, it is generally a beneficial process – the body's natural way of dealing with the infection, bringing relief of pain and pressure, and the release of the infected pus, thereby protecting the ear from further damage. The tympanic membrane generally repairs naturally within a few days. The fact that the ear drum needs to burst is, however, an indication of inadequate drainage through the proper channels which remains unresolved.

Glue ear

Otitis media with effusion (OME), commonly referred to as glue ear, is a chronic accumulation of fluid within the middle ear due to dysfunction of the Eustachian tube. Over several weeks or months, the fluid can become thick and glue-like. It is generally a painless condition but may produce a sensation of fullness in the ear. The main concern is loss of hearing.

Glue ear causes partial deafness and, since it may otherwise be symptomless, may often remain unrecognized. If it is not identified, it can affect a child's learning – not hearing what teachers are saying at school, not picking up information in day-to-day communications with parents and friends, and usually of course the child is unaware that they are not hearing properly. This in turn can affect their behaviour, their responses, and their whole relationship with the world around them – teachers and parents assuming that the child is ignoring them, not paying attention, or misbehaving, rather than realizing that the child is partially deaf.

Grommets

In cases of recurrent ear infection or persistent glue ear, if the condition has not resolved following several prescriptions of antibiotics, tympanostomy tubes (commonly known as grommets) may be inserted – a minor surgical procedure (carried out under general anaesthetic).

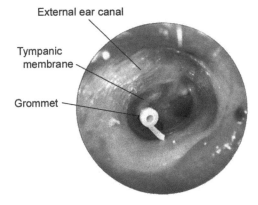

External ear canal

Tympanic membrane

Grommet

35.10 A grommet is a tiny plastic tube inserted into the tympanic membrane

A grommet is a tiny plastic tube which is inserted into the tympanic membrane (Figure 35.10). This enables air to pass through, keeping the pressure on each side equal, enabling the middle ear to function more efficiently. However, grommets also provide a potential channel for infections to enter the ear from outside, so children with grommets may need to take care to avoid possible sources of infection, especially through activities such as swimming. The grommets eventually fall out (usually within a few months or a year) and may need to be replaced from time to time. Grommets may bring relief of symptoms (although not always), and in some cases the child will grow out of their recurrent ear infections. In other cases, the condition will persist – because the natural drainage pathway (the Eustachian tube) has still not been addressed.

Antibiotics

In evaluating the use of antibiotics for otitis media, it is necessary to weigh up the advantages and disadvantages. The majority of middle ear infections are initiated by a virus[6] – for which antibiotics are not effective. It is also generally accepted that the majority of middle ear infections will resolve spontaneously within three days without antibiotics:

> A study published in the November 2010 issue of the *Journal of the American Medical Association* (JAMA) confirms the wisdom of avoiding antibiotics for the treatment of ear infections. This study reviewed 125 previous studies on the effect of antibiotics versus placebo, and found that 80 per cent of children with ear infections would recover within about 3 days without antibiotics.[7]

Antibiotics are therefore primarily prescribed as a *prophylactic*, in case of possible complications.

Antibiotics can have side effects – including vomiting, diarrhoea and rash, as well as destroying good bacteria – and in the long term may have a weakening effect on the immune system; whereas allowing the body to deal with the infection itself is the principal means through which the immune system develops and strengthens.

Persistent use of antibiotics also leads to the development of increasingly resistant strains of bacteria, as has become increasingly recognized in recent years:

> Some studies have shown that children treated with antibiotics tend to develop resistance to antibiotics and have more ear infections than children not treated. This makes sense because antibiotics interfere with the production of white blood cells. When white blood cells are unable to fight infections, then recurrence of an infection is more likely.[8]

The standard recommendation these days is only to use antibiotics immediately in severe cases, and only in children under two years old. Otherwise, the recommendation is to wait for three days, monitoring carefully for any deterioration or complication. Complications are rare. Antibiotics are not generally recommended for glue ear.[9]

Parents may therefore need to decide whether to address their child's ear infections naturally insofar as possible, avoiding antibiotics where possible, and allowing their child's immune system to develop through addressing infections for itself; or to seek antibiotic treatment as a matter of course, to guard against the rare possibility of complications.

Each case needs to be assessed on its own merits, and each parent will need to evaluate their position. Understandably, the tendency is for parents to be fearful of complications (however rare) and to seek medication as a matter of course. (It has also been reported that doctors feel pressurized by parents into prescribing antibiotics even when they are not necessary.)

The alternative is to let the infection take its natural course (knowing that the vast majority of cases pass uneventfully without antibiotic treatment) and to use natural resources to enhance the chances of a simple natural resolution – once again assessing each case on its own merits and monitoring carefully.

Cranio-sacral integration

Cranio-sacral integration can be very helpful in addressing any functional restrictions or contributory factors, and in enhancing the body's natural defences. In an ideal world, every baby and child would receive regular cranio-sacral integration as a matter of course, thereby addressing any underlying predisposition to ear infections and enhancing immunity. In an acute middle ear infection, cranio-sacral integration can also help by relieving congestion, improving drainage and enhancing the body's natural ability to fight off infection.

Homeopathy

Acute infections can of course strike at any time, particularly in babies and children and, since most parents do not have immediate access to a cranio-sacral therapist in the middle of the night or whenever the infection may develop, homeopathy can also be a very helpful resource in dealing with an acute infection.

Ideally, homeopathy will be tailored to the specific needs of the individual and their constitution, but certain specific homeopathic remedies are often used routinely for ear infections, depending on the circumstances and the associated symptoms. Homeopathy can also be helpful in addressing chronic ear infections, and the combination of homeopathy with cranio-sacral integration can be especially effective.

Common homeopathic remedies for ear symptoms include pulsatilla, belladonna, aconite, chamomilla, merc sol, ferrum phos, hepar sulph, phosphorus, lycopodium and silica – depending on the specific symptoms and circumstances.

Symptoms involving the ears may also arise as *referred pain*, without any primary issue in the ear itself. These may often be mistaken for ear infections, resulting in the unnecessary prescription of antibiotics. Disturbances of the teeth can be one possible source of earache, more readily recognized in teething babies, but again often misinterpreted in adults. Conversely, symptoms in the teeth may be the result of ear dysfunctions and can lead to unnecessary dentistry.

Dysfunction of the Eustachian tube

It is generally acknowledged that middle ear infections, particularly the more chronic forms such as glue ear, are primarily due to dysfunction of the Eustachian tube:

The common cause of all forms of otitis media is dysfunction of the Eustachian tube.[10]

But there is no readily available, safe and suitable medical means of addressing this.

As long ago as 1724, French physician and inventor Edmé-Gilles Guyot (1706–1786) developed the first known catheterization of the Eustachian tube when he tried to cure his own deafness by passing a pewter tube from his mouth through the opening of the Eustachian tube in his nasopharynx up into his middle ear.[11]

An operation is possible, but the risk of severing the carotid artery and other damage is significant, and the potential risks are usually considered to outweigh the possible benefits.

This is where cranio-sacral integration plays such a crucial, unique role in addressing chronic ear infections, and is one of the principal reasons why cranio-sacral integration is so exceptionally effective in such conditions. Cranio-sacral integration provides a highly effective means of addressing dysfunction in the Eustachian tube, and it does not carry any risks.

Cranio-sacral approach

As mentioned previously, cranio-sacral integration can be beneficial in the resolution of *acute* otitis media (which may resolve spontaneously anyway). But its value lies primarily in addressing the *chronic* recurrent and persistent cases of infection and glue ear – because they are not readily addressed by other means.

The principal basis of the cranio-sacral approach to chronic ear infections is the release of the Eustachian tube, thereby allowing free drainage and fluent function. This revolves particularly around the temporal bones and the spheno-temporal suture, but inevitably also involves all the surrounding structures, along with any tensions, compressions and restrictions throughout the cranial base area and beyond, and any further underlying causes which may be contributing to the restriction of the Eustachian tube.

It also includes ensuring free drainage of fluids and mucus throughout the cranium, giving attention to the venous sinuses throughout the cranium and therefore the intracranial membranes,

and promoting the body's immune function and its natural ability to address infection.

The cranio-sacral approach will as always involve allowing the inherent treatment process to take its course, addressing whatever restrictions and compressions may be present in the individual circumstances. Within that context, specific attention may be given to release of the suboccipital area, the occipitomastoid sutures and jugular foramina, and particularly ensuring the free mobility of the temporal bones and the spheno-temporal suture along which the Eustachian tube runs.

Much of this tension and restriction around the cranial base is likely to have arisen from the birth process:

The root cause of otitis media is birth trauma.[12]

The *physical forces* involved in birth trauma can lead to compression in the suboccipital area and throughout the base of the cranium, with tightness in the surrounding musculature, contributing to congestion and poor drainage. The *shock effects* of birth (as well as contributing to agitation, restlessness, poor sleep and hyperactivity in babies and children) may also create further tension in the suboccipital region.

Restriction in the subocciput may be further maintained by shock and tension throughout the system, including the heart centre and solar plexus centre, and overstimulation of the sympathetic nervous system.

The temporal area may be medially compressed by the birth process. This may particularly be the case following the use of forceps. Contraction of the intracranial membranes, another consequence of shock, may also draw the temporal bones into medial contraction.

Once again, overall cranio-sacral integration, allowing the inherent treatment process to address the individual circumstances as necessary, enhanced by the practitioner's informed awareness, is likely to enable appropriate resolution of the situation. Comprehensive cranio-sacral integration also includes attention to other potential contributory factors, including investigation of allergies, avoiding dairy products and other mucus-producing foods, and promoting the body's immune function and its natural ability to address infection.

Relevant contacts are likely to include the heart centre, the solar plexus centre, suboccipital release, mastoid tip contact, falx release, spheno-basilar release, temporal contacts, ear hold, energy drives through the ears – and any other contacts as required for the individual circumstances. Ultimately, as always, it is a matter of engaging with the system and identifying its individual needs.

Patulous Eustachian tube

A patulous Eustachian tube is a less common condition in which the Eustachian tube remains open most of the time instead of only opening intermittently. Symptoms include an amplified or echoing sound of one's own voice and breathing, and a sensation of fullness in the ear. The persistent openness of the tube may also increase the likelihood of infectious organisms passing up into the middle ear with consequent increased susceptibility to middle ear infections.

Inner ear infections

Infections can also affect the inner ear, presenting a very different picture. Inner ear infections are less common, but often more serious. They are less common because entry of infectious organisms to the inner ear is less readily accessible. They are more serious because infection of the structures within the inner ear – the organs of hearing and balance – can be far more debilitating, causing more permanent damage to the delicate structures of the cochlea and vestibular mechanism and to the vestibulo-cochlear nerve. Conditions resulting from inner ear disturbance include dizziness, vertigo, labyrinthitis, vestibular neuritis and Ménière's disease.

Dizziness

Dizziness refers to a feeling of unsteadiness or instability. It is an imprecise term which may also be used for various subdivisions of dizziness including vertigo, presyncope (lightheadedness) or disequilibrium (off balance).

Episodes may be brought on by inadequate blood supply to the brain due to a sudden fall in blood pressure, whether from standing up suddenly, or due to a heart condition, or due to restricted arterial flow through the cervical spine, suboccipital region or cranial base. This last factor is perhaps one of the more common but least recognized factors in relation to blood supply to the head and ears. Once other causes such as heart conditions have been eliminated, much can be done to alleviate persistent or recurrent cases of dizziness through the release of tensions and restrictions in the neck, suboccipital region and cranial base, through fascial unwinding, suboccipital release and appropriate cranio-sacral integration, potentially abrogating the need for extensive invasive investigations into cranial nerve or inner ear dysfunction and unnecessary treatment.

Dizziness can also be a side effect of various medications, and can be associated with a great many medical conditions including vertigo, Ménière's disease, vestibular neuritis, labyrinthitis, otitis media, tumours, motion sickness, hypotension (low blood pressure), heart conditions, iron deficiency, hypoglycaemia (low blood sugar), hormonal changes (e.g. thyroid disease, menstruation, pregnancy), anxiety, depression and age-related circumstances.

Vertigo

Vertigo is a subdivision of dizziness. It involves a perception of spinning, with consequent imbalance and unsteadiness. It is often associated with nausea and vomiting, sometimes with tinnitus, hearing loss, and fullness or pain in the ear.

Most common causes of vertigo involve the inner ear and vestibular nerve, and include Ménière's disease, vestibular neuritis, labyrinthitis – and of course transiently from consumption of large quantities of alcohol. Other causes include physical trauma and ototoxic antibiotics. More rarely, the cause can be in the central nervous system, due to tumours or haemorrhage, in which case the effects are likely to be more severe, potentially leaving the patient unable to stand or walk.

The most common cause of vertigo is *benign paroxysmal positional vertigo* (BPPV),[13] which occurs when loose calcium carbonate particles enter the semicircular canals, stimulating the hair cells, thereby creating the sensation of motion. This usually results in brief episodes of vertigo on changing position. It can be helped through repositioning movements such as the Epley manoeuvre in which the head is moved into various positions in order to clear the particles within the semicircular canals. In appropriate cases, it is wise to explore this possibility first, since it is totally non-invasive and, if relevant, may abrogate the need for other treatment.

Labyrinthitis

The labyrinth comprises the vestibular system and the cochlea. Labyrinthitis is usually caused by a virus, often following an upper respiratory tract infection (URTI), and is only rarely due to bacterial infection. It can also arise from stress, allergy, or as a reaction to medication. It may occasionally be due to a herpes virus reactivation.

Symptoms include vertigo, hearing loss, and tinnitus, often accompanied by nausea, vomiting and generalized imbalance, and may include sensations of aural fullness. Chronic anxiety is a common side effect of labyrinthitis and may manifest as tremors, palpitations, panic attacks and depression. A panic attack can be one of the first symptoms of labyrinthitis.

Vestibular neuritis

Vestibular neuritis is inflammation of the vestibular nerve, most commonly due to a viral infection of the inner ear. It has similar characteristics to labyrinthitis but it is by definition specifically affecting the vestibular mechanism and does not involve the cochlea, and therefore does not generally include auditory symptoms.

Cranio-sacral treatment for such conditions involves the usual fundamental approach – encouraging free mobility and function through engagement with the inherent treatment process,

and enhancing the body's inherent ability to address the infection.

Ménière's disease

Ménière's disease is named after the French physician Prosper Ménière who, in 1861, first reported that vertigo was caused by inner ear disorders.

It is a disorder of the inner ear, characterized by recurrent episodes of four symptoms – severe vertigo, together with tinnitus, progressive hearing loss or distorted hearing, and a sense of fullness in the ear.

In its most serious form, classic Ménière's can be a severely incapacitating condition, the extreme vertigo leaving the patient unable to stand up. It may be accompanied by nausea and vomiting. As the disease worsens, hearing loss deteriorates, affecting both ears. Attacks can last minutes, hours, or in some cases persisting for days or weeks on end.

In other cases, it can be a much milder condition, not necessarily involving all four classic symptoms.

It is thought to be caused by an increase in the amount of endolymphatic fluid present in the membranous labyrinth of the inner ear. The reasons why this occurs are unknown. Other possible contributory factors include head injury or infection with a herpes virus. It appears to be aggravated by high salt intake, alcohol, caffeine and tobacco.

Hearing loss

There are many causes of hearing loss, some transient, some permanent, some eminently resolvable, others the result of irreversible damage. In many situations, cranio-sacral integration can be highly effective where other methods have not helped and the prognosis can be very positive. Other circumstances cannot be resolved, perhaps due to cochlea damage. The priority is to identify the nature and cause of the deafness and to differentiate between those which can be resolved and those which cannot.

Catriona's Story

Catriona had been experiencing increasing deafness in her right ear for a very long time. This was not only uncomfortable but was also proving very difficult in her communications with others, both at work and socially, leaving her feeling frustrated, embarrassed, and tending to avoid social activities. Her right ear felt constantly blocked, the world around her sounded muffled. Her right nostril also felt blocked. She blew her nose frequently to try and relieve the congestion, and the whole right side of her head felt heavy and congested. She was not aware of having suffered any ear infections, either recently or in childhood.

Her first course of action was to go to her doctor, who prescribed antibiotics. This did not make any difference, so the doctor then prescribed decongestants. This still did not provide any relief and her deafness and feeling of blockage continued to deteriorate, to her continuing frustration. Further visits to the doctor did not provide any further solutions. By the time she came to cranio-sacral integration her condition had been deteriorating for over two years and, realizing that orthodox medical treatment was not helping her, she had decided to try something else.

Engaging with Catriona's system revealed that the whole right side of her head and face was tight, including the temporal, mandibular, maxillary, nasal, occipital and occipitomastoid areas, and that this tightness extended down through her neck, shoulder and arm and through the right side of her thorax. On enquiry, she reported that her right arm also felt tight and restricted most of the time, especially noticeable when reaching for things.

Her main concern was her hearing, but it was immediately apparent that the symptoms in her ear were part of a much wider picture and were being maintained and perpetuated by the tension she was holding throughout the right-hand side of her body. There was undoubtedly restriction in her head and face which needed to be addressed, but it was also essential from the start that treatment should also involve the release of the tightness through her thorax, shoulder and arm, up through her neck – which was pulling her head and neck into a contracted pattern of tension, tightening the muscles and soft tissues at the base of the skull and contributing to the congestion and poor drainage of her ear.

As the right side of her body released, the cranium became more responsive, and the various restrictions in the temporal bone, occipitomastoid suture, spheno-temporal suture, sterno-cleido-mastoid muscle, suboccipital muscles, Eustachian tube, nasal bones, maxillae and mandible all began to release and settle into greater mobility and balance.

The hearing loss had only become apparent around two years ago, but it was clearly evident from the quality of the tissues that the pattern of tightness and restriction on her right side had been developing for many years prior to that. Since the pattern affecting her ear was so widespread and long-standing and was being perpetuated by her day-to-day activities, progress was slow at first, with little symptomatic relief initially, only transient glimpses of change during the first few sessions, with gradually increasing indications of change as treatment progressed. It took around three months and ten treatments before Catriona's hearing fully returned. This inevitably led to her doubting the effectiveness of the treatment, and she required constant reassurance that the situation was progressing, that underlying changes were taking place, and that the treatment would be successful, in order to ensure that she followed the process through.

Further suggestions regarding self-care were also beneficial – encouraging her to sleep on her left side (in order to encourage drainage of the right ear and to avoid compressing the tight right side), to avoid blowing her nose forcefully (as this was forcing mucus up into her ear and sinuses), to hold her phone on her left side (to reduce the tension that she held in her right arm and shoulder and to avoid the tendency to bend her head and neck to the right), and to be mindful of the way that she used her right arm in day-to-day activities, developing a more relaxed, less intense use of the arm and shoulder.

The changes took time, but after three months her hearing was fully restored – for the first time in over two years – to her great relief. She also felt much more comfortable and at ease in her body generally.

Cases of hearing loss which are due to congestion, head injury, structural disturbance, temporal bone restriction, trauma or meningitis are likely to be eminently responsive to cranio-sacral integration. Cases that are due to persistent exposure to loud noise, cochlea damage, nerve damage or age-related deterioration are unlikely to be resolvable – although in some cases they may be improved.

Causes to consider include ear wax, ear infection, glue ear, mucus congestion, conductive deafness, sensori-neural deafness, cochlea damage, vestibulo-cochlear nerve damage, age-related degeneration of hair cells, damage due to persistent loud noise, damage due to medication, osteoarthritis of the ossicles, structural imbalances due to head injuries or whole-body imbalances, and stress factors.

Conductive hearing loss involves any physical obstruction to the conduction of sound, including ear wax, fluid or mucus congestion, and glue ear.

Sensori-neural hearing loss involves damage to the neurological structures of the cochlea and the cochlear nerve.

Congestive causes

The first step is to check for ear wax in the external auditory canal. This is usually carried out at a GP practice (doctor's surgery) and in most patients this will already have been done.

The symptoms and history will then guide the progress. Where the symptoms and history indicate a history of ear infection, glue ear, mucus congestion and sensations of blockage, whether in babies, children or adults, cranio-sacral integration will usually be the most effective option – establishing free mobility, fluent function, clear drainage, overall cranio-sacral integration and any supportive measures that may be appropriate (such as dietary or lifestyle factors).

Results can sometimes be very quick, particularly where the condition is relatively recent. In more chronic cases, resolution may be slower, because not only will it take longer to clear the congestion, but it may also be necessary to release deeply ingrained long-standing structural imbalances in the ears, the cranium, the face and the body generally (as with Catriona).

Even when the structural restriction has been cleared, the body needs time to drain the congestion fully. Furthermore, in long-standing conditions, even when the structural restrictions and the congestion have cleared, it is necessary for the epithelial cells lining the ear to recover and regenerate, and this can take several weeks, or even months.

Patients may need to be patient

Where symptoms are slow to respond, the cranio-sacral therapist will be able to feel the progress within the quality, symmetry and motion of the cranio-sacral system and will need to provide reassurance to the patient who may be concerned about the persisting symptoms and apparent lack of progress. (In the modern medical culture of symptom relief, people expect instant results.) But patients may need to be patient in awaiting the natural healing of the tissues and the resolution of their symptoms. Even with children, glue ear may have been present for several years and may take time to resolve completely.

Mucus congestion affecting the ears may be due to persistent colds, sinus congestion, allergies, food and pollen sensitivities, excessive forceful nose-blowing, poor drainage of the ears, or structural restrictions. As with any situation, symptoms, history and palpation of the cranio-sacral system, combined with informed awareness, insight and a broad perspective, can unravel the background and identify and address the contributory factors according to individual circumstances.

Cochlea damage

In cases where the patient has been exposed to persistent loud noise, the prognosis is not promising. Persistent loud noise causes damage to the hair cells within the cochlea, and there is minimal potential for regeneration. This applies to those who have worked for many years with road drills and other noisy machinery with inadequate ear protection, and also affects a great many rock musicians. The only solution at this stage is hearing aids.

The hair cells within the cochlea may also degenerate with age, and again there is nothing to be done other than hearing aids – but it is advisable to check that there is no other underlying cause, rather than simply assuming that the deterioration is age-related.

Vestibulo-cochlear nerve damage

If there are indications of disturbed function in the vestibulo-cochlear nerve, it will be relevant to check for cranio-sacral restrictions, including bony compressions, particularly involving the temporal bones, membranous tensions, particularly around the internal auditory meatus and the lower pons, residual effects of meningitis or meningisms, or damage from operations.

The therapist can visualize the nerve pathway and surrounding structures, following the

VII

35

pathway with informed awareness and therapeutic attention, observing changes in quality, symmetry and motion and cranio-sacral responses, identifying any indications of restriction or imbalance, and integrating the local matrix and the wider matrix.

Vestigial effects of meningitis are particularly responsive to cranio-sacral integration, and addressing these effects (even where no history of meningitis is recognized) can sometimes bring dramatic results in apparently unpromising cases.

Ototoxic antibiotics

One common cause of damage to the vestibulo-cochlear nerve is exposure to ototoxic antibiotics, such as gentamicin and streptomycin. These may be prescribed for various bacterial infections at any age.

Gentamicin is commonly given to newborn babies with breathing problems, and is used routinely in newborn babies as a prophylactic antibiotic, since it is effective against many bacteria. It is ototoxic and nephrotoxic. In other words it can damage the ears and the kidneys, and it can lead to hearing loss. Its administration therefore has to be monitored and controlled very carefully to ensure appropriate dosage, blood levels and timing, in order to keep it within the safe therapeutic range. Its ototoxic effects are of course recognized. Levels are prescribed carefully to minimize risk, and babies are monitored carefully for any resulting neurological defects. Adverse effects are rare but a significant risk.

Streptomycin is less widely used, and also carries similar side effects of ototoxicity, nephrotoxicity, foetal auditory toxicity and neuromuscular paralysis.

Acoustic neuroma

An acoustic neuroma is a benign tumour of the myelin-producing Schwann cells on the vestibulo-cochlear nerve (usually the vestibular division). Although benign and slow-growing, as its size increases it may compress not only the vestibulo-cochlear nerve but also the facial nerve. It can also affect the brainstem and cerebellum, with more widespread effects. Symptoms vary, but most commonly involve gradual unilateral hearing loss

and tinnitus, and may also affect the vestibular system and other cranial nerves.

It is generally treated through an operation to remove the tumour. Access to the tumour may be translabyrinthine, retrosigmoid/suboccipital or via the middle fossa. This may leave residual damage to the vestibulo-cochlear nerve and to the facial nerve, leading to Bell's palsy.

Tinnitus

Tinnitus is the perception of persistent sounds in one or both ears. The sounds can manifest as a wide variety of noises – including whining, whistling, ringing, humming or clicking – and can vary from minor background sounds to overwhelmingly loud noise that drives the patient to distraction.

Tinnitus is a common condition affecting around 20 per cent of the population. It has no known cause and there is no established explanation as to how or why it arises, what structures might be involved, or what is happening physiologically or neurologically.

Various factors appear to contribute, but these are so variable from person to person that there appears to be no consistent explanation. These factors include restricted temporal bones, nerve compression, neuritis, vascular disturbances, congestion in the ear, imbalances in the neck, persistent exposure to noise, teeth clenching and grinding, TMJ dysfunction, stress factors, and many others.

Some cases respond very quickly, others gradually, others not at all. As with hearing, it is necessary to evaluate the whole picture, to identify the relevant factors through the symptoms and history, and to distinguish those cases that can be completely resolved and those which can only be helped – always bearing in mind that with tinnitus, even in cases where the perceived sound may not be completely eliminated, it is always possible to help the patient to improve their situation.

As always, the priority is overall cranio-sacral integration, including structural and psycho-emotional factors, with particular attention to the temporal bones and factors influencing the temporal area, and to the release of membranous tension in the tentorium and the intracranial membranes. Sometimes, when balance and integration is restored to the temporal region, the tinnitus will disappear – but the disturbance to the temporal region may be arising from anywhere in the body, so overall integration is necessary, and deeply ingrained patterns throughout the body may tend to pull the body out of balance again, leading to the return of symptoms unless they are addressed fully.

In addressing the local area, it can be helpful to explore the relevant anatomical structure in great detail, visualizing deep inside the temporal bone and elsewhere, following nerve pathways, vascular structures, ear canals, the structures of the inner ear, scanning through the detailed anatomy, identifying any changes in quality, symmetry and motion which might reveal the source of disturbance.

There may be pressure on nerve pathways due to bony impingement, membranous tension, infection, inflammation, and arterial or venous pressure. There are various nerve pathways that could be involved. As well as the vestibulo-cochlear nerve, it may be relevant to explore the nerve to stapedius (a branch of the facial nerve), the nerve to tensor tympani (a branch of the trigeminal nerve) and the many widely distributed branches of the sympathetic supply, including branches to the middle ear, inner ear and tympanic membrane, via the tympanic plexus, some of these travelling with cranial nerve branches, others travelling independently.

As described in Chapter 32 on the autonomic nervous system, sympathetic stimulation can lead to hyper-reactivity of tissues and other nerves, including sensory nerves, so increased sympathetic stimulation in the ears may contribute to tinnitus and may also lead to hyperacusis. Sympathetic stimulus in the ears may arise from disturbance anywhere along its pathway from the upper thoracic spine, through the neck, through the carotid canal (where it may be compressed due to increased pressure in the carotid artery), through the tympanic plexus, or throughout its various branches to the ears.

More general systemic levels of sympathetic stimulation due to stress and trauma may also be affecting the ears and contributing to tinnitus.

Reducing stress levels often proves very helpful in reducing and sometimes eliminating tinnitus; but where stress is a factor, it is also relevant to consider why the stress is manifesting specifically in the ears as tinnitus rather than in any of the many other parts of the body where stress can manifest.

As with hearing, if the tinnitus is due to cochlear damage as a result of persistent exposure to loud noise, it is unlikely that the tinnitus will be completely eliminated. However, with all cases of tinnitus, including permanent nerve damage, there is another valuable aspect of treatment which can play a very significant part in the patient's wellbeing. This is the process of learning to manage and cope with the tinnitus.

One of the significant factors in tinnitus is that patients can sometimes find it so irritating and intolerable that it makes life unbearable and may even lead patients to feel suicidal.

Because tinnitus is so common and often so intractable, finding methods to cope with it is something that has been explored for many years in one form or another. This involves developing a different attitude and response to the tinnitus, a calm, positive response rather than an adverse reaction. I have found that the simplest and most effective means of enabling this is through the practice of Mindfulness – a practice that can readily be introduced to patients during treatment sessions.

Mindfulness is a transformative process with potential for life-changing benefits for the health and wellbeing of the individual. It is a simple yet practical means of maintaining greater tranquillity, clarity and calmness. It provides a means for dealing more harmoniously with the ups and downs of day-to-day life – at home, at work, in personal relationships, in all aspects of life – in the face of whatever life may bring your way. It is more commonly applied generally to life as a whole, but can also be used to help specific conditions such as tinnitus.

The essence of Mindfulness is to develop the ability to observe things as they are, while maintaining a calm, detached, non-judgemental, non-reactive response. This can enable a greatly reduced level of irritability and reactivity to circumstances – physical, mental and emotional. It can be beneficial in addressing specific difficulties but, more significantly, regular practice of Mindfulness brings about an underlying transformation in one's response to life. Life simply becomes calmer, easier, more manageable, more harmonious, more contented, without any consciously identifiable explanation – simply through Mindfulness practice.

With many patients who have used this process, their tinnitus is eliminated, but even where it does not disappear completely, it is common to find that, when seeing the patient for some other condition, months or even years later, when asked how their tinnitus is, they have forgotten that they ever had tinnitus, but on thinking about it, they may reply, 'I suppose it is still there, but I never really notice it.'

Teresa came for treatment in a state of great agitation. She had suffered from severe tinnitus for years. She said that it was there all the time, 24 hours a day, at work and at home, and rapidly getting worse. It was driving her mad and was completely unbearable, and she could not stand it any longer. She had tried numerous different treatments without any benefit.

Within the context of her cranio-sacral sessions, I introduced Mindfulness practice. She was sceptical, doubting that it could have any effect and simply wanting someone to get rid of her tinnitus. But in desperation she agreed to practise the Mindfulness process each day as I had suggested.

When she came back for her second session, I asked how her tinnitus was. She said there had been no change, it was just as bad. I commented that she seemed much calmer about it, at which she looked surprised. I asked how the tinnitus was at this moment and she said that she could hear it if she thought about it.

The next session, Teresa again reported that there had been no improvement. I asked how it was at this moment, and she said that she could not hear it now and that she only noticed it at night or when it was quiet.

At her fourth session, she again reported no improvement, and again replied that she could not actually hear it at the moment.

Since the tinnitus had improved so much and was no longer troubling her, she stopped coming for treatment, never having acknowledged any improvement.

About a year later, she came to see me again because she had hurt her back. I asked how her tinnitus was. She looked surprised and said, 'What tinnitus?'

Hyperacusis

Hyperacusis is a heightened sensitivity to sound. Many of the factors previously mentioned may apply to hyperacusis. It may be brought on by exposure to sudden loud noises or loud music at a party or rock concert, or it may develop for no apparent reason, particularly under stressful conditions. Restoring balanced function of the structures of the ear will often bring resolution, with particular attention to excessive sympathetic stimulus causing hyper-reactivity of the nerves and tissues, and to the stapedius and tensor tympani muscles and their nerve supply.

It may also arise as part of a wider symptom picture of hypersensitivity, in which case it would need to be addressed within that context.

Energy drives to the ears may be especially beneficial.

Alert to other sources

It is also necessary to remain alert to the possibility that earache and other conditions affecting the ears may be arising from the teeth, a tooth abscess, or a NICO cavitation, and that ear symptoms might arise from an acoustic neuroma, or a brain tumour.

Contacts relevant to the ears

Contacts relevant to the ears will depend on the nature of the individual circumstances. The first step is to identify whether the condition is one that is likely to be responsive to cranio-sacral integration, or whether it is due to irreversible damage. Having established that cranio-sacral treatment is appropriate, one can then engage with the system, evaluate what factors are relevant, bearing in mind that ear symptoms, like anything else, can arise from disturbances anywhere in the body, and then allow the inherent treatment process to take its course.

In many cases, the relevant contacts will include standard familiar contacts such as the heart centre, solar plexus centre, suboccipital release, falx release, all the contacts for the temporal area such as the mastoid tip contact, temporal balancing, and ear hold. All of these have been described in *Cranio-Sacral Integration – Foundation*.

The mandibular contact (Chapter 13) is also particularly helpful, enabling release of tension in the muscles of mastication, the TMJ and in the cranial base generally, as well as balancing the temporal bones.

In addition, it can be helpful to introduce energy drives through the ears.

The *heart centre* and upper thorax will be significant in relation to drainage of the cranium and therefore to congestion and drainage of the ears, as well as to immune function, release of stress and shock, the release of tensions transmitted up into the neck, subocciput and head, and disturbances to the sympathetic supply to the head and ears arising from T1/2.

The *solar plexus* will also be relevant to addressing stress and shock (especially from birth trauma) and tensions transmitted up to the cranial base and sympathetic stimulation through the system as a whole.

The *suboccipital release* (Figure 35.11) is always crucial to health generally, and is specifically relevant to conditions affecting the ears, through enabling the free mobility of the whole base of the cranium, assisting the release of the occipitomastoid sutures and enhanced mobility of the temporal bones, releasing the many surrounding muscles and soft tissues in the vicinity of the cranial base, and enabling more fluent drainage of the cranium, which in turn will assist drainage of the ears, and once again addressing disturbances to the sympathetic nerve supply, particularly at the superior cervical sympathetic ganglion.

Enhancing mobility of the *neck and throat* (including fascial unwinding) can address vertebral restrictions in the cervical spine, and is crucial to those same muscular restrictions at the cranial base, with various muscles of the neck and throat attaching to the temporal bones. This will also enhance arterial supply to the head and venous drainage via the jugular veins through release of the carotid sheath, thereby helping to reduce any persistent tendency to throat infections which might spread to the ears. The neck is also relevant to the sympathetic pathway passing up through the cervical sympathetic chain.

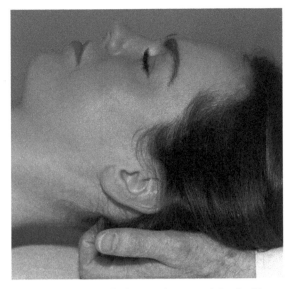

35.11 The suboccipital release is always crucial to health, and is particularly relevant to the ears

The *bowl hold* (Figure 35.12) can, as always, be one of the most significant contacts for overall balance and integration of the cranio-sacral system. The bowl hold is similar to a sphenoid contact, but with the fingers spreading further under the occiput in order to cradle the whole cranial bowl. This is particularly valuable for releasing a solidly restricted cranial base, and therefore very beneficial for many conditions affecting the ears.

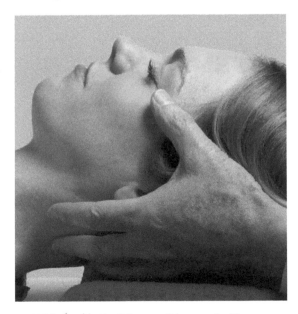

35.12 The bowl hold can be one of the most significant contacts for overall balance and integration of the cranio-sacral system

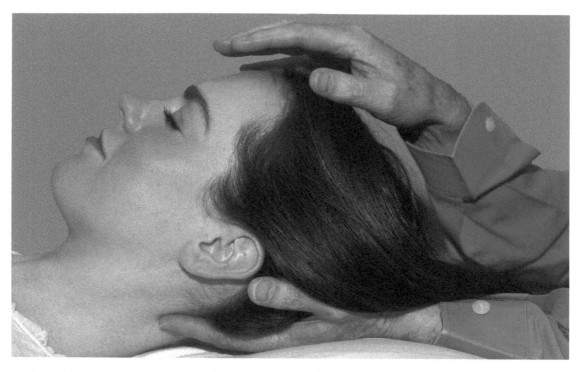

35.13 The falx release is a powerful process for releasing tensions within the intracranial membranes, thereby encouraging drainage throughout the cranium

The *falx release* (Figure 35.13) is helpful for (among other benefits) releasing tensions in the intracranial membranes and for encouraging venous drainage through the venous sinuses, assisting drainage throughout the cranium, including mucus drainage, and helping the body to address infection.

The *temporal bones* are obviously crucial to the function of the ears. Any restrictions to the temporal bones are likely to have adverse effects on the ears, whether through impingement on the Eustachian tube as it runs along the spheno-temporal suture, or to the drainage of the cranium as a whole through the jugular foramina and

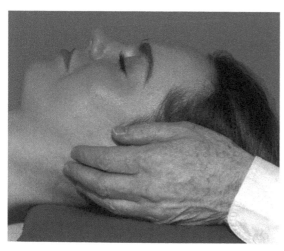

35.14 Temporal contacts are clearly crucial to the function of the ears

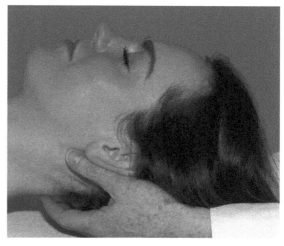

35.15 The mastoid tip contact is particularly significant for releasing the mastoid sutures and jugular foramina, thereby encouraging drainage of the ears and the cranium

occipitomastoid sutures, or affecting cranial nerve pathways, or influencing general cranio-sacral mobility and function. All the usual contacts for the temporal area are likely to be relevant – general temporal contact, mastoid tip contact, ear hold. These contacts can be useful for engaging with the temporal area generally and addressing whatever arises, for releasing the occipitomastoid suture – so commonly restricted, pulling the temporal bones into medial compression and internal rotation and restricting venous drainage through the jugular foramen – and for releasing the spheno-temporal suture, with consequent release of the Eustachian tube. This may specifically be assisted by following the temporal bones into internal rotation until they release into an expansive external rotation, or by enhancing external rotation through a mastoid tip contact, and particularly through the ear hold process (Figures 35.14–35.16).

The *ear hold* can be highly effective in enabling the whole temporal area – bones, muscles, membranes, sinuses, soft tissues – to open out into a wide posterolateral expansion, drawing the temporal bones out from their wedged position between the sphenoid and occiput, releasing the spheno-petrous and occipitomastoid sutures and bringing spaciousness and mobility to the whole surrounding matrix. This expansive decompressive contact is particularly effective once compressive forces and restrictions have been released through the previous temporal contacts.

The *mandibular contact* (Chapter 13) is also very valuable. The mandible exerts a profound influence on the temporal bones through the TMJ, as well as on the muscles of mastication, the various other muscles which attach to the temporal bones, and on all the surrounding structures. Working with the mandible helps to release tension and contraction within the soft tissues at the base of the cranium and around the TMJ, which may be restricting drainage of the Eustachian tube. The bony exit of the Eustachian tube lies immediately medial to the TMJ, so releasing tensions around the TMJ via the mandible can also help to enhance drainage. The mandibular contact can also encourage the temporal bones into external rotation, again assisting in opening the Eustachian tubes (Figure 35.17)

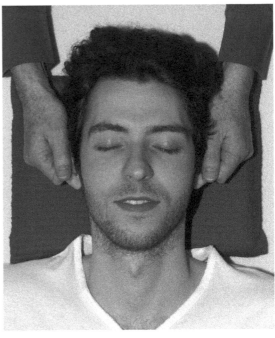

35.16 The ear hold can be highly significant in enabling free mobility of the temporal area

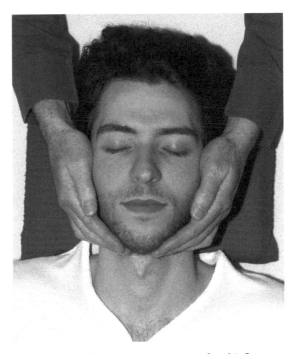

35.17 The mandibular contact exerts a profound influence on the temporal bones through the TMJ and associated structures, and is particularly valuable in encouraging drainage through the Eustachian tube

VII

35

The various contacts for the *muscles of mastication* (Chapter 14) are also relevant, partly in relation to any jaw clenching and tightness in the muscles, which may be contributing to further compression at the base of the cranium and in the ears themselves. Contacts for the medial and lateral pterygoid muscles are also particularly significant, bearing in mind that the lateral pterygoid muscle often has attachment to the malleus within the ear.

Restrictions in the *face* can also contribute to congestion and blockage in the ears, so, particularly where symptoms in the ears are accompanied by congestion in the sinuses and facial area, it is relevant to check the maxillae, palatine bones, vomer, zygomata, nasal bones and ethmoid. It can also be relevant to be aware of the exit of the terminal portion of the Eustachian tube, located posterior and inferior to the inferior nasal concha.

Finally, *energy drives* through the ear canals can be very powerful, whether targeting one ear, or both ears simultaneously. This contact involves placing the middle finger of each hand in the external auditory meatus, with the fingers pointing along the axis of the external auditory canal, engaging with the pulsation of the energy drive, and directing the energy through the ears along the relevant pathways according to individual circumstances (Figure 35.18). The energy drive could initially be directed along the external auditory canal, through the tympanic membrane, and into the middle ear. Attention could then branch off along the Eustachian tube to the nasopharynx, or alternatively proceed through the oval window into the inner ear, to the cochlea, the vestibular mechanism, the semicircular canals and along the vestibulo-cochlear nerves through the internal auditory meatus and into the brainstem. As you project your attention along these pathways, you can visualize the detailed anatomy, identify any areas of restriction, and acknowledge and respond to any changes in quality, symmetry and motion.

Whilst it is of course useful to explore particular structures, identify specific fulcrums of restriction, and utilize these relevant contacts, ultimately it is the overall release of the matrix, local and systemic, which will be most fundamental to fluent function.

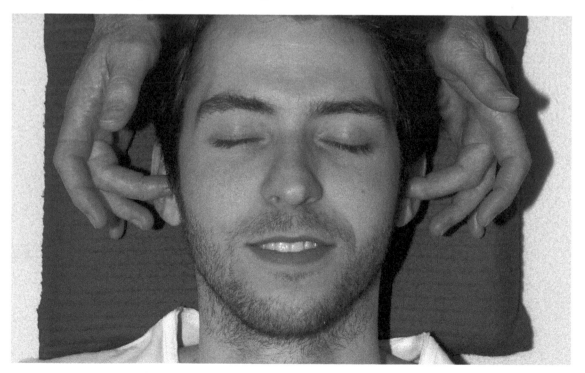

35.18 Energy drives through the ear canals can be very powerful – for the middle ear, for the inner ear, for the Eustachian tube, and elsewhere

Supportive care

In all patients, supportive care beyond the cranio-sacral treatment session can be helpful. This is particularly the case in addressing chronic ear conditions, where lifestyle factors can play a very significant part. This applies to babies and children, and also to adults (as emphasized in Catriona's case).

Supportive care might include:

- avoiding mucus-producing foods, particularly dairy products and refined sugars
- breastfeeding where possible, to promote immune function
- promoting health and immune function through a healthy diet
- strengthening the constitution through homeopathy, particularly where substantial quantities of antibiotics have been used
- for ear infections in babies, propping them up so that they are not lying flat, encouraging gravity to assist the drainage of the Eustachian tube

- in children and adults, regularly throughout the day, encouraging them to hold their nose and mouth closed and blow till they feel a popping or releasing in the ears (the Valsalva manoeuvre). This helps to open the Eustachian tubes, helping them to drain, and allowing pressure in the ears to equalise
- avoiding sniffing, drawing infected mucus back up into the nose, contributing to further congestion and infection
- avoiding blowing the nose too hard while there is infection in the nasal cavity and nasopharynx, thereby forcing infected mucus up the Eustachian tube into the middle ear and also into the sinuses
- avoiding smoking and exposure to passive smoking
- avoiding undue exposure to cold air and to sources of infection – especially at susceptible times
- avoiding swimming while suffering from an infection
- reducing stress levels where indicated.

Part VIII

The Nose, Cheeks, Sinuses and Ethmoid

Chapter 36

The Nose

Introduction

As with everything else, we need to see the nose within the context of the rest of the body.

The nose is inevitably involved in many conditions affecting other structures of the face – sinusitis, ear infections, loss of hearing, recurrent tonsillitis, conditions affecting the eyes and the ethmoid – and needs to be incorporated into treatment of these areas.

Similarly, conditions affecting the nose – chronic congestion, rhinitis, nasal allergies and sensitivities, anosmia – although often viewed locally, need to be understood in relation to the wider picture, particularly in relation to autonomic nerve supply.

Congestion may lead to breathing difficulties and mouth breathing, which may in turn contribute to asthma or dental and gum disease.

Trauma to the nose, whether recent or long-passed, may have ramifications, not only on surrounding structures, but also with more widespread implications throughout the body – structural, neurological or psycho-emotional.

The nasal area may be compressed during birth, particularly at the nasion, commonly causing a deviated nasal septum, and potentially contributing to lifelong nasal symptoms.

Nasal congestion, allergies and sensitivities

Conventional treatments for persistent nasal congestion and rhinitis such as nasal sprays and decongestants are useful for bringing temporary relief, but will usually bring only transient and limited benefits, since they are only treating the symptoms and treating locally. Where nasal congestion is causing significant discomfort, perhaps contributing to sinusitis, earache and hearing loss, a more comprehensive approach is needed.

Common causes of nasal congestion include:

- structural restrictions, causing blockage and limiting drainage and fluent function of the area
- excess mucus production
- disturbances to autonomic nerve supply.

Structural restriction

The nasal cavity is formed from several different bones, and a variety of contacts described in other chapters may be relevant. Release of structural restrictions will inevitably involve engagement both with the nasal area itself and with the surrounding structures of the face and cranium.

Establishing free mobility of surrounding structures can enable more fluent drainage, both of mucus and of vascular pathways. The vascular pathways are significant in enabling the body to address infection and congestion and in promoting immune function. This includes enhancing flow through the venous sinuses, particularly through release of the intracranial membranes, and also through the occipitomastoid sutures, jugular foramina and other structures around the cranial base and suboccipital region.

Mucus production

Excessive mucus production, allergic reactions, and sensitivities to dust, pollens and foods, including hay fever, are often a consequence of autonomic nerve dysfunction. This may involve disturbed parasympathetic nerve supply to the glands of the nose (via the parasympathetic division of the facial nerve), sympathetic overstimulation of the mucous membranes, and sympathetic facilitation of neurological and physiological function throughout the nasal area (as described in Chapter 32).

The pterygopalatine ganglion may be a particularly significant component of these autonomic pathways. Contacts for the palatine bones, maxillae and the pterygopalatine fossa may therefore be relevant.

Jim came to see me because he had suddenly developed hay fever in his mid-forties for the first time in his life, without any apparent cause. He was puzzled as to why this should have arisen. It soon became apparent that the onset had coincided with the break-up of his marriage and the increased sympathetic stimulation from the associated stress.

Hay fever and other nasal, allergic or hypersensitivity symptoms are often relieved through release of sympathetic overstimulation. As always, this can include not only stress factors, but also structural disturbances anywhere along the sympathetic pathway.

This can often be observed on a small scale, since a suboccipital release (thereby releasing pressure on the SCSG and the sympathetic pathway) will often bring immediate relief of nasal symptoms. This simple measure in itself may bring only transient relief, but addressing the underlying patterns contributing to the restriction in the suboccipital region and to overstimulation of the sympathetic pathway can therefore bring more lasting long-term relief.

Nasal disturbances are also likely to be aggravated by spicy foods, salt, refined sugar and other irritants, especially where there is an underlying sympathetic overstimulation.

Immune function

Immune function will inevitably be enhanced through overall cranio-sacral integration. In babies prone to infections or subject to mucus congestion, this will also be helped by breastfeeding.

In babies, children and adults, it can also be helpful to avoid dairy products and other mucus-producing foods, and to avoid smoking (including passive smoking). Dairy products can be particularly relevant in babies and children, in whom milk and dairy-based formula can lead to a substantial increase in mucus production, thereby contributing to recurrent ear infections and nasal congestion, feeding difficulty, breathing difficulty and mouth breathing, with a continuing domino effect of dysfunction, potentially contributing to the development of asthma and sinusitis.

Dairy products are such an inherent part of our diet that it might seem difficult to conceive of life without them, but they do have a significant effect, and eliminating dairy products from the diet – whether in babies or in adults – can produce dramatic changes in health (always of course ensuring adequate replacement in the diet).

Anosmia

Anosmia (loss of smell) may arise simply due to nasal congestion, along with associated reduction in sense of taste. It may also involve the olfactory nerve (Cr I), particularly as a result of pressure on the nerve fibres passing through the cribriform plate of the ethmoid. This may be due to inflammation of the mucous membranes in the roof of the nasal cavity, or tension in the meninges and associated dural sheaths enveloping the olfactory fibres and covering the cribriform plate. Anosmia may also arise as a result of damage to the cribriform plate following an injury. It can also sometimes be induced by emotional shock.

Identifying and addressing the relevant components in each individual case will enable an appropriate response, with attention to the bony structure, membranous tensions and neurological pathways, and focused therapeutic attention to the area as appropriate to the circumstances. As well as the nasal contacts described below, contacts for the ethmoid (Chapter 39) may also be relevant.

Deviated nasal septum

A deviated nasal septum is very common (Figure 35.7). The septum is a very delicate structure, largely consisting of bone as thin as tissue paper. The inferior portion is formed by the vomer, the superior portion by the perpendicular plate of the ethmoid, the anterior portion being formed of cartilage. It is easily compressed and, particularly in early life, prior to ossification, is able to adapt its shape in order to absorb compressive forces between the face and the cranium (the palate and the sphenoid). This is particularly valuable during the birth process, reducing the compressive forces imposed on the sphenoid.

VIII

36

A deviated septum may or may not lead to difficulties. Many people go through life with a deviated septum without any symptoms. Sometimes, specific conditions such as nasal congestion or snoring are attributed to a deviated septum, but there may not necessarily be a connection. Operations to correct a deviated septum may be carried out in the hope of improving breathing difficulties or eliminating snoring, with mixed results.

Cranio-sacral treatment for a deviated septum primarily involves the release of any compressive forces between the face and the cranium, particularly arising from birth, restoring balance and integration to the whole area, so that the septum can naturally settle into a more symmetrical uncompressed state. This is likely to be especially beneficial in a baby or child, where the tissues are more malleable, enabling more balanced growth and development of the face and cranium. It will still be useful in adults, releasing the compressive forces within the matrix and consequently relieving symptoms, but may have less evident effects on the septum itself following the ossification of the vomer during teenage years. It will also be useful to work with the vomer (Chapter 18) and with the ethmoid (Chapter 39).

Birth compression

The nasal area and the nasion may be compressed or disturbed during birth, particularly with a back-to-back presentation. This will of course be part of a wider birth pattern affecting the whole body. A restricted nasion can have profound effects on function and on the whole nature, facial appearance and personality of the individual, and is an area which can sometimes be neglected. In the context of treating the birth pattern as a whole, the nasion may need particular attention. The adapted falx contact described in the chapter on the ethmoid (Chapter 39) may prove beneficial.

Compression of the nasion may lead to ramifications in the ethmoid, the frontal bone, or throughout the cranium and the whole system, contributing to local nasal symptoms or wider repercussions throughout the body.

Medial compression of the whole face and head during birth, whether through the forces of the birth process itself or specifically from the use of forceps, may lead to widespread compression, particularly through the maxillae and zygomata, but also potentially through the frontal, sphenoid and temporal areas, resulting in medial compression of the whole nasal area, with consequent restriction, blockage, congestion and disturbance. Working with the compression and decompression contacts for the maxillae and zygomata (Chapters 16 and 37) may be crucial in such situations, as well as standard contacts for the frontal, sphenoid and temporal areas (see *Cranio-Sacral Integration – Foundation*).

Similar medial compressions can also arise from direct injury to the side of the face.

Direct injury

Working with the nasal area is particularly relevant where there has been direct trauma to the nose, with similar compressive forces as described above, and force vectors into the face and cranium from any number of different directions.

Falling on the face as a young child could set up patterns of restriction which may result in any of the symptoms mentioned above and also establish distorted growth patterns in the face, teeth and cranium. These repercussions are unlikely to be traced to such an apparently insignificant and probably long-forgotten fall, and are more often simply seen as a part of the individual's nature and constitution.

As always, the release of underlying patterns of trauma – physical and emotional – throughout the system, and overall reintegration of the system, are the key to addressing any condition or situation.

Wider ramifications of direct injury

Direct injury to the nose may be transmitted not only through the local structures directly impacted, but also through other associated structures of the face, the cranium and the whole body.

The force of a blow to the nose may push the head back into forceful backward bending, disturbing the relationship of the head on the neck at the suboccipital area, with ramifications throughout the neck, the spine and the rest of the body.

There may also be emotional implications associated with the trauma which may be held into the system – fear in the case of a car accident or fall, and perhaps a combination of fear and anger on being punched or attacked. These emotional ramifications may have widespread effects both physically and on personality, and releasing these effects through cranio-sacral integration can bring profound changes and relief.

Where there is direct trauma to the nose, the nasal area may be the most appropriate point of access for engaging with the physical and emotional components of the trauma throughout the system.

Anatomy

The nasal area is formed and influenced by all its surrounding structures – including the frontal bone, nasal bones, zygomata, maxillae, palatines, vomer and ethmoid, and needs to be viewed and treated within this perspective.

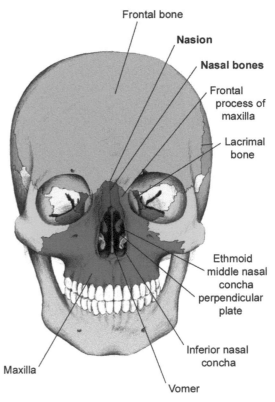

36.2 *The nasal area is formed and influenced by all its surrounding structures*

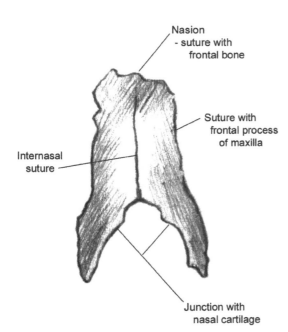

36.1 *The nasal bones are two small slivers of bone, forming the upper part of the nose*

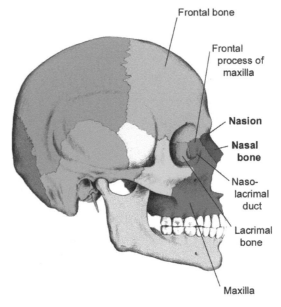

36.3 *The nasal area in situ – lateral view*

VIII

36

The *nasal bones* (Figures 36.1–36.3) are two small slivers of bone, forming the upper part of the nose (the lower portion being composed of cartilage). They articulate with the *frontal bone* superiorly at the nasion and with the *frontal processes of the maxillae* which pass up laterally along the sides of the nose. They also articulate with the *ethmoid* posteriorly. The *nasion* is the junction between the nasal bones and the frontal bone.

Behind the nasal bones, the ethmoid forms a large portion of the nasal cavity, including the roof (formed by the cribriform plate), the lateral walls, the upper portion of the nasal septum, the ethmoid sinuses and the superior and middle nasal conchae (Figure 36.4). The ethmoid is a bone which has profound associations (to be explored in Chapter 39), and the proximity of the nasal bones to the ethmoid therefore presents potential profound ramifications for any trauma to the nose.

The *vomer* forms the lower portion of the nasal septum, so a deviated septum which might be contributing to breathing difficulties or congestion may benefit from treatment through the vomer (Figure 36.4). The *maxillae* form the floor of the anterior nasal cavity and the lower portion of the lateral walls (Figures 36.4 and 36.5). The *palatine bones* form the floor and walls of the posterior nasal cavity (Figure 36.5).

The *nasal conchae* (Figures 36.4 and 36.5), also known as turbinates, together with the nasal hairs (vibrissae), play a crucial role in circulating the air to remove particles of dust and warming the air before it enters the lungs. Mouth breathing, perhaps as a result of chronic nasal congestion, bypasses this crucial process, with potential adverse effects on the lungs, allowing particulate matter to enter the lungs, reducing oxygen absorption and potentially contributing to asthma. The conchae are shell-shaped structures (*concha* means shell in both Latin and Greek). The superior and middle nasal conchae are an integral part of the ethmoid bone.

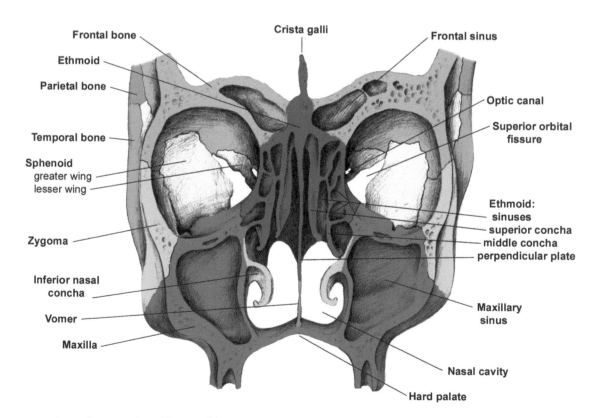

36.4 The nasal cavity is formed by several bones

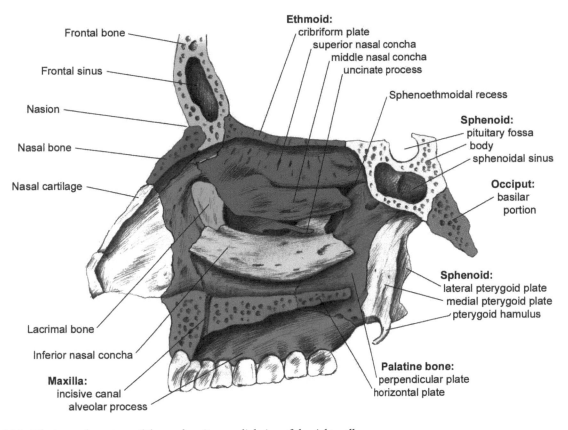

36.5 The internal structure of the nasal cavity – medial view of the right wall

The *inferior nasal conchae* are separate bones attached to the medial walls of the maxillae in the lower part of the nasal cavity. They are closely associated with the drainage holes for the frontal, maxillary and ethmoidal sinuses. They cannot readily be contacted directly, and can best be addressed through general decompression and release of the nasal area, and through maxillary contacts (Chapter 16), with specific therapeutic attention to the conchae.

Choanae

The *choanae*, or posterior nares, are the two spaces connecting the posterior nasal cavity to the pharynx (Figure 36.6). Mucus and other matter from the posterior nasal cavity and sinuses passes through the choanae, in order to drain into the pharynx to be swallowed. This is the natural pathway for drainage of mucus from the nose, but may sometimes be experienced as the discomfort of post-nasal drip. Excessive mucus passing through the choanae may contribute to chronic coughs and a persistent need to clear the throat. The approach in such cases is to address the nasal congestion in the nasal cavity and sinuses and the excess mucus production.

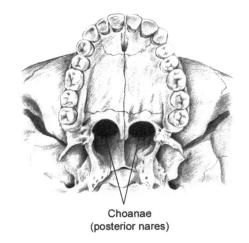

Choanae
(posterior nares)

36.6 The choanae are the two openings connecting the posterior nasal cavity to the pharynx

VIII

36

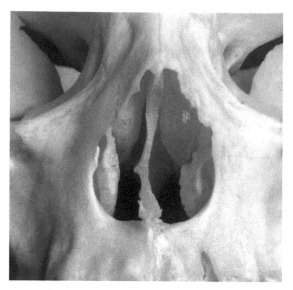 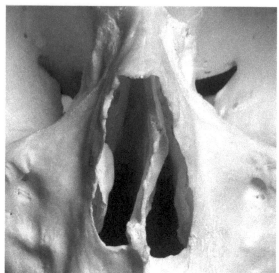

36.7 A deviated nasal septum is very common

Cranio-sacral motion

During the expansion (flexion) phase of cranio-sacral motion, the lateral edges of the nasal bones flare, as if hingeing around the inter-nasal suture. During the contraction (extension) phase, the nasal bones narrow.

Treatment

In treating the nasal area, or any condition affecting the nasal area, the underlying principle, as always, is integration of the whole person by responding to the inherent demands of the cranio-sacral system. Within that context, the approach will of course need to be adapted according to individual needs and local circumstances. This may involve various contacts described elsewhere, and integration of the face and cranium as a whole, with an understanding of the structural relations, neurological connections, immune responses and the role of sympathetic overstimulation.

Within that context, specific contacts for the nasal area may be appropriate and may often be incorporated into the treatment of many different circumstances.

Contacts

Contacts on the nasal area can be taken up, with the practitioner either standing or sitting at the side of the patient's head. If standing, let your arms hang loosely from your shoulders. If sitting, establish a position which does not cause tension in holding up your arms.

Take up contact with one hand over the spheno-frontal area of the cranium. Once you have engaged with your patient's system, take up contact on the nasal bones with the other hand, resting the thumb and middle finger onto the nasal bones, your index finger resting lightly onto the frontal bone, just above the nasion, in order to monitor responses and counterbalance the middle finger and thumb (Figure 36.8a).

Take care to place your finger and thumb close to the midline (in order to ensure that you are contacting the nasal bones rather than the frontal processes of the maxillae), and that your contact is well up towards the nasion (in order to ensure that you are on the nasal bones, rather than on the cartilage below).

As engagement develops, allow the inherent treatment process to evolve, responding to the individual needs expressed by the body. Various patterns of movement or restriction may emerge according to the individual history and circumstances. These can be monitored and engaged with, through the combined interaction between the contact on the nasal area and the contact over the spheno-frontal area.

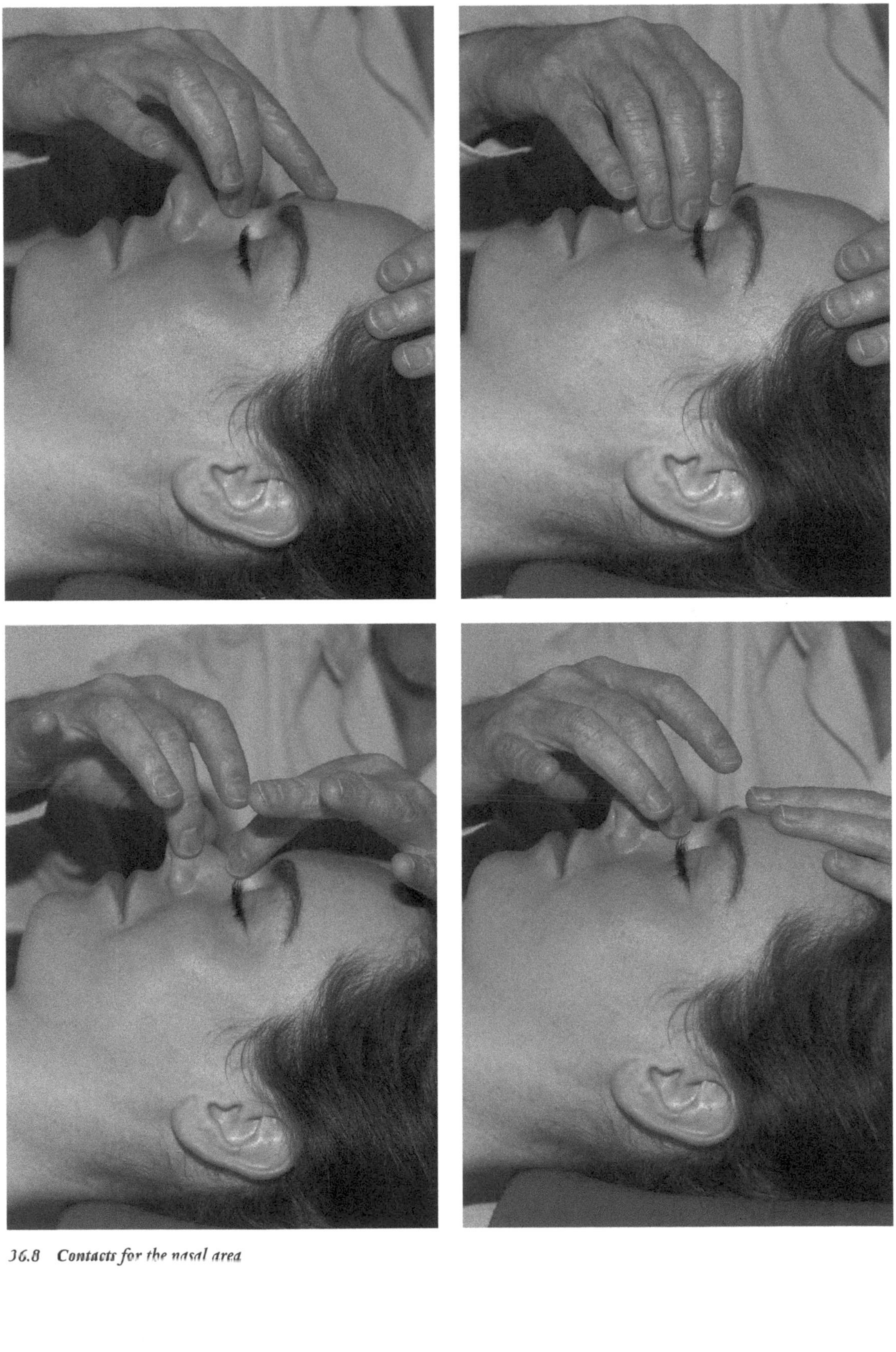

36.8 *Contacts for the nasal area*

VIII

36

Impaction (compression) of the nasal bones up towards the frontal bone, leading to restriction at the nasion and distortion of the nasal area, is a common pattern. This may arise spontaneously during treatment. Alternatively, in due course, you could ask yourself if there is any sense of impaction, whether bilateral or unilateral, allowing the system to respond according to its needs. As always, it is helpful to follow any exploration of impaction with an invitation to disimpaction (decompression) infero-anteriorly, down along the long axis of the nose. Allow the expression of any variations that may arise. You could also be aware of any tendency to forces and restrictions imposed medially or laterally across the nose by blows from the side, or from any direction.

As you engage with the cranio-sacral system through the nasal area, bear in mind the potential repercussions throughout the body of injuries to the nose, identifying connections elsewhere in the system, tracing patterns of restriction, force vectors and whole-body patterns. Visualize through the body, surveying through the system, noting in particular any repercussions of trauma at the subocciput, the neck, the cervico-thoracic junction, the heart centre, the solar plexus and beyond, both physical and psycho-emotional.

This is one of many possible contacts for the nasal area. It may be appropriate to place your fingers along the side of the nose (Figure 36.8b), or to move your contact to whatever focal point or location the system may require. Improvise contacts according to the needs of the moment, maintaining a broad perspective, addressing other surrounding structures as required, incorporating various other contacts as necessary, such as medial compression of the maxillae (Chapter 16) or zygomata (Chapter 37). It can be helpful to try out contacts on yourself to see which points of contact feel most effective.

It is also often helpful to take up contact on the nasal cartilage, especially where this has been displaced by an injury to the nose (Figure 36.8c).

As always, once any local treatment to the nasal area is complete, it is appropriate to continue with overall integration, in order to ensure that any local changes have been integrated and that the system as a whole feels balanced and complete.

Chapter 37

The Zygomata

The zygomata (or zygomatic bones) are the cheek bones, forming the high point of the cheek under the lateral corner of each eye. They also form the lateral and inferior rim of the orbit and part of the lateral wall of the orbit (Figures 37.1 and 37.2).

The Greek word *zygoma* (plural: *zygomata*) means a yoke, and the zygomata were regarded by early anatomists as forming a yoke across the facial structures, similar to a yoke across a pair of oxen (although the two zygomata are not connected medially, being separated by the maxillae and the nasal bones). They are also known as the *malar bones* (from *mala* – Latin for cheek).

Each zygoma consists of a main body with three processes (projections) emerging from the body directed medially, superiorly and posteriorly respectively (Figure 37.3). The medial projection (*the maxillary process of the zygoma*) articulates with the *maxilla* – along the lower rim of the orbit. The superior projection (*the frontal process of the zygoma*) articulates with the zygomatic process of the *frontal bone* – passing up along the lateral rim of the orbit. The posterior projection (*the temporal process of the zygoma*) articulates with the zygomatic process of the *temporal bone* – together forming the *zygomatic arch*. Each zygoma also articulates with the greater wing of the *sphenoid* – together forming the lateral wall of the orbit (Figure 37.2).

Each zygoma articulates with only one facial bone – the maxilla – but articulates with three cranial bones – temporal, frontal and sphenoid – which can be significant in relation to impact transmitted directly from the zygoma into the cranium.

Cranio-sacral motion

During the expansion (flexion) phase of cranio-sacral motion, the zygomata externally rotate, arcing downward and outward. During the contraction phase, they internally rotate, arcing superiorly and medially.

Located at the crossroads between the temporal bones, the frontal bone, and the maxillae, their motion adapts to accommodate all of these other bones:

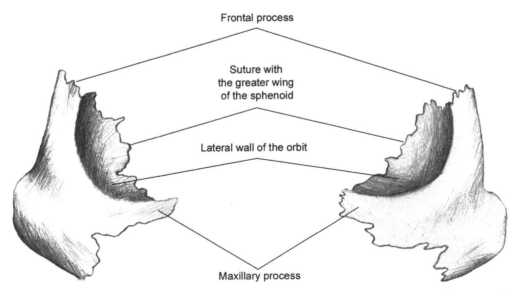

Frontal process

Suture with
the greater wing
of the sphenoid

Lateral wall of the orbit

Maxillary process

37.1   The zygomata – each zygoma consists of a main body with three processes emerging from the body (the temporal processes are not visible in this anterior view; see Figure 37.3)

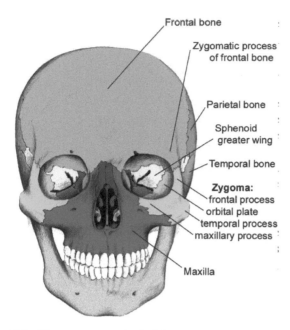

37.2   *The zygomata are the cheek bones*

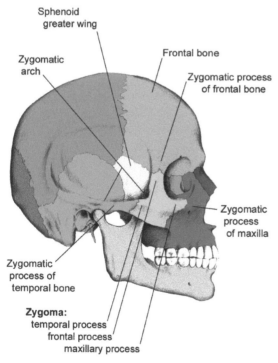

37.3   *Each zygoma articulates posteriorly with the zygomatic process of the temporal bone, together forming the zygomatic arch*

- As the temporal bones externally rotate during expansion, the zygomata are also pushed out into external rotation.
- As the frontal bone arcs forward and down, the zygomata are pushed inferiorly.
- As the maxillae and the rest of the face rise to meet the frontal bone, the zygomata are squeezed outward between the face and the frontal bone.

The result is external rotation, arcing down and out, around *an axis which runs from the nasion to the angle of the jaw.*

Associations

The zygomata are an integral part of the face and may therefore be involved in conditions affecting the eyes, the nose, the ears, the sinuses, the teeth, the TMJ, and the health and function of the face generally. They therefore need to be assessed in relation to any of these conditions.

They may be compressed during birth, or disturbed by dentistry. They may have been restricted as a result of long-forgotten childhood falls, setting up distorted growth patterns which have influenced the patient's whole development and nature. So once again the zygomata need to be in the therapist's awareness with all patients, even where there are no local symptoms or reported injuries.

The most common source of disturbance of the zygomatic bones is direct injury – through being hit in the face, or as a result of a car crash or fall. Their prominent position means that they are particularly susceptible to direct blows. The effects of such impacts can be transmitted into the cranium and, as with injuries to the nasal area, may have repercussions throughout the system, with the head being pushed back into forceful back-bending; and potential ramifications, both physical and emotional, reflecting through the face, the cranium, the suboccipital region, the neck and the whole system.

When working with the zygomata in such cases, it is necessary to bear this in mind, to trace the repercussions or survey such effects throughout the body, and to engage with the complete picture, the whole story, and the combined effects of the trauma on the whole system as one unified experience. Where the zygoma is the site of impact or injury, it may be the most effective and appropriate point of access for engaging with the physical and emotional components of the trauma throughout the system.

Shattered faces

In some cases, the face may have been severely injured in a road accident or fight, with multiple fractures, bones shattered, and widespread damage. Following such accidents, cranio-sacral integration can play a very significant part in restoring the face to a healthy balanced state. Surgery may be necessary to repair the injuries, but cranio-sacral integration can release the traumatic forces imposed on the area and reintegrate the underlying matrix. This can enable the repaired tissues to regrow within a more favourable and conducive therapeutic environment which can in turn enable more successful repair and resolution. Even the best surgery does not address the traumatic forces held within the matrix.

Cranio-sacral integration may be appropriate at the earliest opportunity after the injury, before surgery, in order to release the shock and trauma from the area, reduce pain and discomfort, and establish a more receptive environment which can enable surgery to proceed more smoothly and effectively. At this point, the emphasis is entirely on allowing the underlying matrix to express its needs, release shock, and restore balance and integrity, rather than giving attention to specific bones.

Following surgery, cranio-sacral integration can play a significant part in further reintegration, restoring subtle balance and harmony, and addressing any residual pain or discomfort. This is, of course, not specific to the zygomata but applies to the whole face.

Contacts

The zygomata will as always be treated as part of an overall integrated treatment. Within this context there are various local contacts which can be helpful:

External bilateral contact

Sitting at the patient's head, let your forearms rest on the couch, in such a position that the pads of your slightly curled fingers can sink down through the energy field until they come to rest lightly onto the zygomatic region of the face, resting along the anterior border of the zygomata (Figure 37.4). Take care to keep your contact over the zygomata rather than straying onto the surrounding structures such as the maxillae. In other words keep your contact close below the lateral corner of the eye, not spreading across towards the nose or down towards the mouth. Take care not to weigh too heavily on the face.

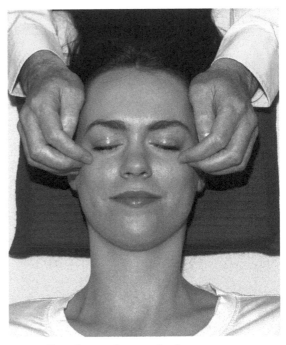

37.4   Bilateral external contact for the zygomata

With this contact, follow the usual process of engagement, allowing the inherent treatment process to evolve, allowing your hands to float fluently with the fluidic movements which you encounter, following the system to points of stillness and release, aware not only of the zygomata, but also of patterns throughout the face and connections through the whole system. Compare the two zygomata in terms of their quality, symmetry and motion. Observe the rate, amplitude and free expression of rhythmic

VIII

37

motion as the zygomata move through internal and external rotation. Observe the connections to surrounding tissues. Observe patterns of restriction or imbalance spreading through the rest of the face, the head and the whole body. Evaluate the degree to which the zygomata seem to be primary factors in such patterns (the original source of the pattern or injury) or to what extent they seem to be merely reflecting primary patterns arising from elsewhere, assessing through their quality and response. Trace the patterns of imbalance to their source, whether local or distant, and allow the system to bring the process to release, resolution and integration.

Some practitioners may find a variation of this contact more comfortable (Figure 37.5). Sitting at the patient's head, let your elbows rest on the couch (to support the weight of your arms, so that your hands and arms can relax completely without weighing heavily onto the patient's face), with your hands hovering above the face, hanging loosely from the wrists. From this loose, relaxed position, allow your fingers and thumbs, loosely bunched together, to come to rest lightly onto the zygomatic region of the face.

Where more specific patterns of restriction are identified, directly affecting the zygomata, more specific contacts may be appropriate:

Contact for engaging with forces of medial compression

The zygomata may be injured by a blow to the side of the face. They may be compressed medially during the birth process, particularly through the use of forceps, or they may be held medially by contractile tensions within the facial muscles.

Where you encounter such forces and where a sense of medial compression or contraction seems to be inviting your hands inwards, it may be useful to rest your fingers bilaterally on the lateral surface of each zygoma (as in Figure 37.4 above). From this position, you can engage with the forces within the face, explore different levels of medial compression and containment, and observe and follow the responses within the system as usual.

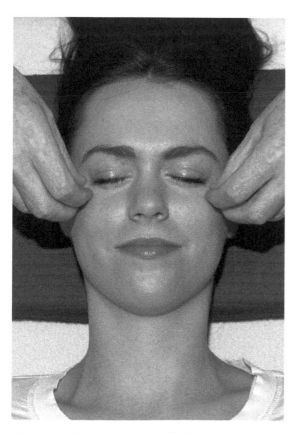

37.5 Alternative external contact for the zygomata

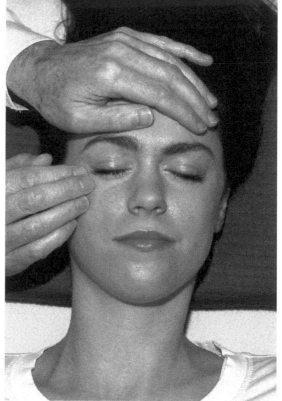

37.6 A fronto-zygomatic contact may be beneficial where there is vertical compression of one side of the head and face

Unilateral fronto-zygomatic contact

This contact is useful where there are forces compressing one side of the head and face vertically, with the zygoma compressed superiorly towards the frontal bone, and the frontal bone compressed inferiorly towards the zygoma, perhaps as a result of a fall on the head, a blow from below, or a traffic accident (Figure 37.6).

Intraoral contact

This is the contact which is most specific to the zygomata, and is particularly useful where specific restriction of the zygomatic bone has been identified, or to integrate the zygomatic bone within the overall facial structure, following a severe facial injury or surgery. It can also be particularly useful in addressing more chronic patterns of restriction in the face, where mobility of one zygoma in relation to its surrounding structures is severely compromised.

Standing at the side of the patient's head, take up contact with one hand over the spheno-frontal area of the cranium (Figure 37.7). Once you have engaged with your patient's system, invite them to open their mouth so that you can take your index finger *inside* the cheek, but *outside* the teeth. Take your index finger up as far as is comfortable inside the cheek and outside the gum so that the tip of the finger is resting under the zygoma. Let the pad of your thumb come to rest lightly on the external surface of the cheek and zygoma, holding the zygoma lightly between index finger and thumb, taking care not to pinch (Figure 37.8).

Engage with the zygoma and allow the inherent treatment process to proceed in its own way, identifying directions of ease and restriction and allowing the process to reach points of stillness and release. As the bone releases and the system settles, evaluate the rhythmic motion, observing gentle internal and external rotation as the system moves into contraction and expansion. Evaluate the range of motion and the motility of the zygoma.

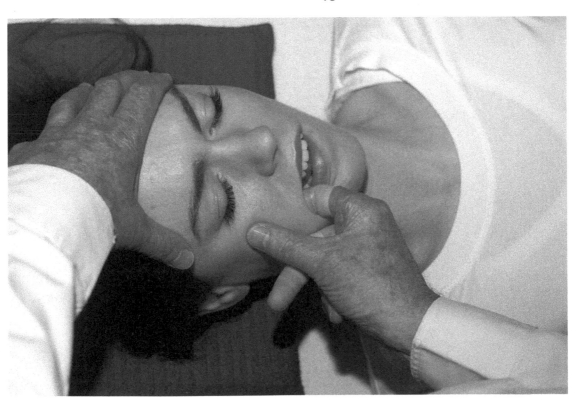

37.7 An intraoral contact for the zygoma can be more specific

VIII

37

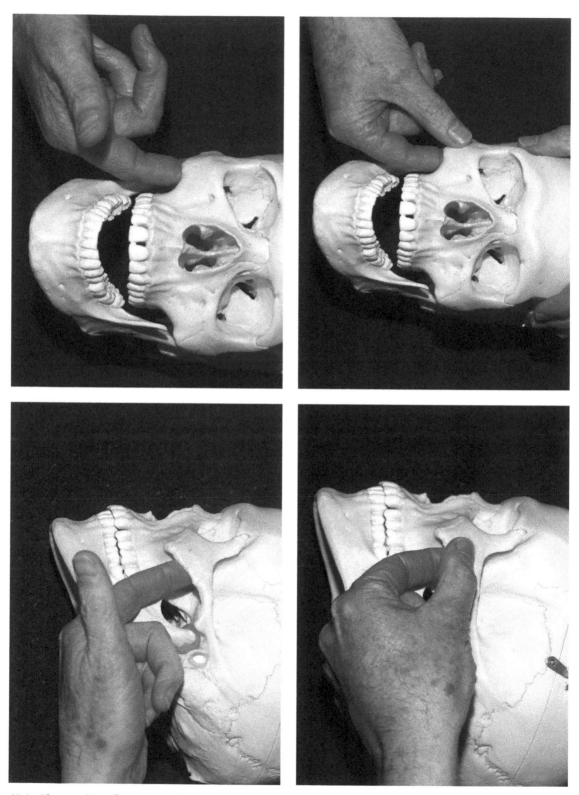

37.8   Finger positions for an intraoral contact on the zygoma

The system may draw spontaneously to Still Points at extremes of contraction or expansion. You can also explore this possibility by observing more closely. The zygoma is more likely to be held in contraction (internal rotation) since blows to the face are more likely to impose forces in this direction. Ask yourself if the zygoma is drawing consistently into internal rotation (superiorly and medially). Allow it to move as far as it wishes, perhaps feeling a build-up of pressure in the system and responses both locally and throughout the system, reaching stillness and eventual release. Upon release, allow the zygoma to settle into its natural rhythmic motion and observe the increased amplitude, mobility and balance of the zygoma, within itself and in relation to your spheno-frontal contact.

Rocking the zygoma

Where a zygoma is significantly restricted, it can also be useful to rock the zygoma, engaging with rhythmic motion, allowing the free regular expression of internal and external rotation, and then enhancing the motion, following the bone more specifically into each phase of motion – like swinging on a swing, with a slight hint of encouragement in each direction at the appropriate moment within each phase, as it approaches the extreme of motion.

This contact may be most commonly used because a specific zygoma on one side has been injured or has been identified as severely restricted. It may therefore not be necessary to work with the other zygoma. However, when the restricted zygoma has been released, the patient may feel that the other side feels less mobile in comparison, so it may be useful to treat the other side as well. It can also be valuable to treat each side and compare the findings and responses.

Having completed any local treatment on an individual zygoma, it is useful to return to the external bilateral contact, to compare and assess the balance of the two zygomata.

It is then, as always, appropriate to continue with the overall integration of the system as necessary.

VIII

37

Chapter 38

The Sinuses

Why are the sinuses so susceptible to dysfunction and pain? One significant factor is the fact that we walk on two legs rather than four. In a quadruped, as in most mammals, the head is held forward and down, and the drainage holes for many of the sinuses are located towards the inferior region of the sinuses – a sensible place for natural drainage through gravity.

When standing on two feet, with our heads held high, the drainage holes for the maxillary sinuses are near the top of the sinuses, which is not helpful in terms of drainage. The result is that mucus and infectious organisms tend to settle at the bottom of the sinuses, unable to drain easily, leading to stagnation, infection, inflammation and pain. Drainage holes for other sinuses are directed more horizontally in the biped, rather than downwards as in quadrupeds, also less helpful for drainage through gravity.

It takes many generations for the body to adapt to change. Our ancestors have been land animals walking on four feet for 400 million years, and we have been standing on two feet for less than 1 per cent of that time, so evolution will need a great deal more time to adapt to this new-found two-legged state.

Sinusitis is a common cause of pain and discomfort, affecting 12–20 per cent of the population. The sinuses where pain is most commonly experienced are the frontal and maxillary sinuses. The sphenoidal and ethmoidal sinuses are also clinically relevant, albeit less commonly a source of pain. We also need to consider the mastoid air cells.

The word 'sinus' means a space. The sinuses with which we are concerned here are the air sinuses – spaces filled with air (not to be confused with the venous sinuses which contain venous blood).

The reason for their existence is not entirely clear, but it is generally considered that these hollow spaces serve the functions of providing greater resonance to our voices, and reducing the weight of the head.

Structure

There are four main pairs of air sinuses – frontal, maxillary, sphenoidal, ethmoidal – all of which drain through small ostia (openings) into the nasal cavity (Figures 38.1–38.4).

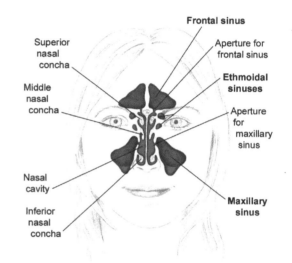

38.1   The air sinuses – anterior view

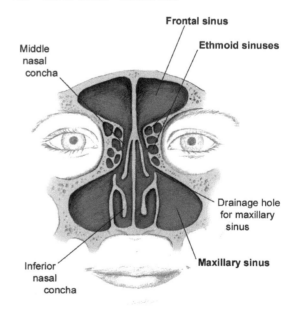

38.2   The sinuses drain through small openings into the nasal cavity

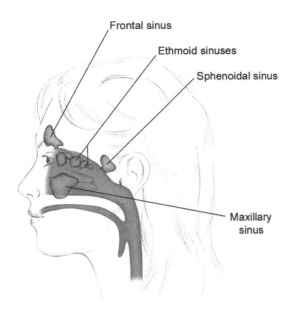

Frontal sinus

Ethmoid sinuses

Sphenoidal sinus

Maxillary
sinus

38.3   There are four main pairs of air sinuses

The sinuses are lined with mucous membranes (respiratory epithelium) containing cilia and producing mucus which can trap and clear inhaled particles and infectious organisms. The cilia within the mucous membranes continuously encourage movement of mucus towards the apertures to encourage drainage. In many of the sinuses, the apertures are very small, limiting the potential for free drainage – particularly when the diameter of the holes is further reduced through congestion and inflammation.

The *frontal sinuses* are located within the anterior inferior portion of the frontal bone, one on each side, of variable size and shape, usually unequal in size, larger in men than in women, with a thin septum between them (Figure 38.4). They drain via the fronto-nasal ducts through the ethmoidal sinuses into the middle meatus of the nasal cavity, between the middle and inferior nasal conchae.

The *maxillary sinuses* are the largest of the air sinuses. They are shaped like pyramids lying on their sides, with the base medially and apex laterally, occupying the space within the body of

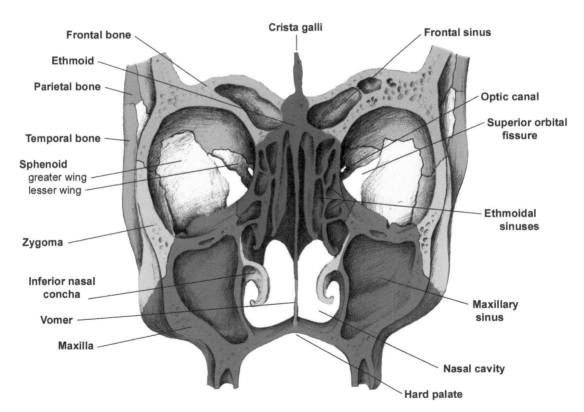

Frontal bone

Ethmoid

Parietal bone

Temporal bone

Sphenoid
greater wing
lesser wing

Zygoma

Inferior nasal
concha

Vomer

Maxilla

Crista galli

Frontal sinus

Optic canal

Superior orbital
fissure

Ethmoidal
sinuses

Maxillary
sinus

Nasal cavity

Hard palate

38.4   Location of the sinuses

each maxilla – below the eyes, above the upper teeth. The roof of each maxillary sinus forms the floor of the orbit. The medial walls form the lateral walls of the nasal cavity. They drain into the middle meatus of the nasal cavity, their apertures situated high in the medial wall of the sinus, well above the floor of the sinus. The aperture is small, and is further reduced by the fact that it is overlapped by the lacrimal bone, the palatine bone and the inferior nasal concha.

The floor of each maxillary sinus lies very close to the upper teeth and is marked by elevations produced by the upper molar and premolar teeth. The roots of the teeth may penetrate the bony floor, terminating just beneath the mucous lining or penetrating into the sinus – with potential for disturbance and pain in the sinuses from tooth infections and dentistry (such as root canal treatment).

The *sphenoidal sinuses* occupy the hollow space within the sphenoid body, the two sinuses divided by a central septum. They drain into the back of the upper nasal cavity (the spheno-ethmoidal recess) directly above the choanae. Their apertures are located high on the anterior walls of the sinuses, again limiting drainage.

The optic nerves, carotid arteries and cavernous sinuses lie immediately lateral to the sphenoidal sinuses and may be at risk from spread of infection.

The *ethmoidal sinuses* consist of a variable number of around twenty small cavities divided into anterior, middle and posterior groups, like a honeycomb. They are located between the eyes, near the top of the nasal cavity. They are the last of the sinuses to develop, only appearing around the age of four years, gradually developing during childhood. They drain into the middle meatus of the nasal cavity between the middle and inferior nasal conchae, along with the frontal and maxillary sinuses.

The bony wall between the ethmoidal sinuses and the orbits is very thin, with potential for infection to spread into the eyes. There is also very little protection above the ethmoidal sinuses, providing potential for spread of infection up through the cribriform plate into the anterior cranial fossa, potentially leading to meningitis or encephalitis.

Drainage

The small size of the apertures (around 3–4mm in diameter), and their location at the top of the sinus in the case of the maxillary sinuses, renders drainage difficult (Figures 38.5 and 38.6). Excessive mucus production can lead to persistent mucus congestion which clogs up the nasal cavity and further reduces the potential for drainage. Inflammation may lead to swelling of the mucous membranes, reducing the effectiveness of the cilia, increasing the production of mucus, and further reducing the size of the already small apertures. Once sinusitis has become established, it can therefore be difficult for the body to clear it naturally.

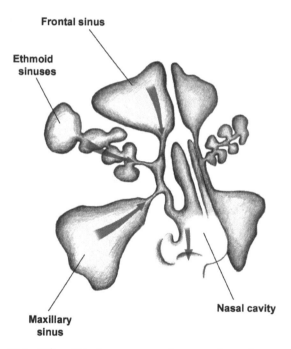

38.5 Cilia within the mucous membranes continuously encourage movement of mucus towards the apertures to encourage drainage

Inflammation of the mucous membranes may arise as a result of infectious organisms, allergies, sensitivities, irritation due to dust particles and other particulate matter and chemical irritants, or in response to neurological overstimulation.

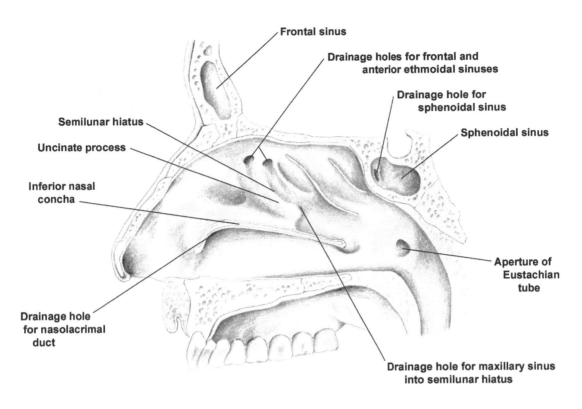

Frontal sinus

Drainage holes for frontal and anterior ethmoidal sinuses

Drainage hole for sphenoidal sinus

Sphenoidal sinus

Semilunar hiatus

Uncinate process

Inferior nasal concha

Aperture of Eustachian tube

Drainage hole for nasolacrimal duct

Drainage hole for maxillary sinus into semilunar hiatus

38.6   Apertures for drainage within the nasal cavity

Colds and other nose and throat infections can spread from the nasal cavity. Mucus and infectious organisms may be pushed into the sinuses by forceful nose-blowing or sneezing. Persistent mucus congestion in the nasal cavity also increases the chances of spread to the sinuses.

Contributory factors

Structural

Certain individuals may be more susceptible than others due to various factors. These include structural restriction affecting the bones of the cranium and face, arising from birth or injury, and restricting drainage. Cranio-sacral treatment to increase free mobility enhances drainage, and enhanced rhythmic motion of the cranio-sacral system also acts as a pump to promote drainage.

Immunity

Low immunity increases susceptibility to colds and other infections. There may also be a susceptibility to allergies, or sensitivities to foods, dust, pollen and other irritants.

Lifestyle

The inhalation of particulate matter or chemical irritants may be work-related if protective masks are not worn where necessary, or may arise from cycling in a polluted city environment without a face mask. Smoking may add further irritation, including exposure to passive smoking. The sinuses may also be affected by excessively dry or excessively humid conditions. Forceful nose-blowing may push mucus from the nasal cavity into the sinuses.

Autonomic nerve stimulation

Parasympathetic nerve facilitation anywhere along the pathway of the parasympathetic branch of the facial nerve (Cr VII), including the pterygopalatine ganglion, may increase mucus production and may also lead to dryness, irritation, inflammation and consequent greater susceptibility to infection.

Sympathetic overstimulation arising from impingement anywhere along its pathway, or as a result of stress factors, may also increase the irritability and reactivity of the mucous membranes.

Approach

In addressing sinus conditions, the priorities are:

- improving drainage by restoring free mobility
- reducing inflammation by promoting immune function
- addressing lifestyle factors
- reducing autonomic nerve overstimulation.

As always, the need is to integrate the whole person rather than merely treating the face, and to ensure drainage and flow of the system as a whole – including the venous sinus system and all other factors that contribute to fluent arterial, venous and lymphatic flow from the face and head, rather than merely focusing on drainage of the sinuses themselves.

The overall approach is therefore the familiar process of general cranio-sacral integration, adapted according to the needs of the individual, with attention to:

- the heart centre (for immune function and stress reduction)
- the solar plexus (for stress factors and reducing sympathetic overstimulation)
- the suboccipital region – to encourage free drainage and arterial, venous and lymphatic flow
- free mobility of the cranium as a whole
- free mobility of the intracranial membranes
- free mobility of the face including the maxillae, palatines, vomer, zygomata, nasals, ethmoid and associated structures
- parasympathetic pathways
- sympathetic supply throughout its pathway.

It is also necessary to address lifestyle factors:

- Dietary – particularly avoiding dairy products, refined sugars, salt and spicy foods.
- Avoiding smoking (including passive smoking).
- Allergies and sensitivities. Along with dairy products, wheat is another very common source of disturbance. A comprehensive evaluation of individual allergies and sensitivities may also be helpful.
- Wearing a face mask where necessary for work-related irritants or cycling in cities.
- Taking care not to blow the nose forcefully. It is preferable to reduce nose-blowing substantially, wiping rather than blowing and, where necessary, blowing only gently.
- If one side of the head is congested, sleeping on the opposite side to encourage drainage, and identifying other activities which may persistently induce tension on one side – such as regularly holding a telephone to the same ear.
- Stress.

Once healthy function has been restored through fluent mobility and drainage, lifestyle factors may become less significant as the body becomes less susceptible to irritants.

It is also relevant to be alert to other less obvious sources of sinus pain, bearing in mind that an infected nerve root or tooth decay in one of the upper teeth may manifest as maxillary sinus pain, and that root canal treatment which penetrates too far up into the bone may also adversely affect the maxillary sinus. Conversely, maxillary sinus infection could cause pain in the upper teeth.

Time to clear and regenerate

When the sinuses have been chronically congested, it is unrealistic to expect instant clearance. Even when mobility and drainage are restored, it will take time for the congestion to clear, and even after that, the damaged respiratory epithelium (mucous membrane) needs to regenerate, so it may take several weeks, even months, to clear completely and restore healthy function.

Contacts

Contacts for addressing sinus dysfunctions include all the contacts for the cranium and face and the cranio-sacral system described previously, according to the needs of the individual. In addition, it may be helpful to apply a gentle pumping action to the relevant areas of the face and cranium.

Mastoid air cells

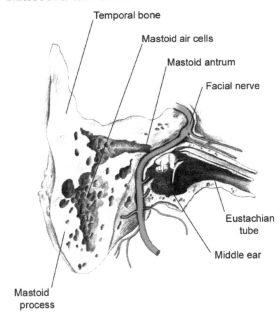

Temporal bone

Mastoid air cells

Mastoid antrum

Facial nerve

Eustachian tube

Middle ear

Mastoid process

38.7   The mastoid air cells are similar sinus-like structures, forming a honeycomb of smaller air spaces within the mastoid portion of the temporal bones

The mastoid air cells are similar sinus-like structures, forming a honeycomb of smaller air spaces within the mastoid portion of the temporal bones (Figure 38.7). These are not directly connected to the other sinuses and do not drain into the nasal cavity. They are located posterior to the middle ear, to which they connect via the mastoid antrum, rendering them susceptible to infection spreading from the middle ear. Mastoiditis can therefore be a complication of recurrent ear infections and glue ear. Because the bony medial walls of the mastoid air cells are very thin, there is potential for mastoiditis to break through these walls into the cranial cavity, leading to meningitis or encephalitis.

Whilst many of the general principles for addressing the sinuses will remain the same for the mastoid air cells, other considerations will be more specific to the mastoid air cells.

In treating mastoiditis, the first priority is to be aware of the possible complication of spread to the cranial cavity, and to monitor carefully for any indications of this. Apart from that, the principles of treatment will be similar to those described for the ear (Chapter 35), clearing infection and accumulated fluids from the middle ear cavity, with specific therapeutic attention to the mastoid air cells and drainage through the mastoid antrum.

Chapter 39

The Ethmoid

The ethmoid holds a very special place within the cranio-sacral process – an area of profound connection to deeper levels of being. This is reflected both in its structure and in its location.

It is a remarkable bone, extremely delicate and intricate. The quality of the bone itself is exceptionally light and fragile, as if it were made of tissue paper. If you take a disarticulated ethmoid bone and place it on the palm of your hand, it is so light that it is as if you are not holding anything at all.

It has an exceptional intricacy and complexity, composed of many apparently disparate pieces, with elaborate curves and a maze of tiny cavities – and yet all combined to form one unified bone.

Its location is elusive – somewhere deep inside the cranium, not readily accessible. It is not visible or contactable on the outside of the skull. No part of it emerges to the surface. It is hidden and intangible, somewhere behind the nose, between the eyes. Even when you look inside the skull, only certain parts of it are clearly identifiable, and it is not easy to gain a clear concept of its overall shape or location. It remains elusive, and when you do isolate a disarticulated ethmoid, its beautiful intricacy has an abstract ethereal quality to it.

It plays an interesting role as a bridge between cranium and face – being a part of both, yet not quite belonging to either.

It is the site of the 'third eye', the seat of intuition, an area through which we might engage with higher levels of consciousness.

All these features reflect its nature and its significance. When we engage with the ethmoid, we are engaging with a profound level of being, a more abstract ethereal level, a subtle elusive intuitive aspect of the patient's nature, the higher self, their connection with the universe.

Anatomy

The ethmoid does of course have a structure, however elusive. It is located between the orbits, in front of the sphenoid body, behind the nasal bones, above the palate, forming a substantial portion of the nasal cavity (Figures 39.1–39.6).

It has a *roof* consisting of the *cribriform plate*, sitting within the ethmoid notch between the two halves of the frontal bone, identifiable through its 'pepper-pot' appearance within the anterior cranial fossa of the cranium (Figures 39.1 and 39.3). (The word *ethmoid* is Greek for sieve, reflecting the sieve-like appearance of the cribriform plate. The word *cribriform* is Latin for sieve-like.)

It has two *lateral walls*, passing down on each side, forming the predominant part of the medial walls of the orbits (with the body of the sphenoid forming the posterior portion, and the lacrimal bones forming the anterior portion) (Figures 39.1 and 39.5).

It is hollow and spacious, with *ethmoid sinuses* in the upper part of the nasal cavity, composed of an intricate honeycomb of spaces separated by tissue-paper-thin dividing sections.

It has no floor, the spaciousness of the ethmoid being bounded inferiorly by the hard palate (formed by the maxillae and palatine bones).

It has a *perpendicular plate*, passing down centrally through the midline of the nasal cavity. This perpendicular plate extends superiorly up through the cribriform plate into the anterior cranial fossa to form the *crista galli*, for the attachment of the falx cerebri. The crista galli develops gradually (like most bony projections) in response to the pull of the falx cerebri. The perpendicular plate extends inferiorly to form the upper part of the *nasal septum*, dividing the nasal cavity into two halves, and continuous with the vomer below (Figure 39.4).

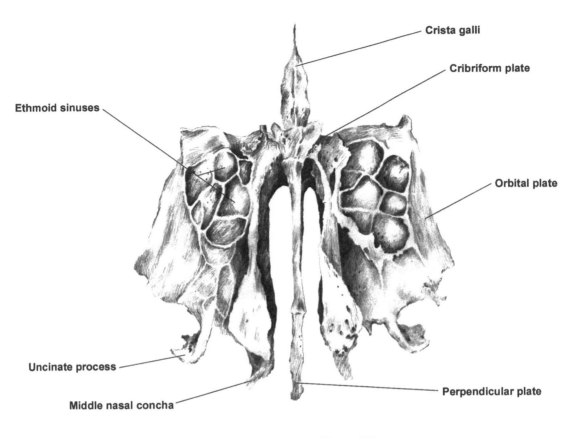

Crista galli

Cribriform plate

Ethmoid sinuses

Orbital plate

Uncinate process

Middle nasal concha

Perpendicular plate

39.1   The ethmoid is an exceptionally delicate, intricate, complex and beautiful bone

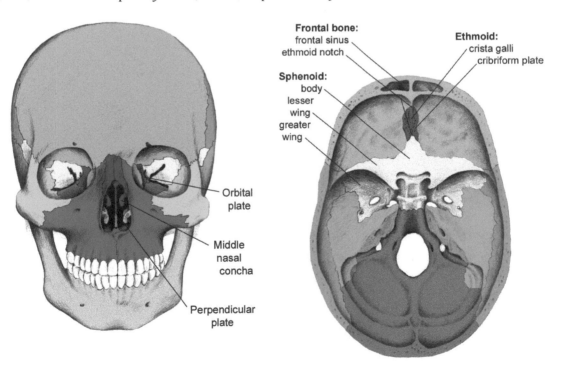

Frontal bone:
frontal sinus
ethmoid notch

Ethmoid:
crista galli
cribriform plate

Sphenoid:
body
lesser
wing
greater
wing

Orbital
plate

Middle
nasal
concha

Perpendicular
plate

39.2   The ethmoid's location is elusive, somewhere behind the nose, between the eyes, and above the palate, forming a substantial portion of the nasal cavity

39.3   The roof of the ethmoid is the cribriform plate, sitting within the ethmoid notch between the two halves of the frontal bone

VIII

39

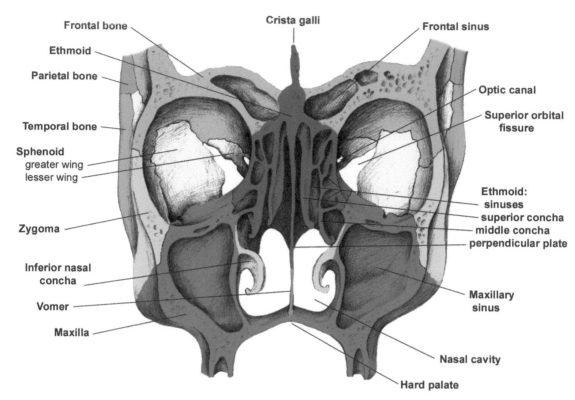

Frontal bone

Ethmoid

Parietal bone

Temporal bone

Sphenoid
greater wing
lesser wing

Zygoma

Inferior nasal
concha

Vomer

Maxilla

Crista galli

Frontal sinus

Optic canal

Superior orbital
fissure

Ethmoid:
sinuses
superior concha
middle concha
perpendicular plate

Maxillary
sinus

Nasal cavity

Hard palate

39.4 *The ethmoid sinuses are composed of an intricate honeycomb of spaces separated by tissue-paper-thin dividing sections*

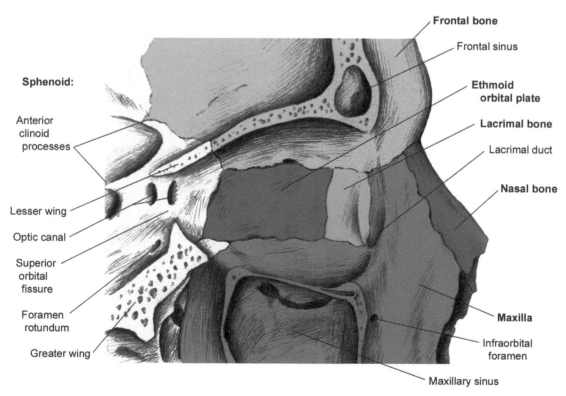

Frontal bone

Frontal sinus

Ethmoid
orbital plate

Lacrimal bone

Lacrimal duct

Nasal bone

Maxilla

Infraorbital
foramen

Maxillary sinus

Sphenoid:

Anterior
clinoid
processes

Lesser wing

Optic canal

Superior
orbital
fissure

Foramen
rotundum

Greater wing

39.5 *The lateral walls of the ethmoid form the medial walls of the orbits*

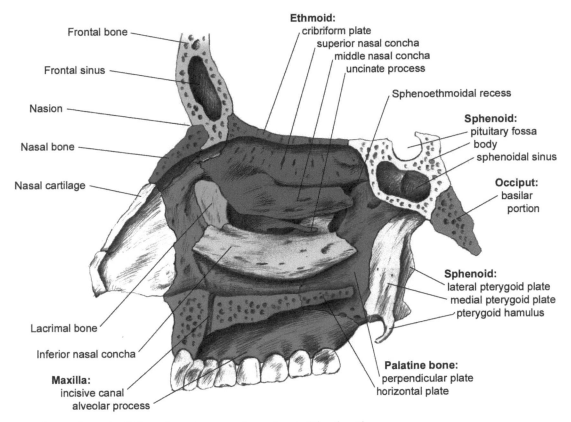

39.6   The superior and middle nasal conchae are an integral part of the ethmoid

From the lateral walls of the ethmoid, the *superior and middle nasal conchae* (turbinates) project medially into the nasal cavity. These are small, intricate, shell-like bony projections whose function is to create turbulence in the air entering the nasal cavity, in order to remove particles and warm the air before it enters the lungs. (The *inferior* nasal conchae are *not* part of the ethmoid, but are separate bones attaching to the medial walls of the maxillae.)

The anterior border of the ethmoid is bounded by the nasal bones, the ethmoid articulating with the nasal bones at the nasion.

The ethmoid therefore makes direct connections with the sphenoid, the frontal bone, the lacrimal bones, the nasal bones, and the vomer; and it receives membranous attachment at the falx cerebri.

Cerebrospinal fluid drainage

The many tiny foramina in the cribriform plate provide a passageway for the fibres of the olfactory nerve (Cr I). Damage to the ethmoid can therefore affect sense of smell.

These same holes also provide a channel for drainage of cerebrospinal fluid from the subarachnoid space, the cerebrospinal fluid draining into lymphatic channels and thence to the venous system. Recent research suggests that this is a more significant channel of drainage than the arachnoid villi.[1,2]

Damage or congestion around the ethmoid may therefore interfere with drainage, leading to reduced flow of cerebrospinal fluid within the cranium and increased intracranial pressure. Immediately below the cribriform plate is the nasal cavity, including the ethmoid sinuses. The nasal congestion of a cold may therefore lead to reduced cerebrospinal fluid flow, both through mucus blockage and through inflammation of the membranous lining of the foramina. This becomes more significant if the nasal congestion is a persistent chronic condition, with potential adverse consequences on mental faculties and clarity of mind.

Structural damage to the cribriform plate, perhaps from a blow to the face or a car accident, could have similar long-term consequences.

Navigating the universal field

It has been suggested[3] that a significant element in migrating birds' ability to navigate their way around the world is a crystalline structure within the ethmoid bone, through which they can interact with the magnetic field, and perhaps with the wider Higgs boson field around them. It is possible that we also have vestiges of this potential, explaining why the ethmoid is associated with deeper intuitive connections to the universe.

Bridge between cranium and face

Another ambiguous feature of the ethmoid is its position between the cranium and the face. It is contained within the ethmoid notch of the frontal bone and, insofar as it receives direct membranous attachment (unlike any facial bone), it is part of the cranium. However, in its cranio-sacral motion, it moves with the mouth parts – maxillae, palatines and vomer – and is an intimately integrated component of these facial structures. It can therefore be seen as a bridge between cranium and face.

Cranio-sacral motion

The ethmoid moves with the mouth parts – maxillae, palatines and vomer. Its anterior portion rises during the expansion (flexion) phase, and falls during the contraction (extension) phase, rotating around a transverse axis through the centre of the ethmoid.

As the sphenoid arcs forward and down during the expansion phase, the sphenoid body pushes the ethmoid forward, the ethmoid rotating in the opposite direction to the sphenoid, on their respective transverse axes, like cogs in a mechanical clock.

Susceptibility

Since the ethmoid is so delicate, its integrity is highly dependent on its surrounding structures –

the maxillae, palatines, vomer, nasals, frontal and sphenoid.

It is easily distorted, whether by birth trauma, facial injuries or cranial compression. Even in adulthood, its delicate tissue-like structure renders it prone to distortion. The ethmoid develops embryologically in three parts and is not fully ossified until the age of five or six years, so at the time of birth it is all the more susceptible to compressive forces and intraosseous distortion. As one of Sutherland's 'speed reducers' (along with the vomer and palatines) it is able to act as a shock absorber and absorb some of these forces, thereby reducing the impact transmitted through to the cranium; but in doing so, its own integrity and function can be compromised.

Compression of the ethmoid area may contribute to sinus congestion and nasal symptoms. It may affect the sense of smell through the olfactory nerve. It may also compromise connections to intuitive faculties and higher consciousness. Releasing and opening up the spaciousness of the ethmoid may help to develop such qualities – a faculty which appears sometimes to be enabled or enhanced by a head injury.

Approach

In working with the ethmoid, the first priority is to release any compressive forces imposed by surrounding structures, in order to restore integrity and free mobility of the cranium as a whole and the local area in particular. This can be enabled by engaging with the system and allowing the expression of the inherent treatment process in response to any forces that arise spontaneously. This might include working with the sphenoid, the frontal bone and the temporal bones, along with any bones of the face that may be indicated by the inherent treatment process and the needs of the individual. It is also particularly relevant to explore medial compression of the ethmoid area through the maxillary and zygomatic compression and decompression contacts described previously (Chapters 16 and 37) and also similar contacts for the frontal area (see *Cranio-Sacral Integration – Foundation*).

It may be relevant to treat the ethmoid area for mundane matters such as nasal congestion, a deviated septum and structural restrictions.

However, the most significant connection with the ethmoid is enabled through engagement with its more profound spacious qualities, its more esoteric intuitive aspects, its sense of connection to higher consciousness, the higher self and the universal field. The initial phase of releasing structural compression and creating space will enable this to some extent. It is then primarily enhanced through settling into deep spaciousness and engaging with the profound ethereal qualities that connect with these higher levels.

Contacts

Some contacts for the ethmoid are more suitable for engaging with its structural aspects, releasing compressions and other restrictions. Other contacts are more suited to engaging with its more profound and spacious esoteric aspects. The more structurally orientated contacts may serve as effective precursors to the more profound contacts. All contacts will of course engage with whatever level the inherent treatment process chooses within the context of the practitioner's level of therapeutic attention.

Contacts for structural integration

Medially compressed ethmoid
– frontal contact

Sometimes, when you engage with this area, you may feel that the ethmoid is squashed between the two medially compressed halves of the frontal bone – particularly as a deeply embedded birth pattern. When you encounter this compressive pattern, it can be helpful to explore these medially compressive forces.

Taking up contact on each side of the forehead with the fingers pointing medially, ask yourself whether there is any sense of medial compression (Figure 39.7). If the system responds positively to this enquiry, you can follow to points of stillness and release, until the whole frontal area opens up into an expansive lateral decompression and the whole cranium and ethmoid space opens up to greater spaciousness.

This is a pattern which can frequently be imposed at birth. Babies often emerge from the birth canal with very narrow heads, and if the birth has been long or traumatic, this narrowness may

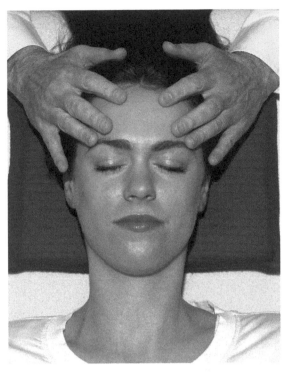

39.7 Engaging with compression of the ethmoid notch through the frontal area

remain imprinted into the cranium throughout life (unless released) and may sometimes be visible in the shape of the head. Such forces could squeeze the ethmoid within the ethmoid notch and leave a sense of contraction and compression – probably experienced as 'normal' by the individual who has lived with that restrictive pattern all their life – and restrict their connection to universal consciousness.

This contact can be a useful precursor to the ethmoid notch spread, enabling a more comprehensive and profoundly effective response.

Medially compressed ethmoid
– maxillary contact

The ethmoidal space may also be restricted by medial compression of the maxillae, in which case it may be beneficial to spread the maxillae, particularly where there is evident medial compression of the maxillary arch, initially allowing the expression of any compressive forces imprinted into the area, subsequently encouraging bilateral decompression, as described in Chapter 16 (Figure 39.8).

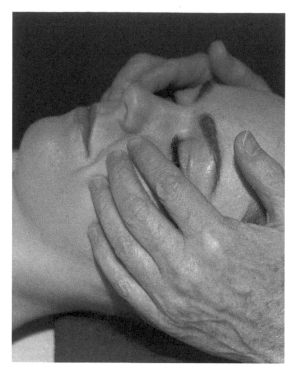

39.8 Engaging with ethmoid notch compression via the maxillae

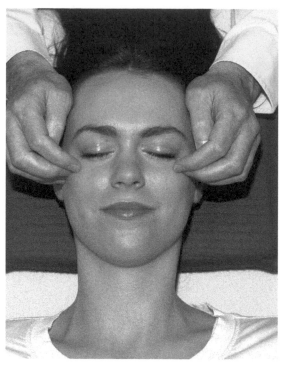

39.9 Engaging with ethmoid compression via the zygomata

Medially compressed ethmoid – zygomata contact

The same principle applies in relation to the zygomata. Exploring medial compression of the ethmoid through a bilateral contact on the zygomata can be particularly effective (Figure 39.9).

Vertically compressed ethmoid

It may also be appropriate at times to address vertical compression of the ethmoid area, where the frontal bone is compressed inferiorly towards the face, and the face compressed superiorly towards the frontal area, whether from a fall on the head, an injury or a birth pattern. Contacts can be improvised between the frontal and the maxillae, or the frontal and the nasal bones (as described previously in Chapters 16 and 36) (Figure 39.10).

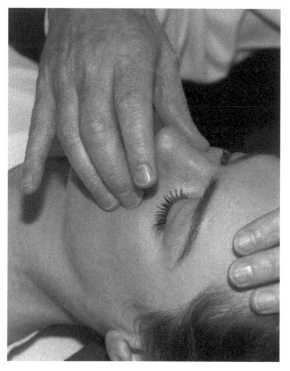

39.10 A maxillary-frontal contact can be beneficial for vertical compressions of the ethmoid area

Ethmoid pump

With these contacts for a vertically compressed ethmoid, a slightly more physical approach can sometimes be beneficial, especially in relieving sinus congestion, improving vascular and lymphatic drainage, and enhancing cerebrospinal fluid flow around the cribriform plate, through a gentle pumping action, the two hands very gently compressing and releasing repeatedly. It is essential to emphasize the need to be *very gentle* – a soft cranio-sacral pumping, rather than a physical pumping.

Contact through the vomer

The vomer contact (Chapter 18), with one hand over the spheno-frontal area and the index finger of the other hand contacting the hard palate at the cruciate suture, provides another useful point of access to the ethmoid, since the vomer articulates directly with the perpendicular plate of the ethmoid. This may be particularly valuable in working with a deviated nasal septum and in addressing the compressive forces held between the cranium and face that may have caused the deviated septum. As the inherent treatment process unfolds, your attention can spread through the ethmoid and its surroundings.

Contacts for more profound engagement

Working with the ethmoid has a sacred quality. It is therefore appropriate to approach it with reverence and delicacy and with awareness of these more profound connections and associations. This can be enhanced not only through all the usual processes of establishing spacious practitioner fulcrums, but also by tuning in to your own ethmoid and your own third eye.

Settling into a deeply spacious meditative state, take your attention to your eyes, letting go of your eyelids, letting go of your eyeballs, sensing the spaciousness of your orbits, allowing that spaciousness to expand to the space between your eyes, above your eyes, behind your eyes and throughout the spaciousness within your cranium. Allow your inner sense of spaciousness to expand out into the spaciousness around you and the spaciousness of the universe around you, feeling the increasing sense of connection with the universal field and universal consciousness. Maintain this engagement with the wider universe as you engage with your patient's ethmoid and its infinite associations and ramifications.

Since the ethmoid cannot be contacted directly, it is necessary to take up contact elsewhere in the system, and project attention through to the ethmoid area. This could be enabled from anywhere in the body – the feet, the sacrum, the cranium, or elsewhere – since it is the focus of your attention rather than the position of your hands which is more significant. In practice, it is often most appropriate to take up contact as close to the ethmoid as is convenient, notably through the sphenoid, the frontal bone, or the falx cerebri – all of which have direct connections to the ethmoid itself.

Contact through the falx cerebri

Take up contact through the falx cerebri (see *Cranio-Sacral Integration – Foundation*), with one hand under the occiput, the other hand over the frontal area. However, in order to make as close a connection as possible to the ethmoid, place the fingers of your frontal hand a bit further down towards the nasion than usual, so that your middle and ring fingers are settling gently into the indentations on each side of the nasion close to the medial corners of the eyes – keeping the contact very light.

As you engage with the system through the falx, let your attention extend from the falx cerebri to the attachment of the falx at the crista galli, from the crista galli down through the cribriform plate to the perpendicular plate, spreading out to observe and engage with all the surrounding structures and tissues, including the lateral walls of the ethmoid, the sphenoid body posteriorly and the lacrimal bones and nasal bones anteriorly. As the inherent treatment process evolves, you can allow the various responses within the system to be expressed. You may encounter specific focal points of restriction or activity which demand your attention. More significantly, particularly as the system settles, you may sink into deep engagement with the soft, light, airy, ethereal qualities of the ethmoid, letting your perception expand out to engage with ever-increasing levels of spaciousness and expansiveness, settling into the profound stillness which often pervades and

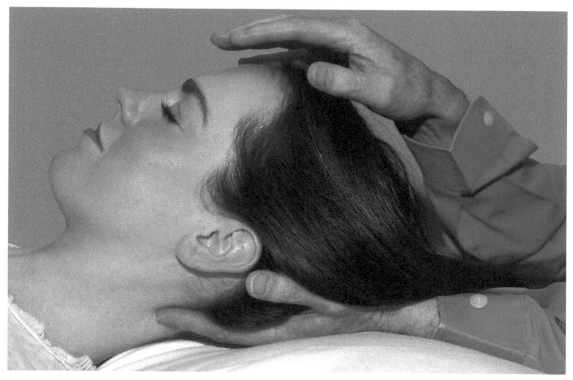

39.11 The falx release is a very powerful means of engaging with the ethmoid through its attachment at the crista galli

characterizes the ethmoid area, connecting with deeper levels of consciousness and engaging with a profound sense of oneness between yourself, the patient and the universal field within which we all exist.

As this process progresses, you may find your upper hand floating off the body on an increasingly expansive fluidic field (Figure 39.11).

Contact through the sphenoid

In the same way, you can take up contact on the sphenoid (see *Cranio-Sacral Integration – Foundation*), with your thumbs at the tips of the greater wings. As you engage with the system, project your attention from your thumbs, along the greater wings, to the body of the sphenoid, then project anteriorly from the sphenoid body to the ethmoid. Engage with the ethmoid as before, in all its aspects – settling into stillness, softness and spaciousness (Figure 39.12).

Ethmoid notch spread

The ethmoid notch spread is one of the most valuable and profound ways to engage with the ethmoid.

For this contact there are many variations and you may wish to adjust your position to find the most comfortable contact. The essence of the contact is to rest your fingers bilaterally on the frontal bone and, once engaged with the ethmoid area, gently visualize the spreading of the two halves of the frontal bone in order to expand the spaciousness of the ethmoid.

One way to take up contact is to lean forward with your elbows spreading out laterally on each side of your patient's head. If you have an adjustable chair, then lowering it to its lowest setting may be helpful. Alternatively, kneeling at the head can be comfortable and effective (and perhaps kneeling is particularly appropriate for this sacred process). This creates a suitable position for visualizing your hands gently drawing apart.

Allow your fingers to come to rest softly onto the frontal area, fingers pointing medially towards the midline, the tips of your fingers not quite touching as they rest lightly on each side of the metopic suture. Allow your fingers to flatten across the forehead, in order to establish as much contact with the frontal area as possible, keeping the contact light and soft (Figure 39.13a). It

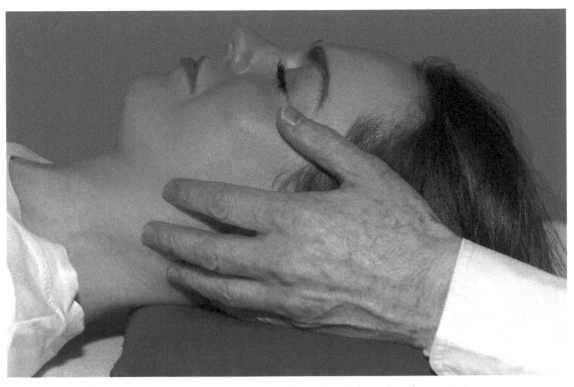

39.12 The sphenoid contact is a valuable means of engaging with the ethmoid due to their close proximity

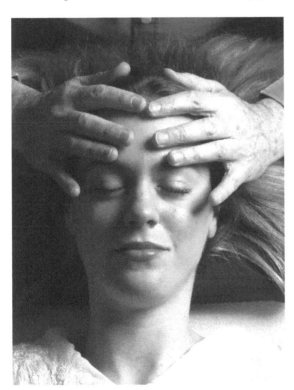

39.13 (a) Ethmoid notch spread

is helpful to place your ring fingers well down towards the nasion in order to be as close as possible to the ethmoid notch (taking care not to invade the patient's eyes).

Alternatively, if you are not comfortable with that contact, you could simply sit at the head as usual (not leaning forward), resting your fingers vertically over the frontal area (rather than transversely), thumbs close together at the midline, the fingers pointing towards the feet (again taking care not to invade the eyes).

A further option is to use your thumbs as the main fulcrum of contact, resting your thumbs vertically along the midline of the frontal bone, with the fingers running down the sides of the head in whatever position is comfortable.

Whichever contact you adopt, as engagement develops, allow the responses within the system. Feel the quality of the area. Connect with the profundity of the ethmoid and its environs.

When appropriate, envisage your hands spreading apart. You might initially be thinking in more structural terms of drawing the two halves of the frontal bone apart, spreading the ethmoid notch, letting your attention sink deeper below and behind the ethmoid notch, envisaging increasingly profound expansiveness.

More significantly, you may find yourself engaging on a more subtle quantum energy field level, feeling your hands softly expanding away from each other, feeling the energy field expanding, the matrix expanding, feeling the spaciousness of the system expanding out into the infinite spaciousness around you (Figure 39.13b).

Grounding

Working with the ethmoid can be a very appropriate way to bring a treatment session to an end, and can leave patients feeling beautifully spacious and serene. In some cases, it may also leave them feeling a bit surreal and ungrounded (in a pleasant way). Following the often profound levels of engagement through the ethmoid, it may be helpful to ensure adequate grounding both for the patient and for yourself, re-establishing connection with the material world, perhaps taking up contact at the feet and introducing grounding processes as necessary.

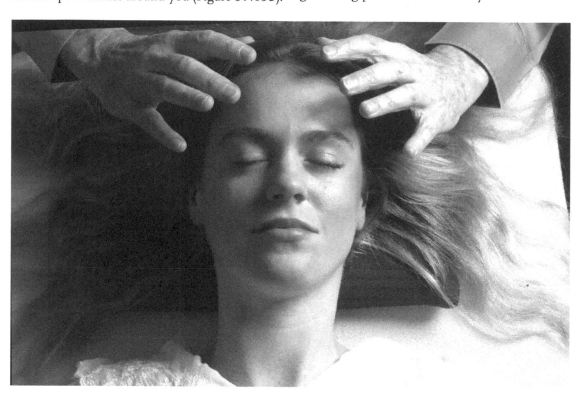

39.13 (b) Floating in a fluidic field of quantum waves and particles

Chapter 40

Conclusion

The face is significant, not only for those with specific facial symptoms, but also potentially for everyone. The face needs to be a part of our awareness in every patient.

Factors involving the face range from the mundane to the ethereal, from simple local symptoms to profound debilitation, from the gross physical to the profoundly spiritual.

Disturbances of the face can have widespread effects on the whole person. Conversely, facial symptoms may arise from anywhere in the body.

In order to enable optimum health, we need to consider the whole person, body and mind, gross structure and subtle matrix, addressing the physical body, addressing underlying trauma and shock throughout the system, and balancing autonomic nervous system function (including both structural and psycho-emotional factors). Within that whole-person perspective, we can address any individual restrictions and disturbances.

Cranio-sacral integration involves engaging with the system and allowing the inherent treatment process to take its course, enhancing the body's natural potential for healing.

Within that context, it is helpful to understand the specific details relevant to particular circumstances, in order to develop an informed awareness that can enhance our therapeutic attention. I hope that this volume has helped in some part to enable that.

Glossary

Abscess an enclosed area of infection and inflammation

Acute a recent or currently active injury or condition

ADHD attention deficit hyperactivity disorder

Adnexa surrounding tissues or structures

Alveolar (Latin: socket) relating to the sockets of the teeth (or the alveoli of the lungs)

Alveolar ridge the bony ridge of the mandible or maxillae within which the tooth sockets are located

Amalgam the most common material used for fillings, composed primarily of mercury and silver

ANS the autonomic nervous system

Ansa cervicalis a nerve loop in the neck, giving off branches to the muscles of the throat

Anterior in front of, forwards, at or towards the front of the body

Arachnoid villi protrusions of arachnoid membrane through the dura of the venous sinuses, through which cerebrospinal fluid can return to the venous blood

Asking the system
- asking questions of the body to see what response arises
- asking questions of yourself to assess more precisely what you are feeling

Asterion
- the meeting point of the squamosal, lamdoid and occipito-mastoid sutures
- the junction between the occiptal, temporal and parietal bones
- located behind the ear on each side of the cranium

Autonomic nervous system the part of the nervous system which regulates involuntary functions such as digestion, heartbeat, pupil constriction and dilation, etc.

Bicuspid a premolar tooth, a tooth with two cusps (points) at the top

Bilateral on both sides of the body

Boson in quantum mechanics, a boson is a particle that follows Bose–Einstein statistics. Bosons make up one of the two classes of particles, the other being fermions

Breath of life
- the natural force which pervades all living things, generating vitality, or aliveness
- it is expressed in the body as rhythmic motion on various levels
- it determines the orderly progression of life, growth, development, health and healing

Bregma
- the meeting point between the sagittal and coronal sutures
- located at the top of the head between the frontal and parietal bones
- the site of the anterior fontanelle (soft spot) in a baby

Bruxism teeth grinding

Caries cavities in teeth due to bacterial damage

Caudad towards the patient's tail

Cavitation (NICO) a deeply buried abscess, an area of ischaemic osteonecrosis within a bone, usually where a tooth has been removed

Cementum a layer of tough bone-like tissue that covers the root of a tooth

Cephalad towards the patient's head

Cerebrospinal fluid the pure fluid which surrounds and bathes the central nervous system

Choroid plexi the vascular structures in the ventricles of the brain, through which cerebrospinal fluid is produced

Chronic long established, a long-established condition

Chronicity the length of time that something has existed

Cisterna (plural: cisternae) a site of accumulation of cerebrospinal fluid within the subarachnoid space – e.g. cisterna magna, lumbar cistern

CNS the central nervous system

Coherence operating as a unified whole

Composite (composite resin) (in dentistry) the white filling material from which white fillings are created, the preferred option due to its lack of mercury and its white appearance

Compression pushed together by external forces

Contraction drawn together by internal forces

Coronal passing across the body from one side to the other (e.g. the coronal suture)

Coronal section a view of the body as if sliced vertically through the body from one side to the other

Cranial base the base of the skull, formed primarily by the occiput and sphenoid

Cranial rhythmic impulse (CRI)
- the cranio-sacral rhythm
- also used by some sources to indicate all levels of cranio-sacral motion

Cranial vault the upper part of the cranium, in contrast to the cranial base

Cranio-facial articulations (cranio-facial joints) the joints of the face and the cranium

Cranio-mandibular joint an alternative term for the temporo-mandibular joint

Cranio-sacral motion the rhythmic movement of the cranio-sacral system at various different rates
- includes cranio-sacral rhythm, middle tide, long tide

Cranio-sacral system

a. the whole person – mind, body and spirit – within the context of their life

b. the anatomical components of the cranio-sacral system – the bones, membranes, fluids and fascia which constitute the anatomical cranio-sacral system

Cranium the bony skull

Crepitus a crackling sound, as heard sometimes when moving the temporo-mandibular joint

Crossbite a lower tooth (or teeth) positioned outside its corresponding upper tooth (instead of inside)

Crown a replacement for an excessively worn or absent tooth

CSF cerebrospinal fluid

Cuspid a canine tooth, a tooth with one cusp (point) at the top

Deciduous teeth primary teeth, baby teeth

Decompression release from compression

Decussate to cross to the opposite side of the body

Diplopia double vision

Dorsal posterior, at the back, on or towards the back of the body

Dura mater the outer layer of the three membranes surrounding the brain and spinal cord, which is itself divided into two layers:
- endosteal dura – the outer layer of dura lining the bone and enveloping the cranial bones
- meningeal dura – the inner lining of dura, enveloping the brain and spinal cord

Dynamic stillness

a. a point of stillness preceding a release, within which subtle dynamic movements such as vibrations, wriggling or pulsation may be felt

b. a profound level of therapeutic stillness where everything becomes still – the deepest phase of the therapeutic process

Dysponesis a functional disturbance

Edentulous without teeth, or with teeth absent

Emotional centres the heart centre, solar plexus centre, pelvic centre, and suboccipital area

• focal points of emotional activity and emotional holding

Endosteum the outer layer of dura lining the bones of the cranium and vertebral column

Energy drive a process for focusing the body's therapeutic forces at a particular fulcrum

Ependyma the thin pia-like membrane which lines the ventricles

Equanimity a state of mental, emotional and spiritual balance

Extension

a. the movement of midline structures during the contraction phase of cranio-sacral motion

b. the movement of the whole system during the contraction phase of cranio-sacral motion

c. opening an angle – e.g. extending (straightening) the elbow

Extension phase the contraction phase of cranio-sacral motion

External rotation the movement of bilateral structures and the body as a whole during the expansion phase of cranio-sacral motion

Facial relating to the face (not to be confused with 'fascial')

Fascia the thin interconnected connective tissue which envelops everything in the body

• surrounding bones, muscles, nerves, blood vessels, organs

Fascial relating to the fascia (not to be confused with 'facial')

Fibrosis the hardening and excessive formation of fibrous tissues

Flexion

a. the movement of midline structures during the expansion phase of cranio-sacral motion

b. the movement of the whole system during the expansion phase of cranio-sacral motion

c. closing an angle – e.g. flexing (bending) the elbow

Flexion phase the expansion phase of cranio-sacral motion

Fluids the various fluids of the body – blood, lymph, CSF, extracellular fluid, etc.

Foramen (plural: foramina) a hole within a bone or between bones

Foramen magnum the large hole at the base of the skull, through which the spinal cord passes up to meet the brainstem and brain

Foramina holes, plural of foramen

Fossa a dip, socket or indentation in a bone, of variable shapes and sizes

Frenotomy (lingual) a minor operation to cut the frenulum when it is overly restrictive

Frenulum the thin membrane which attaches the tongue to the floor of the mouth

Fulcrum (plural: fulcrums or fulcra) a pivotal point around which a system operates

• mechanical fulcrums

• mental and emotional fulcrums

• focal points of resistance around which movement revolves

• practitioner fulcrums – the state of physical, mental and emotional balance from which a practitioner operates

Fundamental principles

• the natural series of stages through which the therapeutic response evolves during the cranio-sacral process

- the orderly process through which the cranio-sacral system enables the therapeutic response
- the components which comprise the inherent treatment process

Ganglion

a. a site of nerve junctions, at which neurological messages are passed from one neuron to another

b. a fluid-filled lump on a tendon, most commonly found in the hand or wrist

Gingivitis inflammation of the surface of the gums around the teeth

Glue ear otitis media with effusion (OME) – a chronic accumulation of sticky fluid within the middle ear

Gomphosis (plural: gomphoses) a type of fibrous peg-and-socket joint, found only between the teeth and their sockets in the maxillae or mandible

Grommet a tiny plastic tube inserted into the tympanic membrane to relieve pressure in the middle ear

Habitus habitual posture or way of holding the body

Higgs boson an elementary particle in the Standard Model of particle physics

Homeostasis a state of dynamic balance, constantly adapting in response to the environment

Hyperacusis an increased sensitivity to sound

Iatrogenic caused by a doctor or by medical treatment

IDD insulin dependent diabetes

Implant a small metal device implanted into the bone of the jaw, as the base for a crown, after a tooth has been extracted

Inertia lack of movement

Inertial fulcrum a focal point of restriction where rhythmic motion is limited

Inferior below, downwards, towards the soles of the patient's feet

Informed awareness awareness of and engagement with patterns expressed by the body, combined with understanding based on background knowledge of anatomy, physiology, pathology, case history, the cranio-sacral process, clinical experience, life experience, personal development, wisdom

Inherent naturally present within

Inherent treatment process

- the inherent therapeutic response of the cranio-sacral system
- the natural tendency of the body to heal itself through the orderly expression of its fundamental principles of therapeutic release
- the natural evolution of the therapeutic process

Internal rotation the movement of bilateral structures and the body as a whole during the contraction phase of cranio-sacral motion

Jugular foramina two foramina in the base of the skull, anterolateral to the foramen magnum, one on each side:

- formed between the occiput and the temporal bones
- through which pass the internal jugular vein and cranial nerves IX, X and XI

Kyphosis

- a forward-bending curve of the spine
- the natural curve of the spine in the thoracic spine and the sacrum

Lamda

- the meeting point between the sagittal and lamdoid sutures
- located at the top of the head between the occiput and parietal bones
- often identifiable through a small indentation

Lamina terminalis

- the anterior wall of the third ventricle
- the fulcrum around which the central nervous system moves in cranio-sacral motion

Lateral at or towards or closer to the sides of the body, or outwards from the midline

Lesion any disturbance to function, whether due to injury, disease, imbalance or any other cause

Lordosis

- a backward-bending curve of the spine
- the natural curve of the spine in the cervical and lumbar regions

Malar bones the cheek bones, another term for the zygomata (zygomatic bones)

Malocclusion the upper and lower teeth not meeting as they should on biting together

Mastication chewing

Masticatory apparatus the various structures involved in mastication (chewing) – jaws, teeth, muscles of mastication, TMJ, tongue, lips, etc.

Matrix (plural: matrices) a flexible environment within which something can grow, develop or exist – a coherent force field

- the embryonic matrix – the force field within which the embryo develops
- the individual matrix – the force field comprising the body and its surrounding aura, consisting of:
  - the internal matrix, the matrix within the body
  - the external matrix, the field around the body
- the universal matrix – the coherent field of forces within which the whole natural world operates as a unified cohesive system, and within which we all exist

ME myalgic encephalomyelitis – a persistent and debilitating post-viral condition

Medial at or towards or closer to the midline of the body

Membrane system the membranes – dura, arachnoid and pia – which enclose the brain and spinal cord, and include the intracranial infoldings

Meningeal dura the inner layer of dura mater

Meninges the triple-layered membranes – dura, arachnoid and pia – which surround the brain and spinal cord, and include the intracranial infoldings

Meningism a milder, often unrecognized, form of meningitis

- symptoms of meningitis without identification of an infectious organism

Meningitis inflammation of the meninges, usually as a result of bacterial or viral infection

- bacterial meningitis, due to bacterial infection, can be rapidly fatal unless treated with antibiotics
- viral meningitis, due to viral infection, usually milder, sometimes persistent, not affected by antibiotics
- the chronic persistent long-term after-effects of meningitis or meningism are often very debilitating, often involving severe headache, neck pain, pain behind the eyes, poor memory, poor concentration, and extreme tiredness; and are usually very responsive to cranio-sacral integration

Molecular web the interconnected network through which every molecule in the body is in continuous communication with every other molecule, enabling coordinated interaction and response, including healing responses, throughout the body

Mucosa the mucous membranes which line various structures such as the nose, mouth and sinuses, and which secrete mucus

Nasion the junction between the nasal bones and the frontal bone, at the top of the nose

Nephrotoxic damaging to the kidneys

Neutral a balanced settled state in which the cranio-sacral system is resting comfortably

- open and receptive, with rhythmic motion being expressed freely and evenly
- a state which indicates and enables engagement or deeper engagement
- a state to which the cranio-sacral system generally returns following a release

NICO (cavitation) Neuralgia Inducing Cavitational Osteonecrosis – a deeply buried abscess, an area of ischaemic osteonecrosis within the bone, usually where a tooth has been removed

NIDD non-insulin dependent diabetes

Occlusal surface the biting surface of a tooth

Occlusion closing the upper and lower teeth together

Ototoxic damaging to the ears

Periodontal ligament (= periodontal membrane) the fibrous tissue which attaches a tooth within its socket

Periodontitis inflammation of the periodontal ligament

Periosteum the membrane (dura) which covers the external surface of bones. In the cranium, the periosteum (on the outer surface) is continuous with the endosteum (on the inner surface) of the bones

Piezoelectric an electrical response generated by pressure

Plaque (dental) a sticky colourless film made of bacteria and the substances they secrete

PNS the peripheral nervous system

Posterior behind, backwards, at or towards the back of the body

Potency the power or strength of the level of vitality within the system

Practitioner fulcrums the state of physical, mental and emotional balance from which a practitioner operates

Primary respiration the expression of the breath of life as rhythmic motion

Process

a. a bony protrusion – e.g. the mastoid process

b. an interaction with the cranio-sacral system through a specific contact (as distinguished from the mere application of a technique)

c. the whole therapeutic process that the patient is going through

d. process work, working with a patient's whole life process – mental, emotional, spiritual, as well as physical

Prone lying on the front, face down

Proprioception awareness of position in space

Proprioceptors the nerve receptors which transmit proprioceptive impulses

Protrusion (of the jaw) positioned anteriorly

Pterion

• the junction at which the frontal, parietal, temporal and sphenoid bones come together

• located at the temple, behind the lateral corner of the eye on each side

Pulp (dental) the soft centre of a tooth which contains blood vessels and nerves

Quantum (plural: quanta) the smallest unit of anything, such as photons of light

Quantum science the basis of modern scientific thinking, initially conceived in the 1920s by Werner Heisenberg, Erwin Schrödinger and Paul Dirac, recognizing that everything in the universe (galaxies, planets, mountains, rocks, plants, animals, humans, oceans, fluids, air, heat, light, thought) is composed of quanta – elementary particles, waves and forces – in a state of constant interaction, through which everything influences everything else, including the observer and the observed

Reciprocal tension membrane system the system of continuously interconnected membranes (dura, arachnoid, pia):

• which surround the central nervous system and form the intracranial infoldings of the falx cerebri, falx cerebelli and tentorium cerebelli

• and which attach to the bones of the cranium and to the sacrum

• so that tensions anywhere in the membrane system are transmitted reciprocally throughout the rest of the membrane system

Reflex arc a rapid response system which enables reflex reactions through connections between sensory and motor neurons at a local spinal cord level, as for instance when you touch something hot

Restoration (in dentistry) restoring the structure of a tooth through the addition of restorative material. Includes fillings, crowns, bridges, veneers, etc.

Retrusion (of the jaw) positioned posteriorly

Rhythmic motion cranio-sacral motion – including cranio-sacral rhythm, middle tide and long tide

Root canal the canal through which blood vessels and nerves enter the pulp cavity of a tooth

Sacrum the tail bone

Sagittal passing between the front and back of the body (e.g. the sagittal suture)

Sagittal section a view of the body as if sliced vertically through the body from front to back

SBJ spheno-basilar joint, same as spheno-basilar synchondrosis

SBS spheno-basilar synchondrosis

Sclerosis hardening

Scoliosis

- an abnormal lateral curvature of the spine – present in many people to some degree
- idiopathic scoliosis – a condition in which a severe and persistent scoliosis of the spine develops spontaneously, commonly starting in teenage and pre-teen years, particularly in girls

Semisupine lying on the back (supine) with the knees bent and the soles of the feet on the surface on which you are lying (a term used in the Alexander technique)

Sinus a space

a. air sinuses – air-filled sinuses within the cranium, prone to infection, leading to sinusitis

b. venous sinuses – spaces within the dural membrane inside the cranium for the collection and drainage of venous blood

Solar plexus the coeliac ganglia and associated neurological structures of the sympathetic nervous system

- an energy centre in the central upper abdomen
- an area where emotion, stress and sympathetic stimulation are often felt

Spheno-basilar synchondrosis the primary cartilaginous joint between the body of the sphenoid and the basilar portion of the occiput

Sphincter a valve-like structure which closes through constriction in order to regulate the passage of food, etc. – e.g. pyloric sphincter, ilio-caecal valve

Squamous flat – e.g. the squamous portion of the temporal bone

Stomatognathic system the various structures of the mouth involved in eating, speaking, etc.

Strabismus squint

Superior above, upwards, towards the top of the patient's head

Supine lying on the back, face up

Sutherland's fulcrum a shifting fulcrum located within the straight sinus, at the junction of the falx cerebri, falx cerebelli and tentorium cerebelli, around which the rhythmic motion of the membrane system operates

Suture

- a fibrous joint between bones of the cranium and face
- the majority of joints between the cranial bones and between the facial bones are sutures

Synchondrosis a primary cartilaginous joint, which ossifies gradually over several years – e.g. the spheno-basilar synchondrosis

System, The the cranio-sacral system

Tartar (dental) a hard substance formed by dental plaque combining with minerals and solidifying

Temporo-mandibular joint (TMJ) the joint through which the lower jaw attaches to the cranium

Therapeutic pulse a pulsation very similar to the arterial pulse, except that it is transient and varies both in intensity and in rate, and generally arises in relation to therapeutic releases

Tinnitus the perception of persistent sounds in one or both ears, including whining, whistling, ringing, humming or clicking

Tissue memory

a. patterns of injury or tension held in the tissues

b. memories of past events arising in conjunction with releases in the tissues

TMJ the temporo-mandibular joint, the joint through which the lower jaw attaches to the cranium

Torticollis a twist of the neck, also known as wry neck

a. infant torticollis – occurs in babies, is often associated with the birth process, and often responds well to the cranio-sacral process

b. acute torticollis – an acute spasm in the neck at any age, frequently associated with sleeping awkwardly, and often very responsive to cranio-sacral treatment

Torus palatinus an abnormal bony protrusion on the roof of the mouth

Traction stretching

Transverse passing horizontally across the body (e.g. the transverse sinuses)

Transverse section a view of the body as if sliced horizontally through the body

Trismus restricted opening of the mouth

Tympanic membrane the ear drum, a membrane located between the external ear canal and the middle ear

Vault hold any contact on the cranium which embraces or contains the cranial vault – e.g. falx contact, temporal contact, sphenoid contact

Vector a line of force passing through or within the body

Venous relating to veins and venous (de-oxygenated) blood

Venous sinuses the system of sinuses (spaces) within the cranium through which venous blood collects in order to return to the heart for re-oxygenation

Vertical dimension the distance between the upper (maxillary) and lower (mandibular) alveolar ridges. Loss of vertical dimension occurs when the upper jaw and lower jaw close together excessively due to the absence of vertical support from the teeth (primarily the molars)

Vibrissae sensitive hairs, such as nasal hairs or whiskers

Endnotes

Chapter 1

1. Smith, J. (2014) *Ear Infections in Children*. Available at www. deaconess.com/MyHealth/MyHealth-Blog/June-2014-(1)/ Ear-Infections-in-Children.aspx, accessed on 6 January 2016.

2. Trigeminal Neuralgia Association UK (n.d.) *What is Trigeminal Neuralgia?* Available at www.tna.org.uk, accessed on 6 January 2016.

3. Attlee, T. (2012) *Cranio-Sacral Integration – Foundation*. London: Jessica Kingsley Publishers.

Chapter 2

1. Laughlin, J. (2005) In L. Chaitow (ed) *Cranial Manipulation – Theory and Practice* (Second Edition). London: Elsevier Churchill Livingstone.

2. Ibid.

3. Ibid.

4. Bjørner, K. (2011) *Lock Foot Syndrome*. Oslo: Kolofon.

5. Laughlin, J. (2005) In L. Chaitow (ed) *Cranial Manipulation – Theory and Practice* (Second Edition). London: Elsevier Churchill Livingstone.

6. Upledger, J. (1987) *Beyond the Dura*. Seattle, WA: Eastland Press.

7. Dentist quoted in: Upledger, J. (1987) *Beyond the Dura*. Seattle, WA: Eastland Press.

Chapter 3

1. Laughlin, J. (2005) In L. Chaitow (ed) *Cranial Manipulation – Theory and Practice* (Second Edition). London: Elsevier Churchill Livingstone.

2. Ibid.

3. Ibid.

4. Ibid.

Chapter 4

1. Laughlin, J. (2005) In L. Chaitow (ed) *Cranial Manipulation – Theory and Practice* (Second Edition). London: Elsevier Churchill Livingstone.

2. Milne, H. (1995) *The Heart of Listening*. Berkeley, CA: North Atlantic Books.

3. Upledger, J. (1987) *Beyond the Dura*. Seattle, WA: Eastland Press.

4. Laughlin, J. (2005) In L. Chaitow (ed) *Cranial Manipulation – Theory and Practice* (Second Edition). London: Elsevier Churchill Livingstone.

5. Ibid.

6. International Academy of Oral Medicine and Toxicology: http://iaomt.org.

7. Echeverria, D., Woods, J.S., Heyer, N.J. *et al.* (2005) 'Chronic low-level mercury exposure, BDNF polymorphism, and associations with cognitive and motor function.' *Neurotoxicology and Teratology 27*, 6, 781–796.

8. Woods, J.S., Heyer, N.J., Echeverria, D., Russo, J.E. *et al.* (2012) 'Modification of neurobehavioral effects of mercury by a genetic polymorphism of coproporphyrinogen oxidase in children.' *Neurotoxicology and Teratology 34*, 5, 513–521.

9. Wojcik, D.P., Godfrey, M.E., Christie, D., and Haley, B.E. (2006) 'Mercury toxicity presenting as chronic fatigue, memory impairment and depression: diagnosis, treatment, susceptibility, and outcomes in a New Zealand general practice setting: 1994–2006.' *Neuro Endocrinol. Lett. 27*, 4, 415–423.

10. Weiner, J.A., Nylander, M., and Berglund, F. (1990) 'Does mercury from amalgam restorations constitute a health hazard?' *Sci. Total Environ. 99*, 1–2, 1–22.

11. Stejskal, J., and Stejskal, V.D. (1999) 'The role of metals in autoimmunity and the link to neuroendocrinology.' *Neuro Endocrinol. Lett. 20*, 6, 351–364.

12. Laughlin, J. (2005) In L. Chaitow (ed) *Cranial Manipulation – Theory and Practice* (Second Edition). London: Elsevier Churchill Livingstone.

13. Magoun, H. (1951) *Osteopathy in the Cranial Field*. Kirksville, MI: Journal Printing.

14. Ibid.

15. Langly-Smith, G. (2012) Lecture.

16. Laughlin, J. (2005) In L. Chaitow (ed) *Cranial Manipulation – Theory and Practice* (Second Edition). London: Elsevier Churchill Livingstone.

Chapter 5

1. Shark Savers. *Shark Teeth*. www.sharksavers.org.

Chapter 7

2. Fonder, A.C. (1977) *The Dental Physician*. Blacksburg, VA: University Publications.

3. *Western Mail* (Cardiff) (19 March 2002) 'Brace Blamed for Illness; SWANSEA: Schoolgirl, 15, Now Recovering.' Available at www.thefreelibrary.com/ Brace+blamed+for+illness%3B+SWANSEA%3A+Schoolgirl, +15,+now+recovering.-a083976316, accessed on 6 January 2016.

Chapter 8

1. McDevitt, W.E. (1989) *Functional Anatomy of the Masticatory System*. London and Boston: Wright.

2. Fonder, A. (1977) *The Dental Physician*. Blacksburg, VA: University Publications.

3. Fonder, A. (1990) *The Dental Distress Syndrome*. Rock Falls, IL: Medical Dental Arts.

4. Selye, H. (1956) *The Stress of Life*. New York: McGraw-Hill.

5. Whatmore, G.B., and Kohli, D.R. (1974) *The Physiopathology and Treatment of Functional Disorders*. New York: Grune & Stratton.

6. Price, W. (1939) *Nutrition and Physical Degeneration: A Comparison of Primitive and Modern Diets and Their Effects*. New York: Paul B. Hoeber, Inc., Harper & Brothers.

7. Guzay, C.M. (1980) *The Quadrant Theorem*. Chicago, IL: Doctors Dental Service.

8. Belli, R. (2011) *A Brief Discussion of Cranial Manipulation and Visceral and Somatic Response*. Available at www.spectrumak.com/resources/spectrum-articles/cranial-manipulation.html, accessed on 6 January 2016.

9. Pert, C.B. (1999) *Molecules of Emotion*. London: Simon and Schuster.

10. Bjørner, K. (2011) *Lock Foot Syndrome*. Oslo: Kolofon.

11. Selye, H. (1956) *The Stress of Life*. New York: McGraw-Hill.

Chapter 14

1. Laughlin, J. (2005) In L. Chaitow (ed) *Cranial Manipulation – Theory and Practice* (Second Edition). London: Elsevier Churchill Livingstone.

2. Upledger, J. (1987) *Beyond the Dura*. Seattle, WA: Eastland Press.

3. Milne, H. (1995) *The Heart of Listening*. Berkeley, CA: North Atlantic Books.

4. Oğütcen-Toller, M., and Keskin, M. (2000) 'Computerized 3-dimensional study of the embryologic development of the human masticatory muscles and temporomandibular joint.' *J. Oral Maxillofac. Surg. 58*, 12, 1381–1386.

5. Upledger, J. (1987) *Beyond the Dura*. Seattle, WA: Eastland Press.

Chapter 15

1. Dentist quoted in: Upledger, J. (1987) *Beyond the Dura*. Seattle, WA: Eastland Press.

2. Upledger, J. (1987) *Beyond the Dura*. Seattle, WA: Eastland Press.

3. Laughlin, J. (2005) In L. Chaitow (ed) *Cranial Manipulation – Theory and Practice* (Second Edition). London: Elsevier Churchill Livingstone.

4. Ibid.

5. Upledger, J. (1987) *Beyond the Dura*. Seattle, WA: Eastland Press.

6. The TMJ Association. www.tmj.org.

7. Ibid.

8. National Institute of Dental and Craniofacial Research (2014) *Temporomandibular Joint Dysfunction*. Available at www.thevisualmd.com.

9. Upledger, J. (1987) *Beyond the Dura*. Seattle, WA: Eastland Press.

Chapter 16

1. Magoun, H. (1951) *Osteopathy in the Cranial Field*. Kirksville, MI: Journal Printing.

2. Dvivedi, J., and Dvivedi, S. (2012) 'A clinical and demographic profile of the cleft lip and palate in Sub-Himalayan India.' *Indian J. Plast. Surg. 45*, 1, 115–120.

3. Ibid.

4. Smile Train. *Cleft Births*. www.smiletrainindia.org.

5. Ibid.

Chapter 17

1. Sutherland, W.G. (1939) *The Cranial Bowl*. Mankato, MN: Free Press.

Chapter 19

1. Upledger, J. (1987) *Beyond the Dura*. Seattle, WA: Eastland Press.

Chapter 22

1. Masaoka, Y., Satoh, H., Akai, L., and Homma, I. (2010) 'Expiration: the moment we experience retronasal olfaction in flavour.' *Neurosci. Lett. 473*, 2, 92–96.

2. Navarrete-Palacios, E., Hudson, R., Reyes-Guerrero, G., and Guevara-Guzmán, R. (2003) 'Biological psychology: lower olfactory threshold during the ovulatory phase of the menstrual cycle.' *Biol. Psychol. 63*, 3, 269–279.

3. Boehm, T., and Zufall, F. (2006) 'MHC peptides and the sensory evaluation of genotype.' *Trends Neurosci. 29*, 2, 100–107.

4. Porter, R.H., Cernoch, J.M., and Balogh, R.D. (1985) 'Odor signatures and kin recognition.' *Physiology & Behavior 34*, 3, 445–448.

5. Weisfeld, G.E., Czilli, T., Phillips, K.A., Gall, J.A., and Lichtman, C.M. (2003) 'Possible olfaction-based mechanisms in human kin recognition and inbreeding avoidance.' *J. Exp. Child Psychol. 85*, 3, 279–295.

6. Werner, P. (n.d.) *A Bear's Sense of Smell*. Sectionhiker.com.

Chapter 25

1. Trigeminal Neuralgia Association UK (n.d.) *What is Trigeminal Neuralgia?* Available at www.tna.org.uk, accessed on 6 January 2016.

2. Ibid.

3. Ibid.

4. Ibid.

5. Theil, D., Derfuss, T., Paripovic, I., *et al.* (2003) 'Latent herpesvirus infection in human trigeminal ganglia.' *Am. J. Pathol. 163*, 6, 2179–2184.

6. Ibid.

Chapter 27

1. Spoendlin, H., and Schrott, A. (1989) 'Analysis of the human auditory nerve.' *Hear. Res. 43*, 1, 25–38.

2. Chen, I., Limb, C.J., and Ryugo, D.K. (2010) 'The effect of cochlear implant-mediated electrical stimulation on spiral

ganglion cells in congenitally deaf white cats.' *J. Assoc. Res. Otolaryngol. 11*, 4, 587–603.

3. Hain, T. (2012) *Gentamicin Toxicity.* Available at http://american-hearing.org/disorders/gentamicin-toxicity, accessed on 6 January 2016.

Chapter 28

1. Upledger, J. (1987) *Beyond the Dura.* Seattle, WA: Eastland Press.

Chapter 29

1. Berthoud, H.R. and Neuhuber, W.L. (2000) 'Functional and chemical anatomy of the afferent vagal system.' *Autonomic Neuroscience 85*, 1–3, 1–17.

2. Porges S.W. (2011) *The Polyvagal Theory: Neurophysiological Foundations of Emotions, Attachment, Communication, and Self-regulation.* New York: W.W. Norton.

3. Upledger, J. (1987) *Beyond the Dura.* Seattle, WA: Eastland Press.

4. *The Vagus Nerve – Physical and Emotional Effects.* https://en.wikipedia.org.

5. Ibid.

6. Darwin, C. (1872) *The Expression of Emotions in Man and Animals.* London: John Murray.

7. Genome Res 19 (2009) *The NIH Human Microbiome Project.*

8. Savage, D.C. (1977) 'Microbial ecology of the gastrointestinal tract.' *Annual Review of Microbiology 31*, 107–133.

9. Gill, S.R., Pop, M., Deboy, R.T., *et al.* (2006) *Metagenomic Analysis of the Human Distal Gut Microbiome.* New York: Science.

10. Nikoopour, E., and Singh, B. (2014) *Reciprocity in Microbiome and Immune System Interactions and its Implications in Disease and Health.* Available at http://ir.lib.uwo.ca/cgi/viewcontent.cgi?article=1038&context=mnipub, accessed on 6 January 2016.

11. Forsythe, P., Bienenstock, J., and Kunze, W.A. (2014) 'Vagal pathways for microbiome-brain-gut axis communication.' *Adv. Exp. Med. Biol. 817*, 115–133.

12. Kok, B., Fredrickson, B., Coffey, K., *et al.* (2013) 'How positive emotions build physical health: perceived positive social connections account for the upward spiral between positive emotions and vagal tone.' *Psychological Science 24*, 7, 1123–1132.

13. Ibid.

14. Darou, S. (2015) *The Vagus Nerve – How Inflammation Can Be Controlled by the Brain.* Available at http://darouwellness.com/the-vagus-nerve-how-inflammation-can-be-controlled-by-the-brain, accessed on 6 January 2016.

15. Ibid.

16. Cohen, J. (2015) *Conditions Which Vagal Nerve Activation Can Help. Thirty-two Ways to Stimulate your Vagus Nerve.* Available at http://selfhacked.com/2015/07/30/28-ways-to-stimulate-your-vagus-nerve-and-all-you-need-to-know-about-it, accessed on 6 January 2016.

17. Papas, H. (2012) *Activating the Vagus Nerve.* Available at https://helenpapas.wordpress.com/2012/11/27/activating-the-vagus-nerve, accessed on 6 January 2016.

18. Cohen, J. (2015) *Conditions Which Vagal Nerve Activation Can Help. Thirty-two Ways to Stimulate your Vagus Nerve.* Available at http://selfhacked.com/2015/07/30/28-ways-to-stimulate-your-vagus-nerve-and-all-you-need-to-know-about-it, accessed on 6 January 2016.

19. Ibid.

20. Speck, D.F., and Bruce, D.S. (1978) 'Effects of varying thermal and apneic conditions on the human diving reflex.' *Undersea Biomed. Res. 5*, 1, 9–14.

21. Goksor, E., Rosengren, L., and Wennergren, G. (2002) 'Bradycardic response during submersion in infant swimming.' *Acta Paediatrica 91*, 3, 307–312.

22. Breatheology (2015) *The Diving Reflex – Your Inner Dolphin.* Available at www.breatheology.com/articles/mammalian-dive-response, accessed on 6 January 2016.

23. Porges S.W. (2011) *The Polyvagal Theory: Neurophysiological Foundations of Emotions, Attachment, Communication, and Self-regulation.* New York: W.W. Norton.

Chapter 32

1. Korr, I. (1970) *The Physiological Basis of Osteopathic Medicine.* New York: Insight Publishing.

2. Upledger, J. (1987) *Beyond the Dura.* Seattle, WA: Eastland Press.

3. Ibid.

4. Attlee, T. (2012) *Cranio-Sacral Integration – Foundation.* London: Jessica Kingsley Publishers.

5. Upledger, J. (1987) *Beyond the Dura.* Seattle, WA: Eastland Press.

6. Sutherland, W.G. (1939) *The Cranial Bowl.* Mankato, MN: Free Press.

Chapter 34

1. Attlee, T. (1992) 'Meningitis, meningism, and subclinical meningitis.' *International Journal of Alternative and Complementary Medicine.*

2. NHS Choices (2015) *Glaucoma.* Available at www.nhs.uk/Conditions/glaucoma/Pages/introduction.aspx, accessed on 6 January 2016.

3. NHS Choices (2015) *Cataracts.* Available at www.nhs.uk/conditions/Cataract-surgery/Pages/Introduction.aspx, accessed on 6 January 2016.

4. Ibid.

5. Bailey, G. (2015) *Cataracts.* Available at www.allaboutvision.com/conditions/cataracts.htm, accessed on 6 January 2016.

6. NHS Choices (2015) *Squint.* Available at www.nhs.uk/conditions/squint/Pages/Introduction2.aspx, accessed on 6 January 2016.

7. Huh, S. (2015) *Toxocariasis.* Medscape. Available at http://emedicine.medscape.com/article/229855-overview, accessed on 6 January 2016.

Chapter 35

1. Waseem, M. (2015) *Otitis Media.* Medscape. Available at http://emedicine.medscape.com/article/994656-overview, accessed on 6 January 2016.

2. Upledger, J. (1987) *Beyond the Dura.* Seattle, WA: Eastland Press.

3. NPS Medicinewise (2013) *Ear Infection (Acute Otitis Media)*. Available at www.nps.org.au/conditions/ear-nose-mouth-and-throat-disorders/ear-nose-and-throat-infections/ear-infection-middle, accessed on 6 January 2016.

4. Rovers, M.M., Schilder, A.G., Zielhuis, G.A., and Rosenfeld, R.M. (2004) 'Otitis media.' *Lancet 363*, 9407, 465–473.

5. Pukander, J., Luotonen, J., Timonen, M., and Karma, P. (1985) 'Risk factors affecting the occurrence of acute otitis media among 2–3 year old urban children.' *Acta Otolaryngol. 100*, 3–4, 260–265.

6. NPS Medicinewise (2013) *Ear Infection (Acute Otitis Media)*. Available at www.nps.org.au/conditions/ear-nose-mouth-and-throat-disorders/ear-nose-and-throat-infections/ear-infection-middle, accessed on 6 January 2016.

7. Torpy, J. (2010) 'Otitis media.' *Journal of the American Medicine Association 304*, 19, 2194.

8. Baker Chiropractic (n.d.) *Ear Infections*. Available at www.bakerchiropractic.org/?s=Ear+Infections, accessed on 6 January 2016.

9. Ibid.

10. Bluestone, C.D. (2005) *Eustacian Tube: Structure, Function, Role in Otitis Media*. Hamilton, London: B.C. Decker Inc.

11. Davison, R. (1962) *Ventilation of the Normal and Blocked Middle Ear: A Review of Mechanisms*. USAF School of Aerospace Medicine. Available at www.dtic.mil/dtic/tr/fulltext/u2/295722.pdf, accessed on 6 January 2016.

12. Fulford, R. (1996) *Dr. Fulford's Touch of Life*. New York: Pocket Books.

13. Woodhouse, S. (2015) *Benign Paroxysmal Positional Vertigo (BPPV)*. http://vestibular.org.

Chapter 39

1. Johnston, M., Zakharov, A., Papaiconomou, C., Salmasi, G., and Armstrong, D. (2004) 'Evidence of connections between cerebrospinal fluid and nasal lymphatic vessels in humans, non-human primates and other mammalian species.' *Cerebrospinal Fluid Res. 2004*, 1, 2.

2. Kapoor, K.G., Katz, S.E., Grzybowski, D.M., and Lubow, M. (2008) 'Cerebrospinal fluid outflow: an evolving perspective.' *Brain Res. Bull. 77*, 6, 327–334.

3. Becker, R.O. (1985) *The Body Electric*. New York: Morrow.

Index

Page references to Figures or Photographs will be in *italics*